SAFETY AND EFFICACY OF RADIOPHARMACEUTICALS

DEVELOPMENTS IN NUCLEAR MEDICINE
Series editor Peter H. Cox

Other titles in this series

Cox, P.H. (ed.): Cholescintigraphy. 1981. ISBN 90-247-2524-0
Cox, P.H. (ed.): Progress in radiopharmacology 3. Selected Topics. 1982.
  ISBN 90-247-2768-5
Jonckheer, M.H. and Deconinck, F. (eds.): X-ray fluorescent scanning of the
  thyroid. 1983. ISBN 0-89838-561-X

Safety and efficacy of radiopharmaceuticals

edited by

KNUD KRISTENSEN
ELISABETH NØRBYGAARD

The Isotope-Pharmacy
The National Board of Health
Copenhagen
Denmark

1984 **MARTINUS NIJHOFF PUBLISHERS**
a member of the KLUWER ACADEMIC PUBLISHERS GROUP
BOSTON / THE HAGUE / DORDRECHT / LANCASTER

Distributors

for the United States and Canada: Kluwer Boston, Inc., 190 Old Derby Street, Hingham, MA 02043, USA
for all other countries: Kluwer Academic Publishers Group, Distribution Center, P.O.Box 322, 3300 AH Dordrecht, The Netherlands

Library of Congress Cataloging in Publication Data

Safety and efficacy of radiopharmaceuticals.

   (Developments in nuclear medicine ; v. 4)
   Includes index.
   1. Radiopharmaceuticals--Safety measures.   2. Drugs--
Effectiveness.   3. Drug trade--Quality control.
I. Kristensen, Knud.   II. Nørbygaard, Elisabeth.
III. Series.   [DNLM: 1. Quality control--Congresses.
2. Radiation protection--Standards--Congresses.
3. Radioisotopes--Congresses.   W1 DE998kf v. 4 /
WN 420 S128 1983]
RM852.S2 1984   615.8'42   83-21938

ISBN-13:978-94-009-6755-7   e-ISBN-13:978-94-009-6753-3
DOI: 10.1007/978-94-009-6753-3

ISBN-13: 978-94-009-6755-7

PREFACE

Safety and efficacy of radiopharmaceuticals are elements of
great importance in nuclear medicine. Since the first meeting
in 1965 in Oak Ridge with the title Radiopharmaceuticals
tremendous developments have taken place. In 1965 the whole
technetium-99m area was just in its very beginning. Safety and
efficacy of the non-radioactive pharmaceuticals have attracted
great attention during the last 10 years and so have similar
aspects of radiopharmaceuticals during the later years.
Regulatory agencies are extending their work also to the
preparation of radiopharmaceuticals at hospitals and to
requirements for registration of radiopharmaceuticals. In a
fast developing field there might be tendencies to
confrontation between interests and there have certainly been
some tendencies to put undue restrictions on the use of radiopharmaceuticals due to the lack of understanding between the
industry and the regulatory authorities and between regulatory
authorities and hospitals. Much of this may have been due to
lack of information and certainly is due to the lack of
fundamental scientific knowledge in many radiopharmaceutical
aspects. A fast and safe introduction of new radiopharmaceuticals and the proper handling of these requires a
lot of development work, but also an understanding of how
general principles from the non-radioactive drug field may be
sensibly transformed into the radiopharmaceutical area. It may
even require compromises between requirements for safety in
different areas such as radiation protection and
pharmaceutical aspects.

Two of the most important areas in these years seem to be
the approval of new radiopharmaceuticals and the preparation
of radiopharmaceuticals at hospitals with the use of kits and
generators. In order to give an up to date survey of these
areas and to include relevant aspects from the registration

procedure for non-radioactive drugs a group of experts were invited to prepare review papers under the two main themes: Development of the documentation for efficacy and safety of radiopharmaceuticals and Design of laboratory facilities for preparation of radiopharmaceuticals at hospitals.

Summaries of these review papers were presented and discussed at the First European Symposium on Radiopharmacy and Radiopharmaceuticals, Elsinore, Denmark. 27. - 30. March, 1983. This meeting was organized by the Danish Society of Clinical Physiology and Nuclear Medicine under the auspicies of the European Joint Committee on Radiopharmaceuticals of European Society of Nuclear Medicine and the Society of Nuclear Medicine, Europe with the support of the Danish Medical Research Council. The Isotope-Pharmacy, The National Board of Health, Copenhagen, provided the secretariate for the meeting.

This book contains the full text of the review papers in part 1 and 2. It also contains in part 3 introductory papers prepared for a panel discussion on Quality control of radio-pharmaceuticals prepared from generators and kits.

It is hoped that the review papers will be useful as reference papers for future development in this field and the editors should like to thank all the authors for their willingness to contribute and for the meticulous care with which they all prepared the reviews.

Thanks are also due to the secretariat staff of the Isotope-Pharmacy: Anne Andersen, Bente Hansen, Inge Kornerup and Irma Østergård who with great care prepared the manuscript for reproduction.

May 1983
Elisabeth Nørbygård
Knud Kristensen

CONTENTS

VIII

CONTRIBUTORS

Neil Bell
University of Strathclyde
Glasgow, Scotland

Per O. Bremer
Institute of Energy Technology
Kjeller, Norway

Jiri Cifka
Nuclear Research Institute
Rez, Czechoslovakia

Yves Cohen
Université de Paris-Sud
Chatenay-Malabry, France

Peter H. Cox
Institute of Radiotherapy
Rotterdam, The Netherlands

Harriet Dige-Petersen
Glostrup Hospital
Glostrup, Denmark

Klaus R. Ennow
National Institute of Radiation Hygiene
Copenhagen, Denmark

Charles Fallais
Institut National des Radioelements
Fleurus, Belgium

Wim B. Huising
Byk-Mallinckrodt
Petten, The Netherlands

Yves Jean-Baptiste
Commisariat a l'Energie Atomique
Saclay, France

Rolf de Jong
Byk-Mallinckrodt
Petten, The Netherlands

Per Juul
Royal Danish School of Pharmacy
Copenhagen, Denmark

David H. Keeling
Derriford Hospital
Plymouth, England

Gerhard Kloss
Hoechst
Frankfurt am Main, Federal Republic of Germany

Knud Kristensen
The Isotope-Pharmacy
Copenhagen, Denmark

Colin R. Lazarus
Guy's Hospital
London, England

Derek E. Lovett
Amersham International plc
Amersham, England

John Mc Afee
Upstate Medical Center
Syracuse, U.S.A.

Jørgen Marqversen
Municipal Hospital
Århus, Denmark

Thomas Müller
The Isotope-Pharmacy
Copenhagen, Denmark

Sten-Ove Nilsson
Karolinska Pharmacy
Stockholm, Sweden

Bertil Nosslin
Malmö General Hospital
Malmö, Sweden

Elisabeth Nørbygaard
The Isotope-Pharmacy
Copenhagen, Denmark

Bente Pedersen
The Isotope-Pharmacy
Copenhagen, Denmark

Gertrude Pfeiffer
Institute of Reactor Research
Würenlingen, Switzerland

Hans Detlev Roedler
Institut für Strahlenhygiene des Bundesgesundheitsamtes
Neuherberg, Federal Republic of Germany

Richard F. Schneider
Upstate Medical Center
Syracuse, U.S.A.

Francis Smal
Institut National des Radioelements
Fleurus, Belgium

Rosemary J. Smith
Department of Health and Social Security
London, England

Gopal Subramanian
Upstate Medical Center
Syracuse, U.S.A.

Maurizio Villa
Sorin Biomedica
Saluggia, Italy

Ole Weis-Fogh
Novo Industry
Bagsværd, Denmark

XIV

Martin G. Woldring
University Hospital
Groningen, The Netherlands

Part 1

DEVELOPMENT OF THE DOCUMENTATION FOR EFFICACY AND SAFETY OF
RADIOPHARMACEUTICALS

INTRODUCTION

A new pharmaceutical is not introduced into general use before it has been tested in a way that an extensive knowledge about its efficacy and safety is available. After the design of a new chemical compound, methods are developed for its description, identification and determination. A stable pharmaceutical form and a production system are developed and a clinical trial through phase 1 to 3 is carried out. At a later stage, phase 4, including a continued surveillance, may be carried out by the manufacturer and also by the registration authorities.

A similar system is considered useful and necessary also for radiopharmaceuticals, taking into account the special properties of these drugs. After a review of design considerations in chapter one the preclinical testing is described in chapter 2 - 8 while the more clinical aspects are dealt with in chapter 9 - 13. Such studies leads to the registration procedure, the official approval, and the paper work involved is reviewed in chapter 14. Adverse reactions and drug interactions are fortunately at a very low level and can only be estimated during the more extended use of the radiopharmaceutical but is, however, of great importance (chapter 15 and 16). The surveillance of the whole system does also include the testing of products on a random basis by the authorities supplemented by hospital reporting of drug defects (chapter 17). Ethical aspects are reviewed in chapter 18. Part one is concluded by a number of chapters on the legal aspects. Some countries have enforced regulations on the licensing of radiopharmaceuticals for many years while others are planning to do so. Examples from different countries are given and problems encountered are discussed (chapter 19 -21). A request was made to all health authorities in Europe about the status of legislation in this field. The replies showed that several countries have introduced new legislation or are planning to do so. In chapter 22 a short summary of the european situation on licensing of radiopharmaceuticals is given.

Discussions at the symposium were informal and touched upon a huge number of subjects. A few subjects were, however, mentioned very often. It is probably characteristic that the field of radiopharmaceuticals now actually is moving against more welldefined chemical compounds particularly in the Tc-99m area. The introduction of newer analytical techniques are just in its beginning and is a precondition for this development. A planned design of new radiopharmaceuticals is, however, very much restricted of the very uncomplete and uncomparable way in which many animal studies are reported. There is an urgent need for standardisation. The cost of developing new radiopharmaceuticals may become prohibitive if too extensive and formal requirements are set up for animal studies. More individual considerations for each type of preparation may be required. The animal experiments may also for other reasons have to be restricted. The radiopharmaceutical area is, besides, the problems faced by drug industry in general, also faced with the radiation problem. This may lead to the discussion of the ethics of carrying out comparative studies and the use of reference groups. It was obvious that many findings in the clinical use cannot at present be explained by analytical methods either because patient factors may be involved or because quality control methods often are very crude. The wellknown problem of "carrierfree" or low level of substances handled, is still bothering us.

The cost-effectivenes of production and control systems were also in focus. In part 3 particularly the quality control aspect and the divided responsibility between the hospital and the kit and generator manufacturer is dealt with.

A very general problem were approached from many sides: How can we best reach a sensible level for the requirements for safety and efficacy. At what level do we set our standards? How much money is the society prepared to spend on extra safety? Who will take the responsibility? This problem is of course in nature a political one but at its basis it requires scientific information, on which risk estimates may be based.

1. STRUCTURE DISTRIBUTION RELATIONSHIP IN THE DESIGN OF Tc-99m RADIOPHARMACEUTICALS

GOPAL SUBRAMANIAN, J.G. MCAFEE, R.F. SCHNEIDER

1. INTRODUCTION

The origin of Quantitative Structure Activity Relationship (QSAR) in medicinal chemistry and drug design can be traced back to the year 1870 when Crum-Brown and Fraser (1) advanced the idea that for any drug,

Biological Response (activity), BR= f (S)

where f (S) is a function of chemical structure. They suggested that it should be possible to develop a mathematical formulation of QSAR by making changes in the chemical structure and relating these changes to the biological response or activity of the drugs so designed. The real barrier at that time was to define changes of chemical structure in numerical terms.

Since then, QSAR studies of drugs have been very significantly advanced mainly through notable works of Corwin Hansch (2) and Free and Wilson (3). Hansch's group was among the first, if not the first, to demonstrate that structure activity relationships can be quantified using substituent constants and regression analysis, thus:

Δ BR = f (Δ electronic + Δ steric + Δ hydrophobic + Δ polarity)

The changes in biological response, Δ BR, can be related to changes in measurable parameters of the drug due to different substituents.

Thus, constants such as π, σ , ES and MR (referring to the above measurable parameters) from model systems can be used to seek solutions to the above relationship using a matrix of equations. A whole library of such constants for more than 2000 QSARs involving 20000 compounds are available (4,5,6,7). A rigorous treatment of Hansch analysis is given by Tute (8).

More of such analysis for several types of drugs can be found in monographs and reviews by Purcell (9), Dietrich (10), Katz (11), Wells (12), Norrington et al (13) and Stuper et al (14).

Availability of computers (14) make these types of analysis easier. A new approach using a manual method for systematic new drug design has been recently reported by Austel (15).

For radiopharmaceuticals, these types of QSAR studies are rather scarce. The radioactive tracer drugs do not produce any measurable biological activity (except due to radiation intended for therapeutic effects) and we can only measure (if at all) their Quantitative Structure Distribution Relationship (QSDR). Scheibe (16) has nicely summarized a mathematical treatment for new radiotracer design based on QSDR analysis. A recent monograph by Spencer (17) discusses QSDRs of a variety of radiopharmaceuticals.

There are fundamental differences between therapeutic drugs and Tc-99m labelled radiopharmaceuticals. Pharmaceuticals have a definite molecular structure whereas the identy of Tc-99m labelled drugs is often unknown. In addition, Tc-99m radio-pharmaceuticals may contain impurities (reduced hydrolysed Tc-99m, free pertechnetate, etc) which can vary from day to day or batch to batch and obscure marginal differences in bio-distribution. The quality of Tc-99m labelled drugs also varies with the quality of Tc-99m pertechnetate used in labelling. The pH, presence of oxidizing agents, quantity of alumina and organic solvents (such as of MEK for Tc-99m extraction) influence the ultimate quality of the labelled compound. Before we attempt to correlate biodistribution with physical/chemical properties of the Tc-99m labelled drug, we have to make sure that the animal distribution data are reliable (18). The choice of animal species (model) for studying the biodistribution should be appropriate to the intended clinical use of the particular radiopharmaceutical. A recent symposium (19) addressed this important problem in some detail.

The biodistribution of radiopharmaceuticals usually depends on the following parameters:
1) molecular structure of the parent compound

2) type of chelate formation (1:1, 2:1 ligand to metal ratio, etc)

3) net charge

4) size (Stokes radius) and geometrical configuration

5) lipophilicity

6) molecular weight

7) protein binding

8) in vitro and in vivo stability

These data are not available for most of the Tc-99m compounds discussed in this review.

In the literature on QSAR studies of therapeutic drugs the constant π is related to lipophilicity as

$$\pi_x = \log P_x - \log P_c$$

where π_x = change in the measure of lipophilicity due to structural change x.

         P_x = (octanol/water) partition coefficient of compound with structural addition x.

         P_c = (octanol/water) partition coefficient of compound of parent compound C without x.

π values are considered important determinants of biological activity. Individual π_x values or similar constants for a variety of substituents are available in the literature (7.20). Recently a correlation between the lipophilicity of Tc-99m labelled radiopharmaceuticals used in hepatobiliary studies and their π values has been reported by Loberg (21). Unfortunately for many other Tc-99m complexes lipophilicity information is not available.

In this review we shall analyze three classes of Tc-99m labelled radiopharmaceuticals for SDRs based on their biodistribution in experimental animals. No rigorous mathematical treatment will be considered.

2. TC-99m LABELLED HIDA DERIVATIVES

2.1. Introduction

Loberg (22) and coworkers first described new Tc-99m labelled hepatobiliary agents utilizing the iminodiacetic acid (IDA) functional group for chelation of Tc-99m and a lidocaine backbone structure for hepatobiliary localization. Since that

time, several others (23, 24, 25, 26b) prepared a variety of
analogs of HIDA (O-dimethyl compound) and studied their
biodistribution in mice, rats, rabbits or monkeys. Compounds
with superior biological distribution were then evaluated in
humans. Recently these developments were reviewed in detail
(21, 27, 28). Defining the structure distribution
relationships studies of this group of compounds also has been
attempted (29, 30, 31). In this review, we shall present the
available animal biodistribution data and analyze their
SDRs.(Structure-Distribution Relationships)

The biodistribution data at 30 minutes after I.V. injection
in mice (25), rats (26a) and rabbits (23, 32) are shown in
Tables 1, 2 and 3 respectively. Scintigraphic images of
several groups of compounds are seen in Figures 1-5 (33).

Table 1. <u>DISTRIBUTION OF HIDA DERIVATIVES IN MICE AT 30 MIN.</u>
(DATA FROM CHIOTELLIS, 25)

SUBSTITUENTS ON PHENYL RING					% DOSE IN WHOLE ORGAN			
R2	R3	R5	R4	R6	BLOOD	LIVER	GIT	BLADDER
CH_3	H	H	H	CH_3	0.7	7.2	60.9	12.8
H	H	H	H	H	1.1	4.7	31.5	43.3
C_2H_5	H	H	H	C_2H_5	2.8	4.8	60.9	13.6
H	H	H	H	nC_4H_9	1.6	7.4	73.3	5.5
H	H	H	nC_4H_9	H	4.2	17.5	50.0	6.9
H	H	H	iC_4H_9	H	1.6	7.4	73.3	5.5
H	H	H	tC_4H_9	H	1.6	9.2	69.2	7.8
H	H	H	H	nOC_4H_9	2.2	16.6	49.9	19.4
H	H	H	nOC_4H_9	H	1.6	9.9	61.0	4.8
H	H	H	iOC_4H_9	H	1.6	8.0	76.4	4.4
H	nOC_4H_9	H	H	H	1.1	5.4	76.0	2.3
H	H	H	nOC_4H_9	CH_3	1.7	7.2	69.9	4.5
H	H	H	H	nOC_6H_{13}	4.7	7.9	55.1	5.3
H	H	H	nOC_6H_{13}	H	1.7	44.7	51.5	2.0
H	H	H	iOC_3H_7	H	1.7	6.3	42.3	31.2
H	H	H	OC_3H_5 ALLYL	H	2.4	2.2	48.1	23.2
H	H	H	H	COOH	5.6	8.3	34.2	28.3
H	OH	H	COOH	H	4.8	9.3	12.0	49.1
H	H	H	NTA AMIDE	H	3.2	1.1	3.8	55.1

Table 2. <u>DISTRIBUTION OF HIDA DERIVATIVES IN RATS AT 30 MIN.</u>

(DATA FROM MOLTER, 26)

<u>SUBSTITUENTS ON PHENYL RING</u>   OCTANOL   %DOSE IN WHOLE ORGAN

WATER

R2	R3	R5	R4	R6	P.C.	BLOOD	LIVER	GIT	KIDNEY	BLADDER
CH_3	H	H	H	HC_3	0.038	1.3	0.8	84	5.1	7.7
C_2H_5	H	H	H	C_2H_5	0.14	1.18	2.5	79	4.5	5.6
C_3H_7	H	H	H	C_3H_7	0.42	3.2	9.3	62	5.8	6.2
H	H	H	CH_3	H	0.38	1.5	2.4	62	4.7	16.3
H	H	H	C_2H_5	H	0.94	0.9	1.6	79	2.8	9.7
H	H	H	iC_3H_7	H	1.74	1.3	2.0	87	2.8	8.4
H	H	H	nC_4H_9	H	4.35	3.2	4.0	83	3.0	2.8
H	H	H	H	tC_4H_9	2.17	2.0	2.8	81	2.2	4.9
H	H	H	nC_5H11	H	32	0.5	12.5	85	1.0	0.13
H	H	H	C_6H_5	H	4.7	1.9	4.7	86	1.0	0.79
H	H	H	OCH_3	H	0.003	1.4	1.6	53	6.4	20.1
H	CH_3	KCH_3	H	H	0.19	1.3	1.3	62	5.9	8.4
CH_3	H	H	CH_3	CH_3	0.075	1.3	1.6	81	3.3	2.9
CH_3	H	CH_3	OH_3	H_3	0.037	1.7	1.7	81	2.3	5.7
H	H	H	F	H	0.096	1.0	1.9	64	4.4	15.6
F	H	H	F	H	0	1.6	2.7	54	4.8	21.5
F	F	H	H	H	0	1.5	3.1	53	8.3	18.4
F	F	F	F	F	0	0.7	3.8	82	1.6	1.8

The kinetic data obtained in the rabbit (23) are reported in Figures 6-10.

2.2 Animal Species Differences

A comparison of the biodistribution in three species of animals are shown in Table 4 below for the 2,6 diethyl and 4-n butyl HIDA. The biliary excretion seems to be the highest in the rat for both compounds. The n-butyl compound is excreted in the bile by the rat in proportionally higher concentrations than in the mouse or rabbit. This fast liver clearance in the rat for n-butyl derivative has not been observed in other animals or in man.The rabbit data for both compounds on the other hand closely resembles those obtained in man. It is

Fig. 2

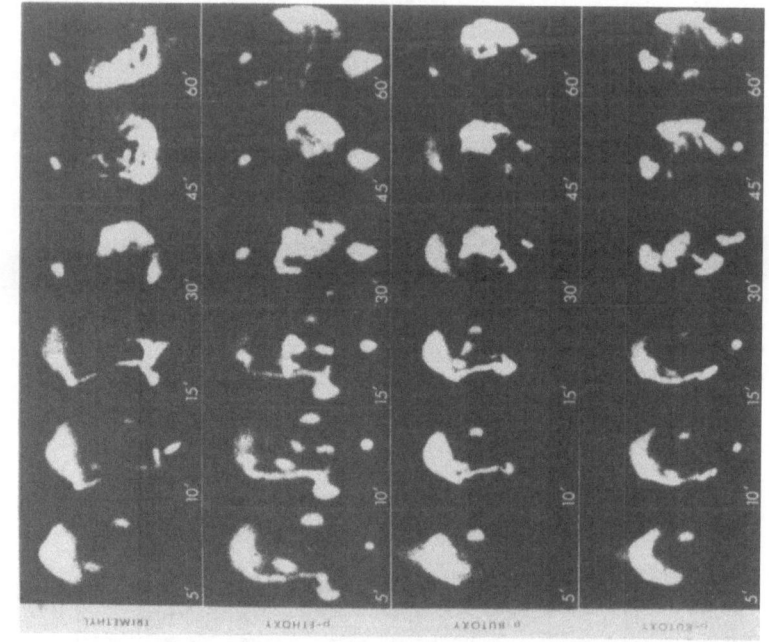

Fig. 1

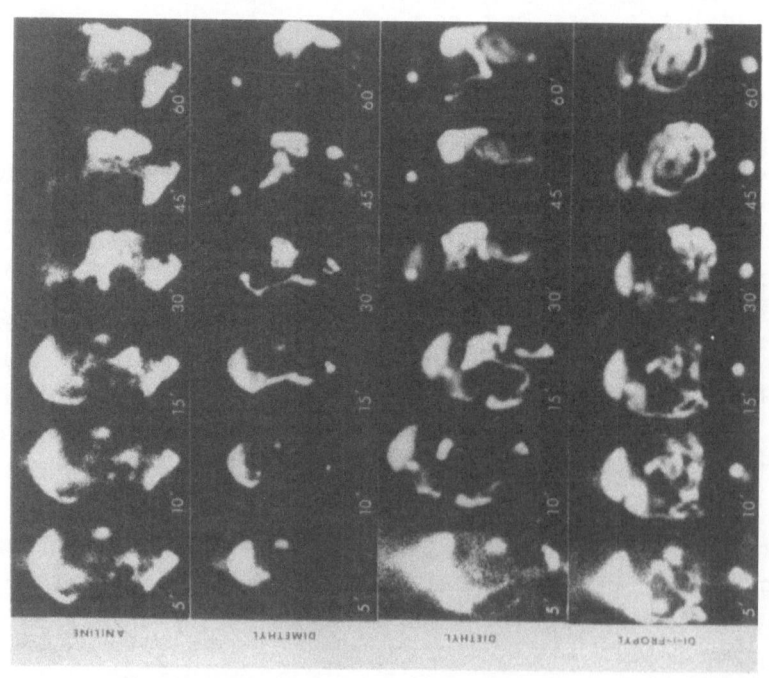

FIG. 1-5: Anterior images of rabbits obtained with wide field gamma camera. Each animal received 1-3 mCi Tc-99m and 2-3 mg of the compound

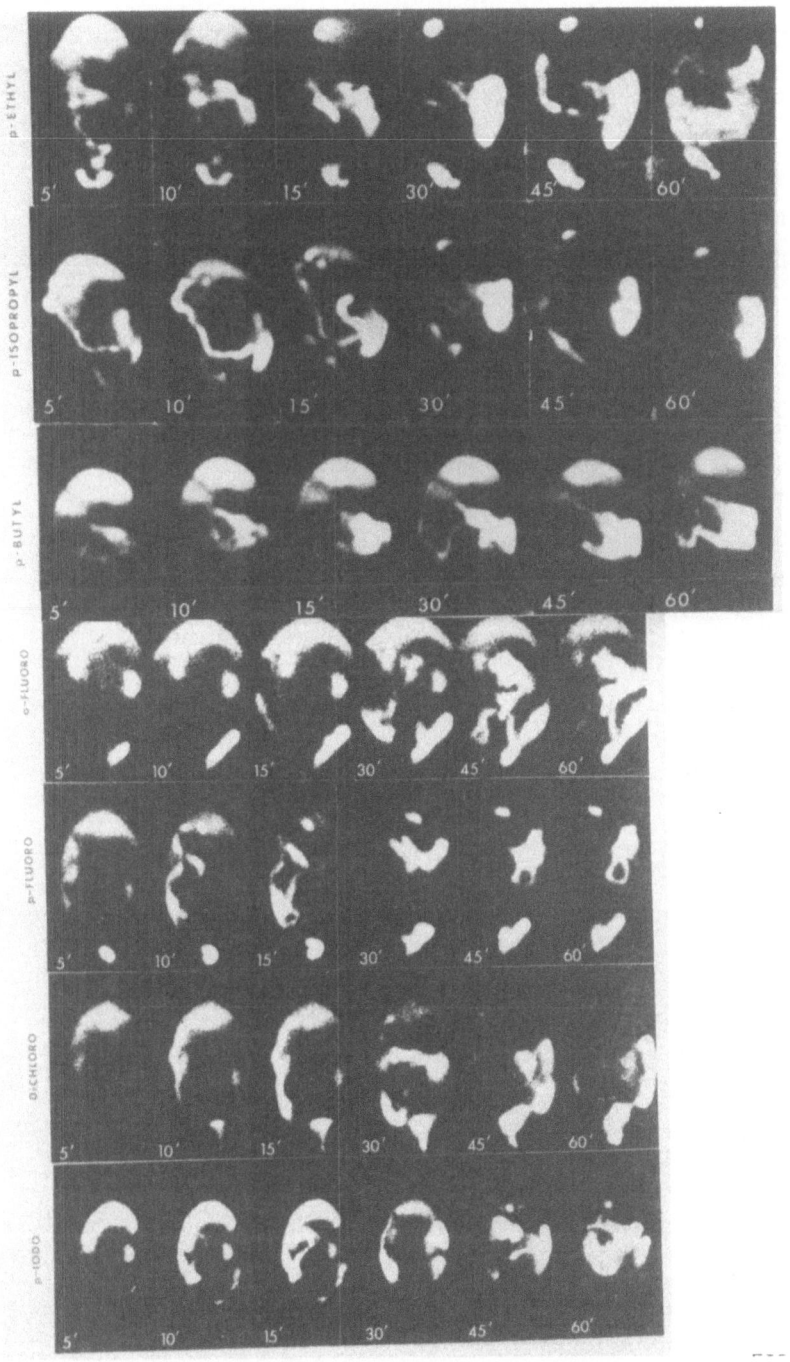

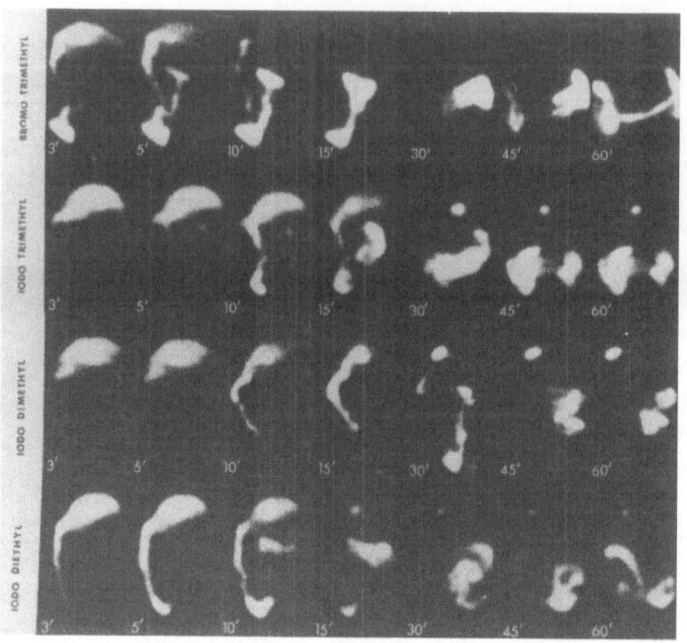

FIG. 5

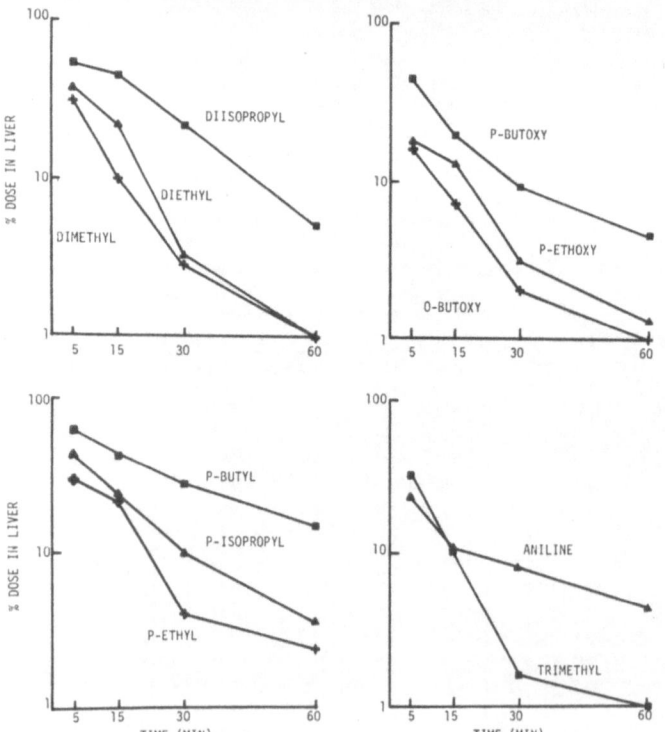

FIG. 6

13

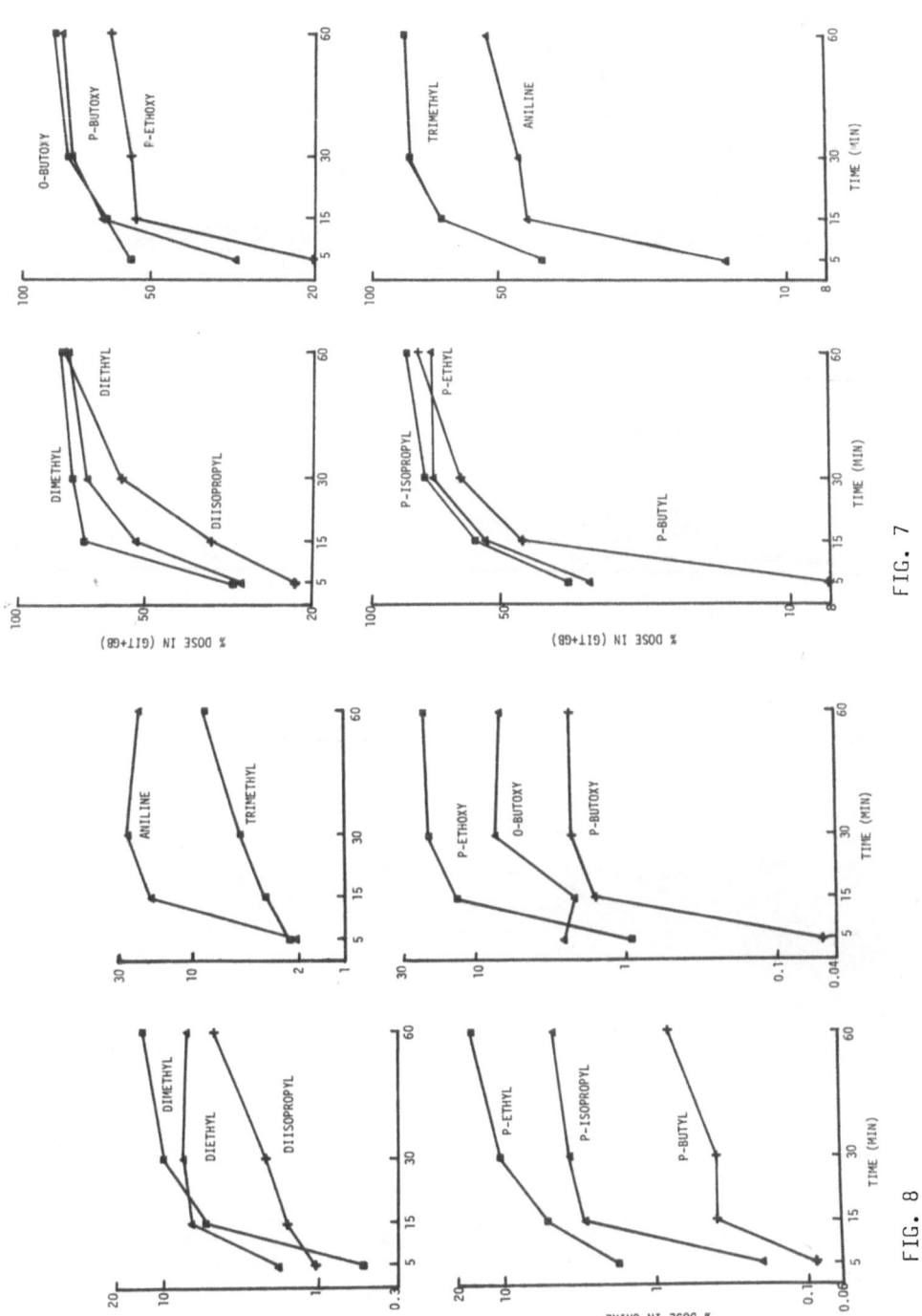

FIG. 7

FIG. 8

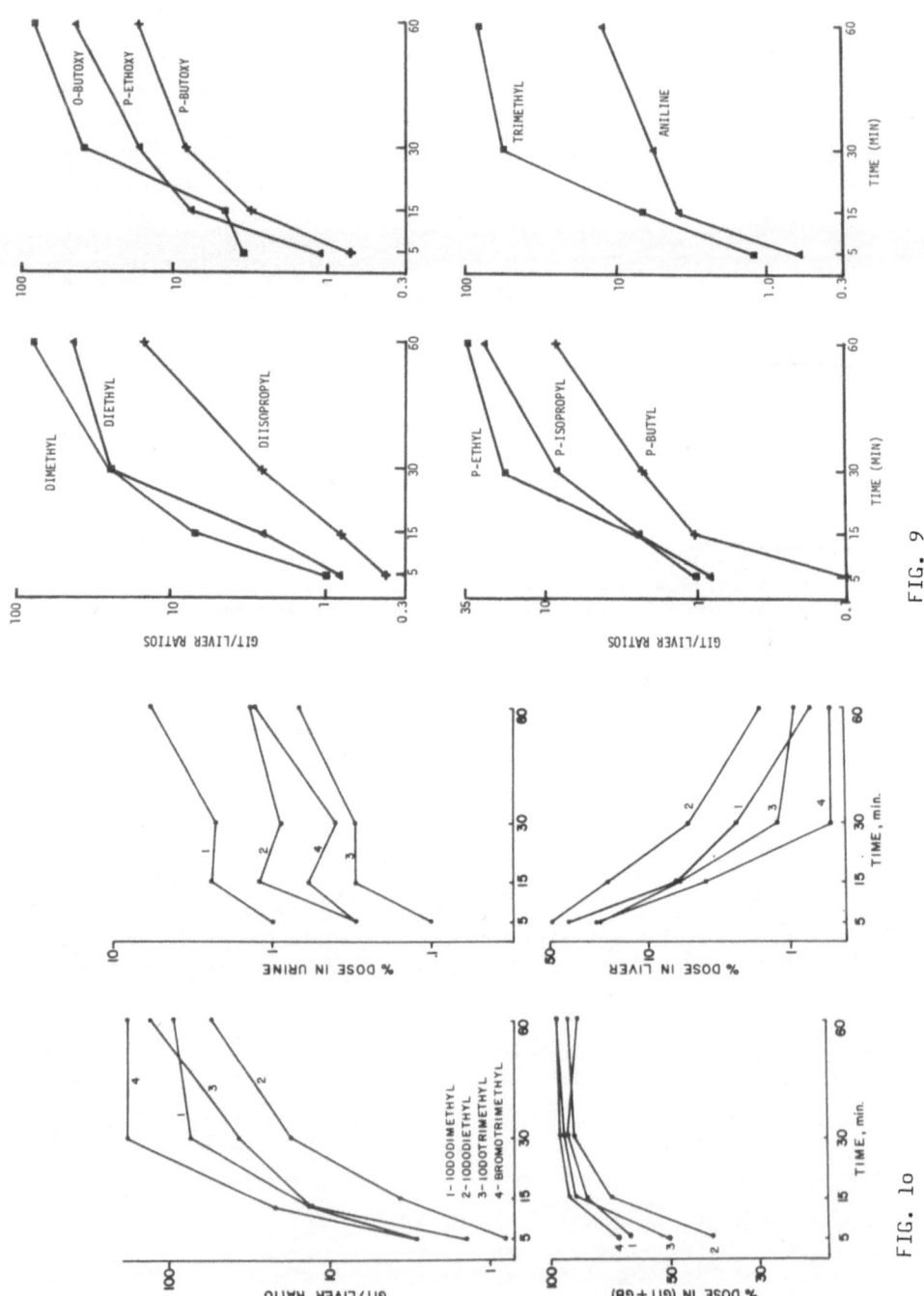

FIG. 9

FIG. 1o

Table 3. <u>DISTRIBUTION OF HIDA DERIVATIVES IN RABBITS AT 30 MIN.</u>
(DATA FROM SUBRAMANIAN, 23)

SUBSTITUENTS ON PHENYL RING				OCTANOL SALINE P.C.	% DOSE IN WHOLE ORGAN				
R2	R3 or R5	R4	R6	P.C.	BLOOD	LIVER	GIT	KIDNEY	BLADDER
H	H	H	H		5.9	8.2	43.5	22.2	4.4
H	H	C_2H_5	H		1.9	4.0	72.2	10.5	3.2
H	H	iC_3H_7	H		1.7	10.0	72.9	3.5	2.7
H	H	nC_4H_9	H		1.8	30.8	67.7	0.4	2.0
H	H	nOC_4H_9	H		1.7	10.4	79.1	2.4	1.4
H	H	H	nOC_4H_9		2.8	2.1	82.7	6.9	0.9
H	O	OC_2H_5	H		4.7	3.4	60.2	20.3	2.2
CH_3	H	H	CH_3		2.4	2.9	74.9	10.0	1.4
CH_3	I	H	CH_3	0.229	0.4	1.2	90.1	2.3	0.3
C_2H_5	H	H	C_2H_5		1.3	3.3	80.8	3.9	1.0
C_2H_5	I	H	C_2H_5	1.604	0.9	5.1	88.1	0.9	0.6
CH_3	H	CH_3	CH_3		2.7	1.7	81.8	5.1	1.0
CH_3	I	CH_3	CH_3	0.744	0.4	2.4	90.8	0.3	0.4
CH_3	Br	CH_3	CH_3	0.368	0.2	0.5	93.6	0.4	0.2
iC_3	H	H	iC_3H_7	0.920	4.8	22.4	59.8	2.2	2.1

generally accepted that biodistributions of radiopharmaceuticals should be performed in higher mammals whenever possible.
For our SDR analysis we shall compare groups of data from
individual animal species.

Table 4. <u>SPECIES DIFFERENCE: HIDA COMPOUNDS</u>

ANIMAL	BLOOD	LIVER	GIT	KIDNEY	URINE
		2,6 DIETHYL			
MOUSE	3.0	5.2	62	–	13.5
RAT	1.8	2.5	79	4.5	5.6
RABBIT	1.3	3.3	75	1.0	10.0
		P – n – BUTYL			
MOUSE	3.2	18.0	50	–	5.9
RAT	3.2	4.0	83	3.0	2.8
RABBIT	1.8	30.9	68	2.0	0.4

<u>2.3 Partition coefficient and biodistribution</u>

In the literature on therapeutic drugs, QSAR studies always
correlated lipophilicity with biological activity. Often a

parabolic relationship was demonstrated between a measured biological response and constant, the logarithm of partition coefficient differences. In SDR studies of radiopharmaceuticals no such attempt has been made. Figure 11 was constructed to demonstrate that there is no real correlation between measured partition coefficient (octanol/water, octanol/saline, ethylene chloride/water) and urinary excretion of Tc-99m HIDAs. Another attempt was made to find a relationship between liver clearance rate and partition coefficient. The results are shown in Figure 12. There seems to be no significant change in the liver clearance rate (as measured by t1/2 in min) up to a partition coefficient value of 1. However, there is a linear relationship between t1/2 and logarithm of the partition coefficient values 1 to 32. These results indicate that highly lipophilic compounds clear from the hepatocytes at a slow rate.

2.4 Molecular weight and biodistribution

Burns (29) demonstrated a direct relationship between structure and biliary (urine) excretion among several HIDA derivatives. The natural logarithm of the molecular weight to charge ratio, $\ln(mw/Z)$, was linearly related to the net biliary excretion. Among his compounds, only two contained hydrophilic groups. In figure 13, we present a similar plot between urinary excretion (at 30 min) and $\ln(mw/Z)$ for all reported compounds in three animal species. In this group of compounds only three radiopharmaceuticals had hydrophilic substituents on the phenyl ring. From these data one can surmise only a vague linear trend of correlation between urinary excretion and $\ln(mw/Z)$. In Figure 14, we present liver and GI tract concentrations and urinary excretion (both at 30 min) plotted against $\ln(mw/Z)$ for individual animal species. Among three species, only the data from the rabbit show any correlation at all.

Thus, it is very difficult to pinpoint one or two general physical parameters of Tc-99m HIDA compounds responsible for high hepatic uptake, clearance or urinary excretion even though some trends could be observed suggesting vague

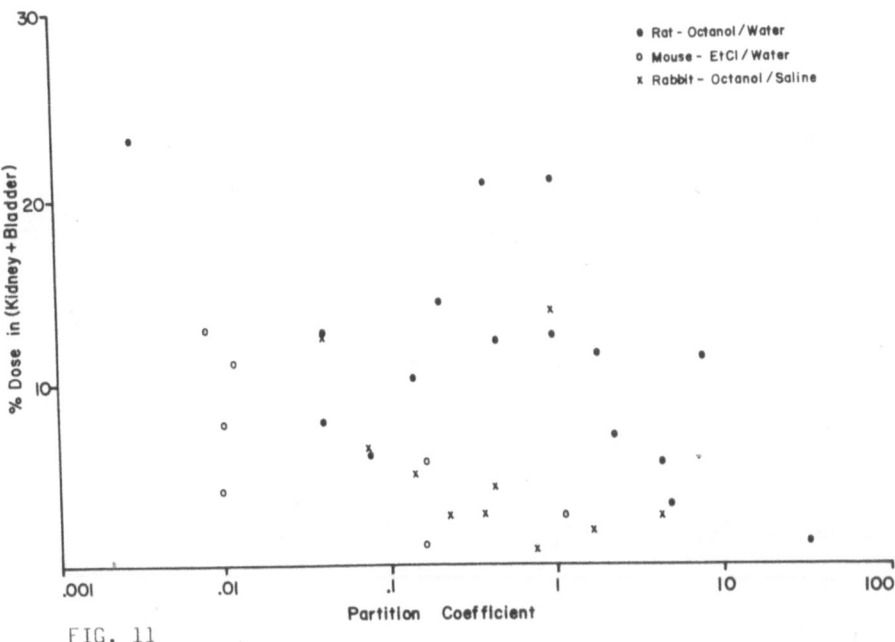

FIG. 11

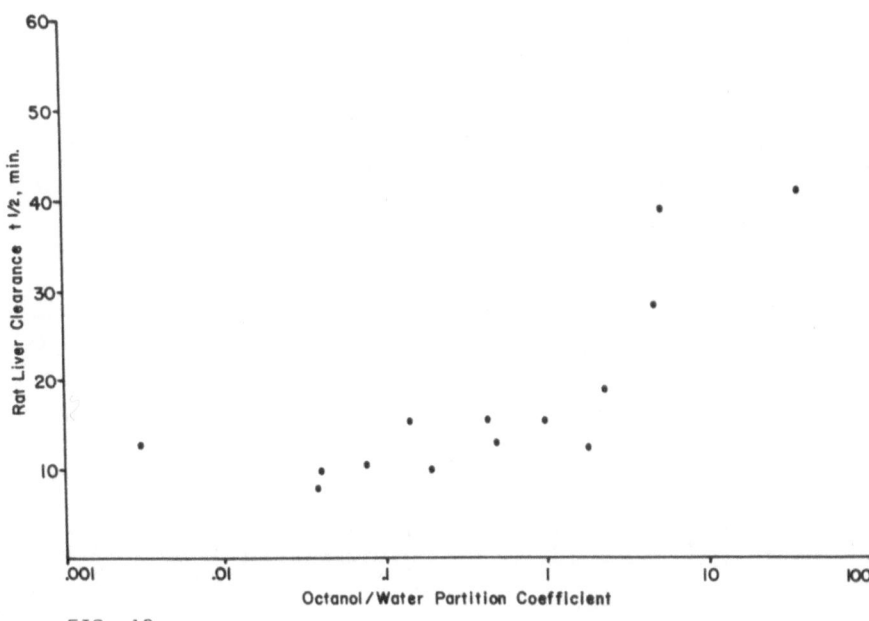

FIG. 12

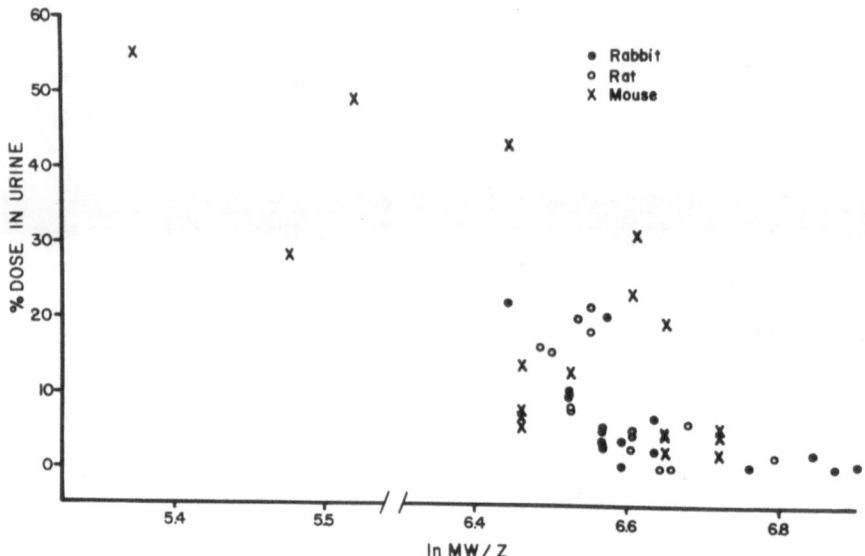

FIG. 13

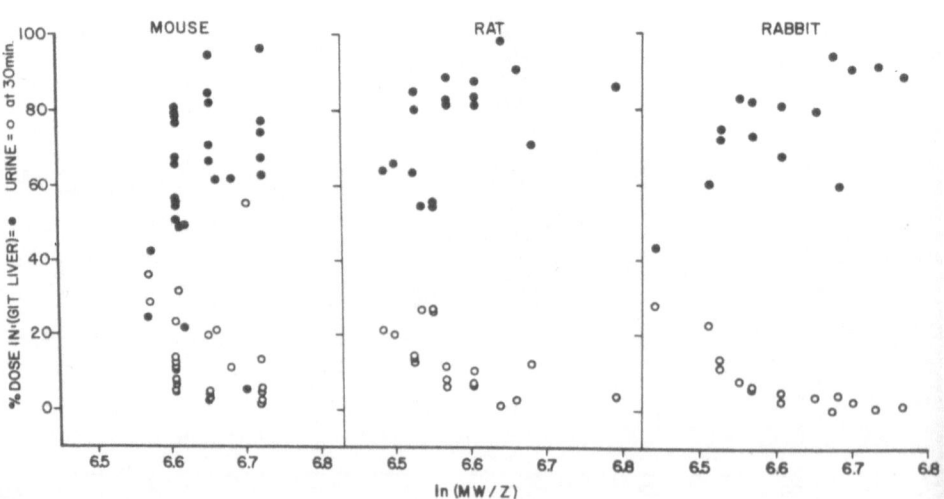

FIG. 14

correlations. To further test the theory that there is a linear correlation between hepatobiliary excretion and ln(mw/Z) parameter we synthesized sulfonic acid and sulphonamide derivates of HIDA and evaluated them in the rabbit by imaging studies using a gamma camera and by biodistribution. The results are shown in Figure 15 and Table 5:

Table 5. <u>DISTRIBUTION OF p-SUBSTITUTED HIDA IN RABBIT</u>

PERCENT DOSE AT ONE HOUR

ORGAN	NONE	$-SO_3H$	$-SO_2NH_2$
BLOOD	5.5	7.8	5.9
LIVER	4.4	3.4	3.2
GIT & GB	52.9	5.1	15.3
KIDNEYS	3.3	4.6	3.8
URINE	23.2	59.1	49.5
MUSCLE	3.3	7.5	8.9

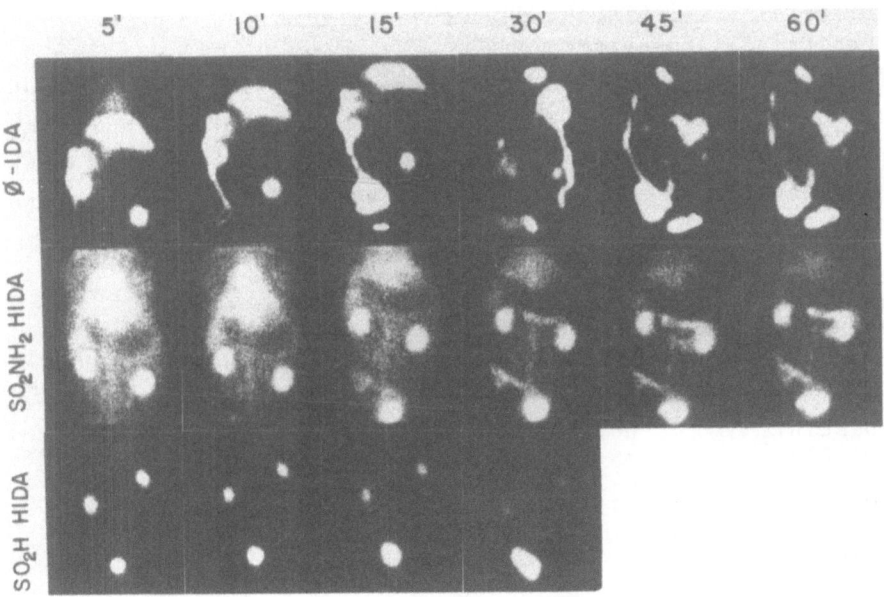

FIG.15: Posterior images of rabbits obtained with gamma camera. Each animal received 1-3 mCi of Tc-99m and 0,5-3 mg compound

For comparison purposes unsubstituted phenyl HIDA was included in the study. The unsubstituted compound is predominantly

excreted in the bile as shown both in the scintigraphs in
Figure 15 and in Table 5. The para substituted sulfonic acid
and sulfonamide derivatives show comparable excretion in the
urine with only marginal differences in biliary excretion,
both distinctly different than the unsubstituted phenyl
derivative. Both the sulfonic acid and sulphonamide compounds
have similar molecular weights but differ in their net charge
by -2 units. The sulphonamide is not ionized at plasma pH
values and the net charge is the same as that of the phenyl
derivative. The higher molecular weight sulphonamide did not
show biliary excretion even equivalent to the phenyl compound.
This may be due to increased specificity for sulfonamide
groups in the kidney. Therefore it can be safely said that
molecular weight has only marginal effect on the biliary
excretion of Tc-99m HIDA derivatives.

2.5 Structural differences and biodistribution
Positional Isomerism:

In this section we will examine the effect of various
substituent groups (on the phenyl rings of HIDAs) on the
biodistribution. Van Wyk et al (34) evaluated six different
dimethyl substituted isomers in rabbits. Their results are
shown below in Table 6. There is a definite steric effect.

Table 6. POSITIONAL ISOMERISM
RABBIT 20 MIN

	TRANSIT EFFICIENCY	TRANSIT TIME MIN.	%DOSE IN BLADDER
2,6 DIMETHYL	66	4	14
2,3 DIMETHYL	75	3	9
2,4 DIMETHYL	64	3	16
2,5 DIMETHYL	71	2	10
3,4 DIMETHYL	69	2	9
3,5 DIMETHYL	82	2	16

2,3 dimethyl, 2,5 dimethyl and 3,4 dimethyl derivatives had a
faster transit time in the liver and a lower urinary excretion
than the other three compounds. The meta substituted
derivatives are considerably better than the ortho substituted
compounds. This conclusion is in contradiction with the data

obtained in rats as shown in Table 7. No significant
differences between 2,4,6 trimethyl, 2,4,5 trimethyl compounds
can be demonstrated except for small differences in liver
transit time.

Table 7. <u>POSITIONAL ISOMERISM</u>

COMPOUND	RAT LIVER t 1/2 MIN	BLOOD	% DOSE AT 30 MIN LIVER	GIT	URINE	GIT/LIVER
2,6 DIMETHYL	9.5	1.3	84.1	84.1	7.7	101
3,5 DIMETHYL	9.9	1.3	62.1	62.1	8.4	48
2,4,6 TRIMETHYL	10.4	1.3	81.0	81.0	2.9	51
2,4,5 TRIMETHYL	7.7	1.7	80.6	80.6	5.7	48

Similar isomer effect has been demonstrated for butyl group
substitution on the phenyl ring. The data from Chiotellis (25)
are shown in Table 8. Between the n-butyl, i-butyl and t-butyl
isomers no significant difference in urinary excretion could
be found. However, both t-butyl and i-butyl derivatives showed
a higher hepatic excretion into the bile than the n-butyl
compound.

Table 8. <u>SIDE CHAIN ISOMERISM PARA POSITION</u>

COMPOUND	MOUSE % DOSE AT 30 MIN BLOOD	LIVER	GIT	URINE	GIT/LIVER
-n-BUTYL	4.2	17.5	50.0	6.9	2.86
-i-BUTYL	1.6	7.4	73.3	5.5	9.91
-t-BUTYL	1.6	9.2	69.2	7.8	7.52
REPEAT:					
-n-BUTYL	3.2	17.1	49.7	5.9	2.81
-t-BUTYL	0.8	10.0	69.3	7.1	6.93

2.6 Increased molecular weight and biodistribution

The effect of higher molecular weight (by increasing the
chain length at the paraposition on the phenyl ring) on the
biodistribution in the rat and rabbit is shown in Tables 9 and
10.

Table 9. SIDE CHAIN LENGTH: PARA POSITION

COMPOUND	RAT LIVER t 1/2 MIN	BLOOD	LIVER	GIT	URINE	GIT/LIVER
$-CH_3$	12.7	1.5	2.4	62.3	16.3	26
$-C_2H_5$	14.7	0.9	1.6	78.5	9.7	49
$-iC_3H_7$	11.7	1.3	2.0	86.8	8.4	43
$-nC_4H_9$	27.6	3.2	4.0	83.3	2.8	21
$-nC_5H_{11}$	41.0	0.5	12.5	85.4	0.1	7
$-tC_4H_9$	18.4	2.0	2.8	80.4	4.9	29

% DOSE AT 30 MIN.

Table 10. SIDE CHAIN LENGTH: PARA POSITION

RABBIT   % DOSE AT 30 MIN.

COMPOUND	BLOOD	LIVER	GIT	URINE	GIT/LIVER
$-H$	5.9	8.2	43.5	24.7	5.3
$-C_2H_5$	1.9	4.0	72.2	10.5	18.1
$-iC_3H_7$	1.7	10.0	72.9	3.5	7.3
$-nC_4H_9$	1.8	30.8	67.7	0.4	2.2

These data clearly demonstrate that increased molecular weight (by para substitution) significantly diminishes the urinary excretion in both rat and the rabbit. However, para substitution by long normal chain aliphatic group also increases the lipophilicity resulting in diminished liver clearance rate. The $i-C_3H_7$ group has similar liver t 1/2 as $-CH_3$ group because of its isomerism. If an $n-C_3H_7$ group has been substituted, the liver t 1/2 would have been significantly higher than that of the $-C_2H_5$ group. A similar explanation could be given for the liver t 1/2 differences between $n-C_4H_9$ group and $t-C_4H_9$ group. This isomerism effect has also been pointed out in Table 8.

Table 11. SIDE CHAIN LENGTH: 2,6 POSITION

COMPOUND	RABBIT			% DOSE AT 30 MIN.	
	BLOOD	LIVER	GIT	URINE	GIT/LIVER
2,6 DIMETHYL	2.4	2.9	74.9	10.0	26
2,6 DIETHYL	1.3	3.3	80.8	3.9	25
2,6 DIISOPROPYL	4.8	22.4	59.8	2.2	2.7

HALOGEN SUBSTITUTION IN META POSITION

3 IODO 2,6 DIMETHYL	0.37	1.2	90.1	2.33	75
3 IODO 2,6 DIETHYL	0.85	5.1	88.1	0.94	17
3 IODO 2,4,6 TRIMETHYL	0.40	2.4	90.8	0.34	38
3 BROMO 2,4,6 TRIMETHYL	0.17	0.5	93.6	0.42	187

The effect of increased molecular weight at the ortho position
on the biliary excretion in the rabbit is shown in Table 11
along with data on new halogen substituted HIDA derivatives
(35,36,26). Similar to the para substituted derivatives, the
ortho substituted compounds also show a decrease in urinary
excretion with the increase in molecular weight. The liver
clearance seems to be slower for the o-diisopropyl compound
compared to the other two derivatives. The newer halogen
substituted compounds show dramatic differences compared to
the previous generation of HIDAs. All the four halogen
derivatives in Table 11 show superior biological
characteristics and present as almost ideal compounds for
clinical use. Similar results can be expected for the iodine
derivatives also. Based on the above analysis Table 12 lists
compounds acceptable for clinical use.

Table 12. ACCEPTABLE COMPOUNDS FOR CLINICAL USE

OLD	NEW
2,6 DIETHYL	3 IODO 2,6 DIMETHYL
2,6 DIISOPROPYL	3 IODO 2,6 DIETHYL
4 - ISOPROPYL	3 IODO 2,4,6 TRIMETHYL
3,4,5 TRIMETHYL	3 BROMO 2,4,6TRIMETHYL
4 - n - BUTYL	
4 - n - PENTYL	
2 - HEXYLOXY	

The 4-n-butyl, 4-n-pentyl and 2-hexyloxy derivatives have slower liver clearance rates than to other compounds in this list.

It is well known that compounds with molecular weight less than 500 are not excreted in the bile but are filtered out by the kidney when there is no strong in vivo protein binding (37,38,39). The Tc-99m HIDA derivatives are formed by complexation between two HIDA molecules and one Tc-99m atom (40). The net molecular weight of derivatives reported so far range from 680 to about 95o and these complexes usually carry a single negative charge. The high molecular weight compounds are those developed with halogen containing diortho or 2,4,6 trimethyl derivatives. Lipophilicity data for these compounds indicate that the liver clearance time increases with increase in lipophilicity. No good correlations could be found between protein binding (26a) and biliary excretion. Obviously there must be a of range lipophilicity and protein binding values for optimum hepatobiliary excretion. These data are not yet available even for the "optimized" derivatives. Thus the QSDR for Tc-99m HIDAs discussed above still seems to be empirical. Further investigation in this area is necessary.

3. Tc-99m LABELLED DIPHOSPHONATES

Bone imaging is one of the most frequently performed diagnostic tests in nuclear medicine. Since the introduction of Tc-99m skeletal complexes a wide variety of new phosphate compounds has been introduced. These developments have been reviewed previously (41, 42) At present, the Tc-99m diphosphonates are the preferred agents for bone imaging. In this review we shall attempt to search for any QSDR for these compounds. It is difficult to compare the results from various investigators because their data were obtained in different species and were reported in different formats. Biodistributions have been performed in mice, rats, rabbits and dogs, and bone concentration data are reported as percent

Table 13. <u>DISTRIBUTION OF DIPHOSPHONATES IN THE RAT</u>

<u>SUBSTITUENTS</u>   <u>% DOSE/GM AT 2 HRS</u>

R_1	R_2	FEMUR	BLOOD	LIVER	KIDNEY	FEMUR BLOOD	REFERENCE
H	H	1.03	0.025	0.021	0.827	41	(44, 45)
H	H	1.48	0.043	0.027	0.701	34	(44, 45)
H	H	3.00	0.015	0.036	0.658	200	(49)
H	OH	3.01	0.018	0.046	0.276	167	(48)
H	OH	2.58	0.021	0.098	0.929	123	(44, 45)
CH_3	OH	1.13	0.052	0.035	0.796	22	(44, 45)
CH_3	OH	3.0	0.034	0.023	0.615	88	(43)
CH_3	OH	2.04	0.116	0.135	2.184	18	(47)
CH_3	OH	1.87	0.050	0.038	–	37	(47)
CH_3	H	1.26	0.029	0.016	0.882	43	(44, 45)
CH_3	CH_3	0.76	0.053	0.029	0.668	14	(44, 45)
OH	OH	1.14	0.062	0.051	3.614	18	(44, 45)
C1	C1	0.69	0.054	0.025	0.720	13	(44, 45)
	C = O	0.96	0.071	0.214	2.693	14	(44, 45)
H	$CH_2-\phi$	0.77	0.214	0.062	1.361	4	(44, 45)
H	CH_2COOH	3.7	0.02	0.035	0.417	185	(49)
H	CHCOOH	3.8	0.019	0.041	0.425	200	(49)
CH_2-CH_2-COOH	$\overset{CH_2COOH}{\underset{\vert}{CH_2CH_2COOH}}$	2.9	0.06	0.052	0.517	48	(49)
OH	$CH_2CH_2NH_2$	3.2	0.03	0.075	0.617	107	(49)
H	$N-(CH_3)_2$	2.9	0.02	0.047	0.408	145	(49)
H	$N-(CH_3)_2$	1.8	0.064	0.095	0.568	28	(47)
H	NH_2	1.1	0.043	0.045	–	26	(47)
H	$NH-CH_3$	2.68	0.105	0.103	0.721	26	(47)
H	$\overset{+}{N}-(CH_3)_3$	1.31	0.192	0.143	1.747	7	(47)
H	$NH-(CH_2)_3-CH_3$	1.90	0.045	0.045	–	42	(47)
H	$NH-\phi$	2.67	0.486	0.408	2.804	6	(47)
H	$NH-\phi-Cl$	1.66	0.652	0.091	2.926	3	(47)
H	$NH-(CH_2)_2-\phi$	2.24	0.163	0.111	2.14	14	(47)
H	N⬡	1.81	0.047	0.111	0.524	39	(47)

dose in organ, percent dose per gram or percent dose per 1% body weight. Table 13 contains a summary of all the Tc-99m diphosphonate biodistribution data obtained from rats from several investigators (43,44,45,46,47,48,49). The rat is not an ideal model of the adult human skeleton because skeletal growth does not stop in this species. The cortical bone of the adult rats and other smaller animals is mostly endosteal, containing very little primary osteon bone. It does not contain any secondary osteon bone except in healing lesions and lacks the secondary haversian systems of the adult skeleton of larger animals and man (50). Moreover, osteogenesis is induced poorly and slowly in rats and mice compared with man and larger animals (51). It is difficult to intercompare biodistribution data in rats between investigators even for the same compound. A close examination of Table 13 shows that for MDP, the % dose/gm value for femur from different authors varies from 1.03 to 3.0; for EHDP it varies from 1.13 to 3.0. All the data in Table 13 have been converted to the given format using the reported weights of animals used and organ weights from rats of different body weights (data obtained in our laboratory and shown in Table 14). The Hoechst brochure does not provide weights of rats used in their study. We assumed a body weight of 15o gm to calculate % dose/gm values for the liver and kidneys.

Table 14. ASSAYED ORGAN WEIGHTS IN RATS

WT OF RATS	LIVER	KIDNEYS(2)	WHOLE FEMUR
152.9 g (148 - 159)	6.13 g	1.19 g	0.462 g
PERCENT (WT/BWT)	4.01	0.778	0.302
256.4 (240 - 264)	11.12 g	2.13 g	0.714 g
PERCENT (WT/BWT)	4.34	0.831	0.278

Unterspann used 250 gm weight rats and expressed his data as percent dose in whole skeleton assuming skeletal weight is equivalent to 25 times that of a single femur. We converted these values using the femur weights shown in Table 14. Blood weight was assumed to be 6% of the body weight.

Table 15. <u>DISTRIBUTION OF DIPHOSPHONATES IN THE RAT   2 HRS.</u>

(DATA FROM WANG 44,45)

R_1	R_2	% DOSE/GM FEMUR	BLOOD	FEMUR/BLOOD
H	H	1.48	0.043	34
H	OH	2.58	0.021	123
CH_3	OH	1.13	0.052	22
CH_3	H	1.26	0.029	43
CH_3	CH_3	0.76	0.053	14
OH	OH	1.14	0.062	18
C1	C1	0.69	0.054	13
C=O		0.96	0.071	14
H	$CH_2\text{-}\phi$	0.77	0.214	4

The distribution data in rats from Wang (44,45) for 9 different diphosphonates are shown in Table 15. Of these compounds, HMDP with a single OH group on the central carbon seems to concentrate highest in the femur and also has a low blood level. The dimethyl (2,2 propylene diphosphonate), carbonyl and dichloro compounds exhibit considerably lower bone uptake than MDP. The benzyl derivative not only shows poor skeletal uptake but has a high blood level as well.

As explained by Wang (44,45), the relatively higher bone uptakes of MDP and HMDP may be due to keto-enol tautomerism. However, Unterspann (47) disputes this claim pointing out that similar uptake was not observed with his aminomethane derivatives. His explanation is that in addition to keto-enol tautomerism, steric hindrance also plays a very important role in bone uptake of diphosphonates. Unterspann's data are summarized in Tables 16 and 17.

Table 16. <u>DISTRIBUTION OF DIPHOSPHONATES IN THE RAT 2 HRS.</u>

(DATA FROM UNTERSPANN 46,47)

% DOSE/GM

R_1	R_2	FEMUR	BLOOD	FEMUR/BLOOD
H	$N-H_2$	1.1	0.043	26
H	$N-CH_3$	2.68	0.105	26
H	$N-(CH_3)_2$	1.8	0.064	28
H	$\overset{+}{N}-(CH_3)_3$	1.31	0.192	7

Table 17. <u>DISTRIBUTION OF DIPHOSPHONATES IN THE RAT 2 HRS.</u>

(DATA FROM UNTERSPANN, 46,47)

% DOSE/GM

R_1	R_2	FEMUR	BLOOD	FEMUR/BLOOD
H	$NH-H$	1.1	0.043	26
H	$NH-CH_3$	2.68	0.105	26
H	$NH-(CH_2)_3-CH_3$	1.90	0.045	42
H	$NH-\phi$	2.67	0.486	6
H	$NH-\phi-Cl$	1.66	0.652	3
H	$NH-(CH_2)_2$	2.24	0.163	14

In his study of a series of aminomethyl derivatives, Unterspann clearly demonstrates that a secondary binding site (-C-NH-R) such as an imino group on the central carbon of the diphosphonate increases skeletal binding. Saturation of the nitrogen, or quaternisation drastically reduces bone uptake. However, if the R group on the imino nitrogen is liphophilic (e.g. long alkyl, phenyl, phenethyl groups) the bone uptake is also drastically reduced and results in substantial increases in blood levels. Protein binding may be the cause for the increased blood concentrations. These results clearly illustrate that steric hindrance on the central carbon interferes with bone uptake of diphosphonates. The data from the Hoechst brochure are summarized in Table 18.

The percent per gram femur values for all compounds are considerably higher than those reported by other investigators. This increase may be attributed to the small size (age) of the rats (100-150 gm body weights used in this study). We cannot compare these results with anyone else's. However, intercomparisons are possible. Of the six diphosphonates, DPD, containing succinic acid on the center carbon showed the highest skeletal accumulation, followed closely by the diphosphonate containing the acetic acid group.

Table 18. <u>DISTRIBUTION OF DIPHOSPHONATES IN THE RAT   2 HRS.</u>
(DATA FROM HOECHST, 49)

		% DOSE/GM		
R_1	R_2	FEMUR	BLOOD	FEMUR/BLOOD
H	H	3.0	0.015	200
H	CH_2COOH	3.7	0.02	185
H	CHCOOH | CH_2COOH	3.8	0.019	200
CH_2CH_2COOH	CH_2CH_2COOH	2.9	0.06	48
OH	$CH_2CH_2NH_2$	3.2	0.03	107
H	$N-(CH_3)_2$	2.9	0.02	145

However, the compound containing two propionic acid groups on the central carbon of the diphosphonate did not concentrate in the skeleton as well as the DPD complex. Moreover, its blood level is three times higher than DPD. Inspite of the very high bone uptake, the DPD femur/blood ratio is not better than that of MDP. The high bone uptake of DPD may be attributed to its very low in vivo protein binding and high extraction ratio in the bone. These are only speculations and no published data are available to verify this explanation.

From the foregoing analysis, it can be concluded that for high normal skeletal uptake, the diphosphonate should contain a secondary binding site such as -OH, -NH- groups on the central carbon atom, without steric hindrance. The presence of carboxylic groups may reduce in vivo protein binding; however this group should be far enough away from the central carbon such that no secondary chelation between the carboxylic group and phosphate moiety is possible. If these conditions are met, the diphosphonate concentrations is high in normal bone.

Clinical bone imaging studies are performed to delineate abnormal bone from normal skeleton. The abnormal bone concentration of the Tc-99m bone imaging agent is usually higher than normal bone. Therefore any new skeletal imaging agent should provide a better contrast between abnormal and normal bone. The selection of a new bone agent should be based on its lesion detection ability. In recent years new bone imaging agents like HMDP, DPD (48,49,52,53) have been introduced which achieve somewhat higher concentration in normal bone than MDP. To compare these agents in their lesion detection ability, our laboratory evaluated them in rabbits with experimental bone lesions (54). The structural formulae of these agents are shown in Figure 16. Table 19 presents their biodistribution data as Tc-99m/Sr-85 ratios along with the Sr-85 distribution data (from 36 animals) for intercomparison purposes.

The average normal bone concentrations of HMDP, DPD are considerably higher than those for MDP. Other compounds concentrated in the normal skeleton to either equal or less levels than MDP. The compound DMAD showed lower normal skeletal uptake than MDP but almost equivalent abnormal bone uptake thus giving a better lesion/normal bone ratio. The increased lesion uptake could explained as follows: 1) The single pass extraction of DMAD in the normal skeleton may be less than that for MDP. 2) The uptake in a bone lesion depends on its blood flow and surface area The longer the compound circulates without excessive renal excretion, the higher is its concentration in the lesion.

The reverse of the above theory may hold true to the failure of DPD and HMDP to demonstrate high lesion to bone ratios. These results indicate that compounds with high normal bone uptakes need not necessarily concentrate to a higher degree in the lesions. The results obtained with DMAD in our investigations have been confirmed in clinical studies. However, DMAD showed higher blood and soft tissue levels than MDP in patients. At the present time, in comparison with other compounds Tc-99m labelled MDP remains as the best "compromise" agent which visualizes both normal and abnormal bones well. The only agent with better lesion/bone detectability was DMAD.

Structure distribution relationships of Tc-99m diphosphonates discussed above should be considered only as a preliminary report. There are several parameters which influence bone agent distributions. Serum protein binding (not just albumin), renal and bone extraction ratios, in vivo

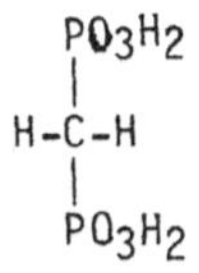

$$PO_3H_2$$
$$|$$
$$H-C-H$$
$$|$$
$$PO_3H_2$$

MDP

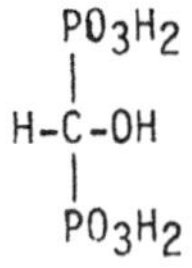

$$PO_3H_2$$
$$|$$
$$H-C-OH$$
$$|$$
$$PO_3H_2$$

HMDP

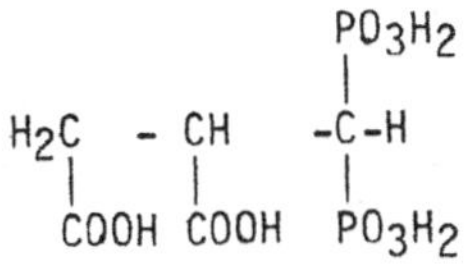

$$PO_3H_2$$
$$|$$
$$H_2C \quad - \quad CH \quad -C-H$$
$$| \quad \quad | \quad \quad |$$
$$COOH \quad COOH \quad PO_3H_2$$

DPD

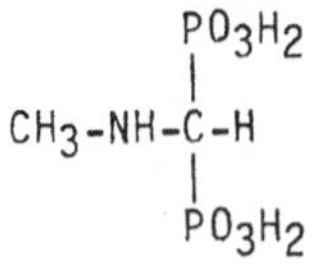

$$PO_3H_2$$
$$|$$
$$CH_3-NH-C-H$$
$$|$$
$$PO_3H_2$$

NMMDP

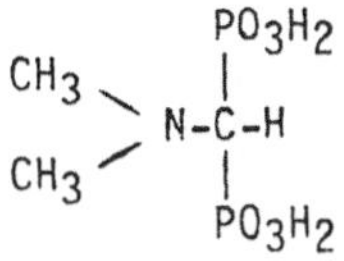

$$PO_3H_2$$
$$CH_3 \quad \quad |$$
$$\diagdown \quad N-C-H$$
$$CH_3 \quad \diagup \quad |$$
$$PO_3H_2$$

DMAD

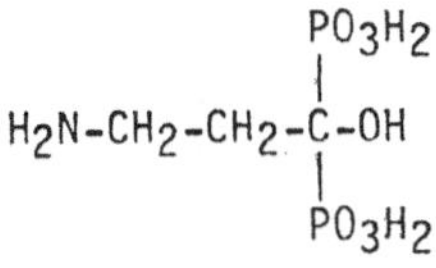

$$PO_3H_2$$
$$|$$
$$H_2N-CH_2-CH_2-C-OH$$
$$|$$
$$PO_3H_2$$

APD

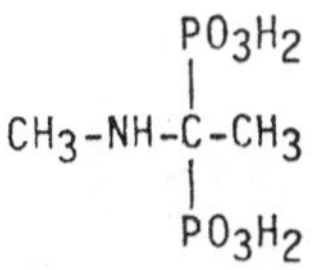

$$PO_3H_2$$
$$|$$
$$CH_3-NH-C-CH_3$$
$$|$$
$$PO_3H_2$$

NMEDP

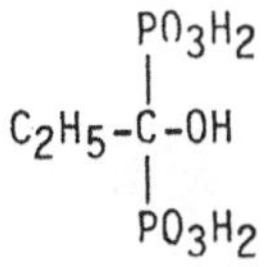

$$PO_3H_2$$
$$|$$
$$C_2H_5-C-OH$$
$$|$$
$$PO_3H_2$$

HPD

$$PO_3H_2$$
$$|$$
$$CH_3-C-H$$
$$|$$
$$PO_3H_2$$

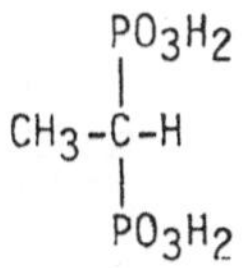

1,1 EDP

Fig. 16 Structural formulae of new Diphosphonates evaluated.

Table 19

DISTRIBUTION OF Tc-99m DIPHOSPHONATES AND Sr-85 IN RABBITS

SIMULTANEOUS STUDY 3 HRS POST INJECTION

Tc-99m/Sr-85 RATIOS

ORGAN	MDP (6)ˣ	HMDP(6)	DPD (6)	NMMDP (6)	DMAD (6)	APD (6)	1,1EDP (4)	NMEDP (3)
BLOOD	0.338	0.388	0.358	0.272	0.319	0.285	0.344	0.675
MUSCLE	0.16	0.289	0.741	0.142	0.183	0.153	0.145	0.338
AVE.BONE	0.805	1.560	1.287	0.818	0.515	0.820	0.542	0.465
CALLUS/TIBIA	1.41	1.08	1.03	1.36	2.00	1.19	1.78	1.58

ORGAN	SR-85 1% BWT	%DOSE
BLOOD	0.515	2.2
MUSCLE	0.150	8.4
AVE.BONE	9.25	40.0
CALLUS/TIBIA	3.2	–

x Ratios were calculated for individual animals and then averaged. (Numbers in brackets indicate the number of animals used for each compound.)

stability, carrier effect and pH of the labelled compound all seem to influence the biological behaviour of Tc-99m bone agents. Few such data are available even for the commonly used diphosphonates. It is clear that considerable new data are needed before one can develop SDRs for Tc-99m diphosphonates in a rigorous manner.

4. Tc-99m LABELLED RENAL TUBULAR EXCRETION AGENTS

Radioiodine labelled orthoiodohippurate (Hippuran) is the agent of choice for renal tubular excretion studies in man. The undesirable physicial properties of Iodine-131 and the cost and limited availability of Iodine-123 prompted a continuing search for a Tc-99m labelled agent to replace Hippuran.

Davison et al (55, 56) introduced a new class of chelating agents containing an ethylenediamine backbone coupled to mercaptoacetyl groups. Thus Tc-99m labelled N,N[1] bis (mercaptoacetamido) ethylenediamine (Tc-99m DADS) became the first promising renal tubular excretion agent. This compound was later investigated in detail by Fritzberg et al (57). They found that this new agent also localized in the liver and was excreted in the bile to the intestines, thus obscuring renal images. In experimental animals, as much as 10% of the injected dose concentrated in the above organs. Later clinical studies also confirmed this observation (Klingensmith (58, 59). Jones et al (60) present further details on this complex. To improve the biological distribution of the Tc-99m DADS complex, Fritzberg (61) prepared a modified complex of DADS incorporating a carboxyl group on the ethylenediamine backbone (CO_2 DADS). The proposed structures of this Tc-99m complex are shown in Figure 17. There are two isomers possible. Fritzberg (61) separated these two isomers by HPLC and found that one of the isomers (peak A) exhibited superior renal tubular excretion. Our laboratory prepared the same complex and determined its biological distribution by imaging studies in rabbits which are shown in Figure 18 comparing it with Tc-99m DTPA and I-131 hippuran. Further evaluation of this complex in higher mammals indicated a species difference. In Figure 19,

Tc-CO₂-DADS

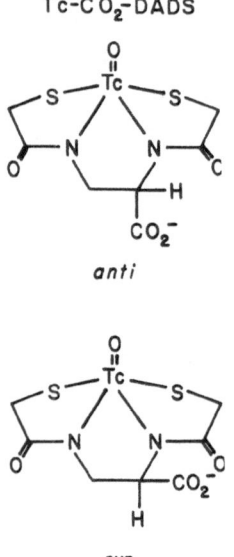

anti

syn

F.IG. 17

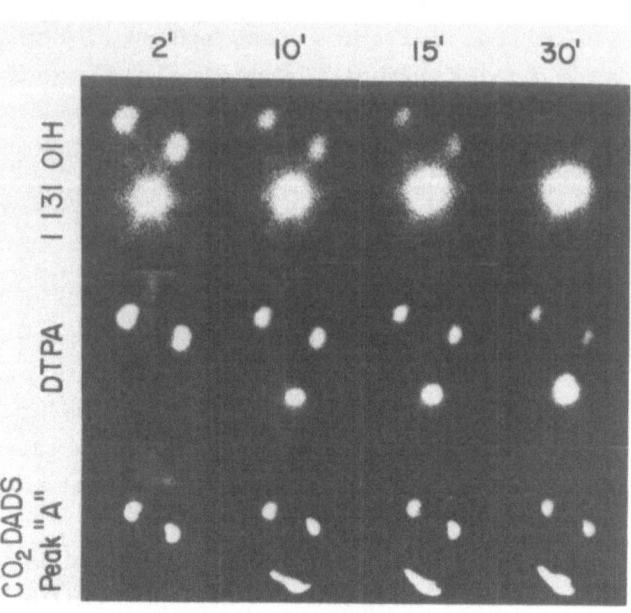

Fig. 18: Posterior images of rabbits obtained with gamma camera (1-3 mCi of Tc-99m or I-131)

Fig. 19:

Posterior images obtained with gamma camera 1-3 mCi Tc-99m for each animal

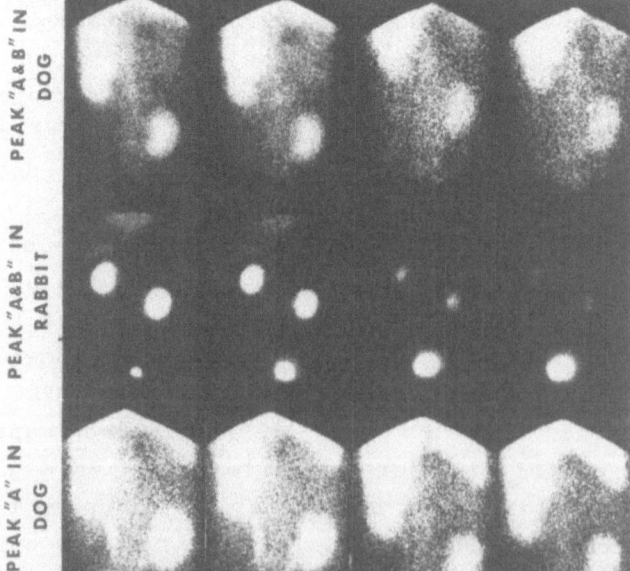

the scintigraphic images of dogs injected with A) Tc-99m CO_2DADS as prepared B) peak A of Tc-99m CO_2DADS are shown, along with rabbit images obtained with the original mixture (peak A & B). There is a dramatic difference in biodistribution between the rabbit and the dog for this compound.

The biodistribution of Tc-99m - CO_2 DADS peak A was performed in rabbits together with I-131 Hippuran. Results are shown in Table 20.

Table 20. DISTRIBUTION OF RENAL AGENTS IN RABBITS

ORGAN	30 MINUTES			60 MINUTES		
	Tc-99m DTPA	C.DADS	^{131}I HIP	Tc-99m DTPA	C.DADS	^{131}I HIP
BLOOD	11.2	2.3	2.5	5.6	0.6	0.9
KIDNEYS	4.1	12.4	3.4	2.1	6.0	1.0
URINE	43.5	70.0	72.6	73.0	86.7	94.5
MUSCLE	14.4	2.8	4.7	5.0	1.1	1.5
GIT & STOM.	5.3	1.9	2.8	2.7	1.2	1.3
LIVER	2.4	1.7	1.0	1.1	1.2	0.4

The blood clearance data obtained from rabbits are shown in Figure 20. These results indicate that the blood clearance of ^{99m}Tc-CO_2 DADS is similar to that of Hippuran. But when compared to Hippuran, there is a delayed urinary clearance of the Tc-99m complex. There is a holdup of activity in the kidney which eventually clears. Klingensmith et al (58, 59) in preliminary clinical evaluation in normal patients demonstrated that Tc-99m-CO_2 DADS peak A was cleared from the kidney like Hippuran.

While Tc-99m CO_2 DADS peak A is an excellent renal tubular excretion agent, it has to be prepared and then separated by HPLC after labelling for use in the clinic. HPLC separation equipment is not ordinarily available in most of nuclear medicine laboratories. Similar compounds which do not require HPLC separation should be valuable. With this idea, our laboratory synthesized a variety of analogs of the original DADS compound. The structural formulae of this new series of compounds are shown in Figures 21 & 22. They contain methyl, hydroxyl, oXo, phenyl, carboxyl, hydroxy phenyl or sulfo substitutes on the ethylenediamine backbone. A new synthetic

36

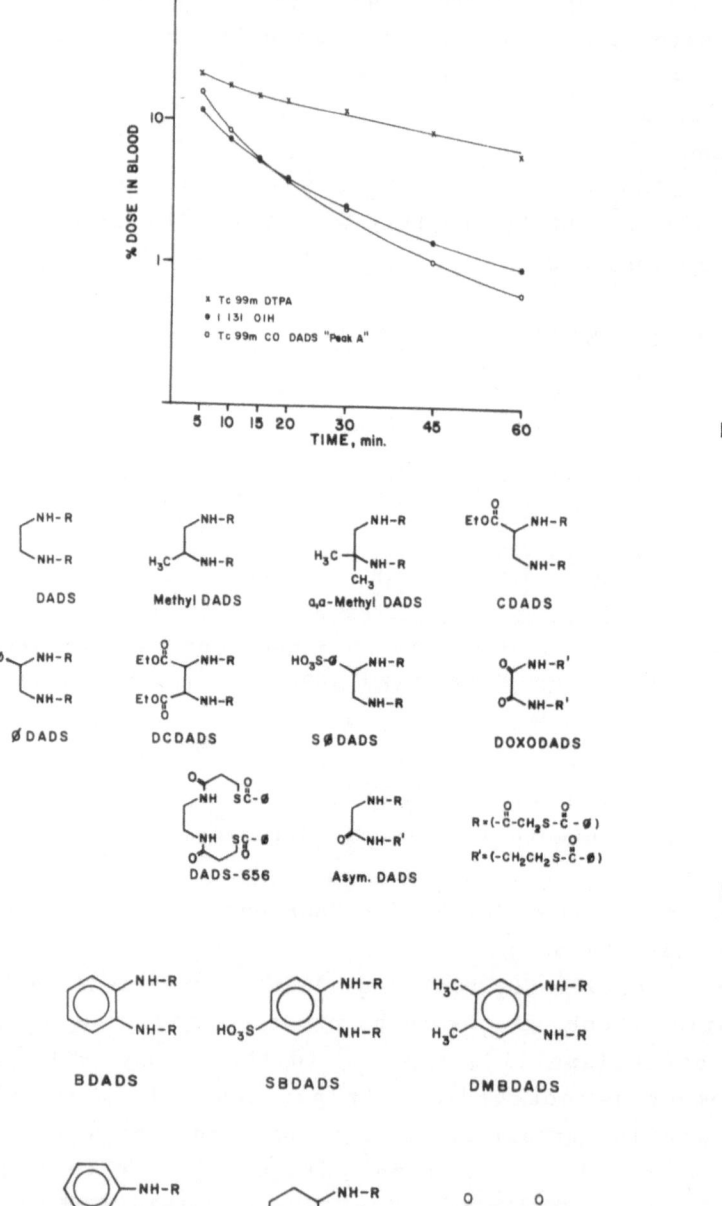

FIG. 2o

FIG. 21

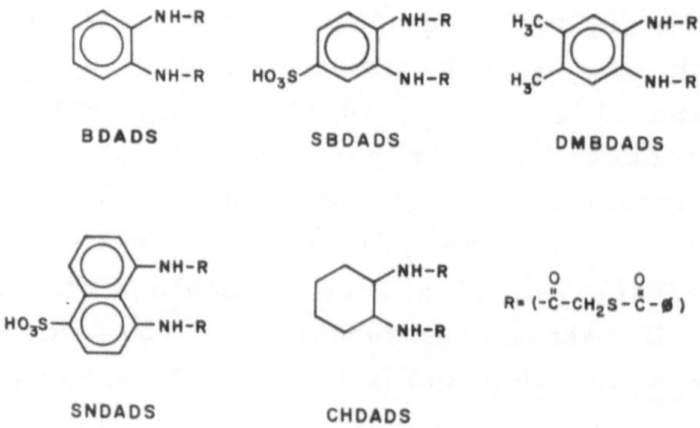

FIG. 22

method was used for the preparation of these compounds (62). These compounds were labelled with Tc-99m following the tin reduction method (61), checked for free TcO_4 by HPLC. With all of these compounds sequential posterior images of rabbits were obtained up to 60` post injection using a gamma camera. These images are shown in figures 23, 24 and 25. Unfortunately none of the newer DADS derivatives were better than CO_2 DADS peak A. This result should have been anticipated. The partition coefficient (Octonal/phosphate buffer) of these new ^{99m}Tc-labelled complexes were considerably higher than that for the CO_2 DADS, and some showed considerable protein binding. Further work on this area is necessary.

FIG. 23-25: Posterior images of rabbits obtained with widefield gamma camera. Each animal received 1-3 mCi Tc-99m containing 0,5-1 mg of the compound.

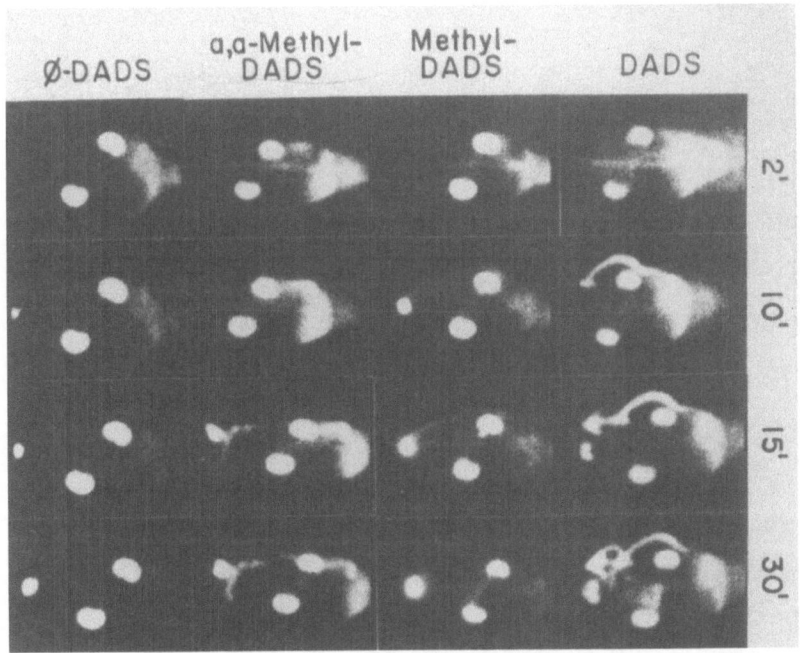

FI(

38

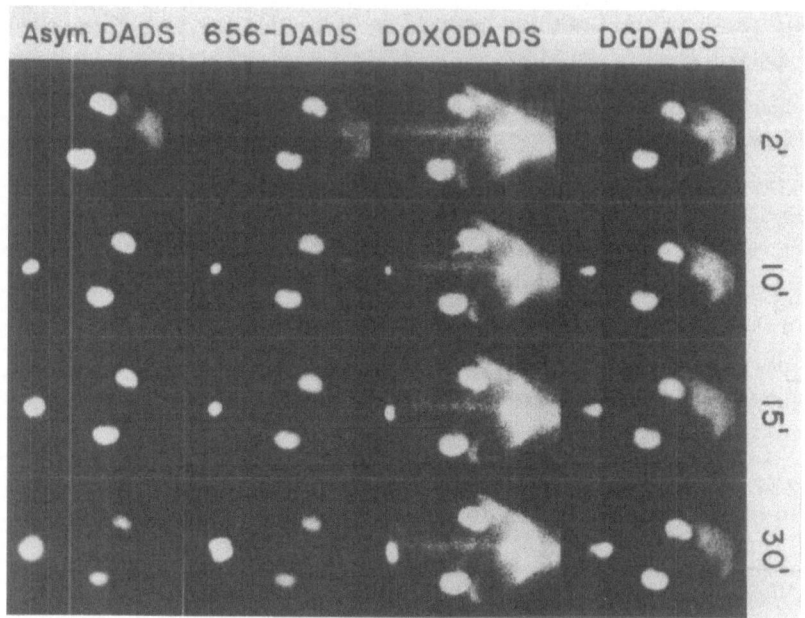

FIG. 24

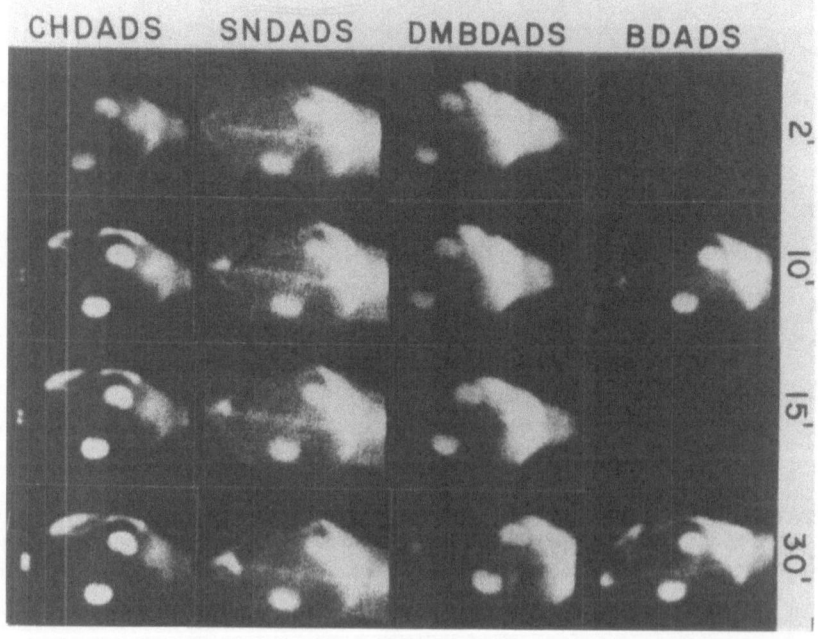

FIG. 25

7. SUMMARY AND CONCLUSIONS

We have analyzed the available data on a wide variety of Tc-99m labelled compounds developed for use in hepatobiliary imaging, bone scintigraphy and renal tubular function studies. But no rigid QSDR`s can be established for these radiopharmaceuticals. There are several fundamental problems which need to be solved. For many Tc-99m complexes we do not know their actual chemical structures or their physico-chemical properties. Lipophilicity (partition co-efficients) data, requiring minimum effort to collect, are not available for many labelled derivatives. The net charges on many of these Tc-99m complexes have not been reported even though these data could have been easily obtained. Data on protein binding, in vivo stability also are not available for most of the Tc-99m compounds. The available animal biodistribution data are not reliable for determining QSDR`s, which can be extended to human studies. The species differences in biodistribution seems to be a major problem. Unless a concerted effort is made by all investigators in this area of research and the basic required data for establishing QSDR`s are collected for each and every radiopharmaceutical, no meaningful chemical structure - biodistribution relationships of practical value can be established.

We have just begun to understand the chemistry of Tc-99m as it applies to radiopharmaceuticals. We have a lot more to learn about chemical structures of new molecules, their physico chemical properties as they are related to biodistribution. We hope that symposia of this type will kindle enthusiasm in this area of radiopharmaceutical research.

ACKNOWLEDGEMENTS

The projects described in this publication was supported in part by grants from the National Cancer Institute CA 32853 and CA 32848, USPHS.

The authors wish to thank C. Zapf Longo, E. Palladino and T. Feld for their technical assistance in the above projects.

40

REFERENCES
1. Crum-Brown & Fraser. Trans Roy Soc Edingburg. 1870.
2. Hansch C, Fujita T. A method for the correlation of biological activity and chemical structure. J A C S 1964;88:1616 Also J A C S. 1962;86:5175.
3. Free S M Wilson J W. A mathematical contribution to structure activity studies. J Med Chem 1964;7:395.
4. Hansch C, Dunn III W J. Liniear relationship between liphophilic character and biological activity of drugs. J Pharm Sci 1972;61:1-19.
5. Hansch C Clayton J M. Liphophilic character and biological activity of drugs II. The parabolic case. J Pharm Sci 1973;62:1-21.
6. Hansch C, Leo A, Unger S H et al. Aromatic substituent constants for structure activity correlations. J Med Chem 1973;16:1207-1216.
7. Hansch C, Leo A. Substituents constants for correlation analysis in chemistry and biology. J. Wiley & Sons, New York. 1978.
8. Tute M S. Principles and practice of Hansch Analysis. A guide to structure-activity correlation for the medicinal chemist. In Harper, N J and Simmonds, A B editors Advances in Drug Research, Vol. 6. Academic Press, New York. 1971:1-77.
9. Purcell W P, Bass G E and Clayton J M. Strategy of drug design. John Wiley and Sons, New York. 1973.
10. Dietrich S W, Dreyer N D, Hansch C et al. Confidence interval estimaters associated with QSAR. J Med Chem 1980;1201-1205.
11. Katz R, Osborne S F and Ionescu F. Application of the free-Wilson technique to structurally related series in homologues. QSAR studies of narcotic analegetics. J Med Chem 1977;20:1413.
12. Wells P R. Linear free energy relationships. Academic Press, New York. 1968.
13. Norrington F E, Hyde R M, Williams S C et al. Physicochemical-activity relations in practice I.A. rational and self consistent data bank. J Med Chem 1975;18:604.
14. Stupper A J, Brugger W E, Jurs P C. Computer assisted studies of chemical structure and biological function. John Wiley and Sons, New York. 1979.
15. Austel V. A manual method for systematic drug design. Eur J Med Chem Chim Ther 1982;17:9-16.
16. Scheibe, P O. Radiotracer design using mathematical models. In: Colombetti LG, editor. Principles of radio-pharmacology, Vol. 1.C. R. C. Press, Bocaraton, Florida. 1979:173-188.
17. Spencer, R P. Radiopharmaceuticals: Structure activity relationships. Grune and Stratton, New York. 1980.
18. Woodard H R, Bigbee R E, Freed B et al. Expression of tissue isotope distribution. J Nucl Med 1975;16:958-959.
19. Lambrecht R L, Echelman W C. Appropriate animal models for radiopharmaceuticals. Springer-Verlag, New York 1983.
20. Kubinyi H. Lipophilicity and biological activity. Drug transport and drug distribution in model systems and in

21. Loberg M, Nunn A D, Porter D W. Development of hepatobiliary agents in Freeman L.M. and Weismann H.S. editors. Nuclear Medicine Annual 1981 Raven Press, New York. 1981:1-33.
22. Loberg M D, Cooper M, Harvey E et al. Development of new radiopharmaceuticals based on N-substitution of iminodiacetic acid. J Nucl Med 1976;17:633-638.
23. Subramanian G, McAfee J G, Henderson R W et al. The influence of structural changes on biodistribution of Tc-99m labelled N-substituted IDA derivatives. J Nucl Med 1977;18:624.
24. Wistow B W, Subramanian G, Van Heertum R L. et al. An evaluation of Tc-99m labelled hepatobiliary agents. J Nucl Med 1977;18:455-461.
25. Chiotellis E, Varvarigou A. Tc-99m labelled N-substituted carbamoyl iminodiacetates: Relationshipbetween structure and biodistribution. Int J Nucl Med Biol 1980;7:107.
26a Molter M, Kloss G. Properties of various IDA derivatives. J Lab Compounds Radiopharm 1981;18:56-58.
26b Subramanian G, Schneider R F et al. Synthesis and evaluation of new Tc-99m labelled iodine substituted acetanilido imidodiacetates.IVth intl.symp.radiop.chem. Julich,West Germany, Radioanalytical Chem. In Press.1982
27. Loberg M D, Porter D W and Ryan J W. Review and current status of hepatobiliary imaging agents. In: Radiopharmaceutical, Vol. II. Society of Nuclear Medicine, New York. 1979:519-43.
28. Chervu L R, Nunn A D, Loberg M D. Radiopharmaceuticals for hepatobiliary imaging. Sem Nucl Med 1982;12:5-17.
29. Burns D, Marzilli L, Sowa D et al. Relationship between molecular structure and biliary excretion of technetium-99m HIDA and HIDA analogs. J Nucl Med 1977;18:624.
30. Jansholt A, Vera D R, Krohn K A et al. In vivo kinetics of hepatobiliary agents in jaundiced animals. In: Radiopharmaceuticals, Vol. II, New York, Society of Nuclear Medicine, 1979:555-564.
31. Jansholt A L, Sheibe P O, Vera D R et al. Correlation analysis of substituent effects on the pharmacokinetics of hepatobiliary agents. J Lab Compounds Radiopharm 1981;18:198-200.
32. Subramanian G, McAfee J G, Henderson R W. The influence of structural changes on Biodistribution of Tc-99m labelled and N-substituted IDA. Proc Soc Nucl Med Europe 1978;18:133-135.
33. Subramanian G. (1983) Unpublished results.
34. Van Wyk A J, Fourie P J, Van Zyl W H et al. Synthesis of five new Tc-99m-HIDA isomers and comparison with Tc-99m-HIDA. Eur J Nucl Med 1979;4:445-448.
35. Nunn A D, Loberg M D. Hepatobiliary agents, in Spencer RP (ed): Radiopharmaceuticals, Structure-Activity Relationships. New York, Grune & Stratton, 1981:539-548.

36. Nunn, A D et al. The development of a new chole-scintigraphic agent Tc-SQ 29962 using a structure distribution relationship approach. J Nucl Med 1981;22:51.
37. Firnau G. Why do Tc-99m chelates work for chole-scintigraphy? Eur J Nucl Med 1976;1:137-139.
38. Levine W G. Biliary excretion of drugs and other xenobiotics. Ann Rev Pharmacol Toxicol 1978;18:81-96.
39. Milburn P M. Factors in the biliary excretion of organic compounds, in Fishman WH (ed): Metabolic Conjugation and Metabolic Hydrolysis, Vol. II. New York, Academic, 1970:1.
40. Loberg M D, Fields A T. Chemical structure of Tc-99m labelled N-(2,6-dimethylphenylcarbamoylmethyl) iminodiacetic acid (Tc-HIDA). Int J Appl Radiat Isotopes 1978;29:167-173.
41. Subramaniag G, McAfee J G, Blair R J, et al. Radiopharma-ceuticals for bone and bone marrow imaging. A review: In "Medical Radionuclide Imaging", Vol.II, Proceedings of a Symposium, Oct. IAEA Vienna. 1976:83-104.
42. Hosain P, Wang T S T. Bone imaging compounds with special reference to structure-affinity relationship. In Radio-pharmaceuticals: Spencer R P editor. Structure Activity Relationships. Grune & Stratton, New York 1981:521-39.
43. Yano, Y, McRae, J Van Dyke D C. Technetium-99m labelled stannous ethane-1-hydroxy 1, 1 diphosphonate: J Nucl Med 1973;14:73-78.
44. Wang T S T, Mojdehi G E, Fawwaz R A et al. A study of the relationship between chemical structure and bone localization of Tc-99m-Sn diphosphonic acids. J Nucl Med 1979;20:1066-1070.
45. Wang T S T, Fawwaz R A, Johnson L J et al. Bone seeking properties of Tc-99m carbonyl diphosphonic acid, dihydroxy-methylene diphosphonic acid. J Nucl Med 1980;21:767-770.
46. Unterspann S. Experimental examinations of the suitability of organoaminomethane bis phosphonic acid for bone scinti-graphy by means of Tc-99m in animals. Eur J Nucl Med 1976;1:151-154.
47. Unterspann S, Finck W. Chemical Structure and pharmaco-kinetics of Tc-99m labelled aminomethane diphosphonic and derivatives. Eur J Nucl Med 1981;6:527-530.
48. Bevan J A, Tote A J, Benedict J J. A radiopharmaceutical for skeletal and acute myocardial infarcct imaging. J Nucl Med 1980;21:961-970.
49. Hoechst, Frankfurt, W. Germany, DPD Brochure 1981.
50. Enlow D H. A study of the post-natal growth and remodeling of bone and Functions of the Haversian System. Am J Anat 1962;110:79-83 and 269-282.
51. Pritchard J J. General histology of bone in Bourne eds. The biochemistry and physiology of bone, 2nd ed., Academic Press, New York. 1972.
52. Schwarz A, Kloss G. Technetium-99m-DPD. A new skeletal

53. Hale T I, Jucker A, Vgenopolous K et al. Clinical experience with a new bone seeking 99mTc-radiopharmaceutical. Nuc Compact 1981;12:54-55.

54. Subramanian G, McAfee J G, Thomas F D et al. A comparison of Tc-99m complexes of newer diphosphonates with methylene diphosphonate for skeletal imaging. (submitted for publication). 1983.

55. Davidson A, Sohn M, Orvig C. A tetradendate ligand designed specifically to coordinate technetium. J Nucl Med 1979;20:641.

56. Davison A, Jones A, Orvig C. A new class of oxotechnetium (+5) chelate complexes containing TcON$_2$S$_2$ Core. Inorg Chem 1981;20:1629-1632.

57. Fritzberg A R, Klingensmith W C, Whitney W P. Chemical and biological studies of Tc-99m N, N`Bis (mercaptoacetamido) - ethylene diamine: A potential replacement for I-131 iodohippurate J Nucl Med 1981;22:258-263.

58. Klingensmith W C, Gerhold J P, Fritzberg, A R et al. Clinical comparison of Tc-99m N-N` bis (mercaptoacetamido) ethylene diamine and (-131$_I$) ortho-iodohippurate for evaluation of renal tubular function. J Nucl Med 1981;23:377-380.

59. Klingensmith, W C et al. (1982, 1983) personal communication.

60. Jones A G, Davison A, LaTegola M R et al. Chemical and in vivo studies of the anion o x o (N,N`-ethylene bis (2-mercaptoacetamido)) technetate V J Nucl Med 1982;23:801-809.

61. Fritzberg A R, Kuni C C, Klingersmith W C et al. Synthesis and biological evaluation of Tc-99m N-N`-Bis (mercaptoacetyl)-2,3 diaminopropanoate. A potential replacement for I-131 iodohippurate. J Nucl Med 1982;23:592-598.

62. Subramanian G, Schneider R F, McAfee J G et al. An evaluation of 16 new Tc-99m compounds for renal tubular

2.   PHYSICAL/CHEMICAL DESCRIPTION

JIRI CIFKA

1. INTRODUCTION

The purpose of this paper is to review the methods having
been used for description of the safety and efficacy of a
radiopharmaceutical   (RPh).   Since   the   group   named
"radiopharmaceuticals" is quite inhomogeneous in the chemical
and physical properties of its individuals it is useful to
explain why and when the particular methods are being used,
i.e. to explain the methodical approach.

It   must   be   emphasized   that   there   is   a   substantial
difference   between   the   nonradioactive   and   radioactive
injections.   The   former   are   prepared   from   well-defined
substances by dissolving them in pure well-defined solvents,
while   the   latter   are   prepared   from   a   reaction   mixture
remaining after the labelling processes. So called labelling,
i.e. incorporation of the radionuclide into a radiopharmaceutical is always a more or less complex chemical process. Past
the labelling, reaction mixtures are directly processed into
the injections, either without or after purification. That is
why in the case of RPhs only the solutions are subjected to
physical and chemical description.

Many RPhs contain the radionuclide with no carrier added.
The total chemical concentration of the radioactive and the
stable isotope is then too low for methods normally applied in
physical chemistry research of compound structures. Model
experiments will aid to the solution of these problems but
there   are   at   least   two   phenomena,   i.e.   adsorption   and
coprecipitation which make conclusions less unambiguous. To a
certain extent it is curious that the verification of model
experiments comes from comparison of biological behaviour,

i.e. from the method of much higher variability than the method verified.

The terms "labelling", "labelled molecule"," compound labelled with" etc. are still confusing. In this review the individual RPhs will be classified into subgroups with respect to the changes of original substances caused by radionuclide incorporation.

This paper will not review physical methods for the determination of emitted radiation. The decay data on radionuclides occurring in RPhs are now well known and sufficient for the calculations of the absorbed dose. More precise characterization of the decay data is a matter of basic research and new results will probably fit in the range of experimental errors. The determination of radionuclidic impurities will be reviewed in chapter 3.

2. INJECTIONS

2.1. Injection solutions of low molecular up to macromolecular substances

Radiopharmaceuticals differentiate in the site of radionuclide in the molecule.

2.1.1. Radionuclide is on the site in the molecule normally occupied by its stable isotope. Only in this case the "labelled molecule" has all the chemical and physical properties of nonradioactive molecule. We can further classify RPhs into three subgroups.

a) Solutions of substances containing C-11, N-13, or O-15. At the present time the use of these compounds in nuclear medicine is limited to the hospitals equipped with a cyclotron. In general, chromatographic methods are considered as a sufficient tool for identity and purity tests, since the basic properties of nonradioactive molecules are well known.

b) Solutions of organic substances containing in the molecule other elements than, C, H, O, N. Radiopharmaceuticals containing radioiodine had been partially derived from nonradioactive x-ray contrast substances. The properties of these substances have been described in detail during the last sixty years. The evidence must be given that the incorporation

of radioiodine does not change the original molecule
(insertion of second iodine into monoiodine compound,
oxidation or hydrolysis of labile group). Radiochromatographic
methods are used for identity tests as well as for the purity
control. The content of the substance in the injection is
determined spectrophotometrically and this method can also be
used for its identification. It is always useful to describe
the properties and the purity of nonradioactive substance to
be labelled. In several cases the nonradioactive substance
cannot be obtained commercially in a sufficient quality. This
is the case of Rose Bengal. The substance should contain only
tetraiodo-tetrachloro fluorescein, however, less iodinated
derivatives are always present. As a consequence, the
radioiodinated substance is again a mixture. The hepatobiliary
transit of various iododerivatives considerably differs.
Therefore WHO Recommendations (1) require the Rose Bengal to
contain more than 70% of the activity in the tetra-
iododerivative.

In general, the activity in the form of an inorganic iodine
is being considered as the only radiochemical impurity. Its
content must be less than 3 - 5%, to ascertain that the
radiation dose to thyroid is low. In special diagnostic
methods, e.g. the measurement of effective renal plasma flow,
the percentage of inorganic iodine must be kept below 1% and
therefore the I-125 iodohippurate is used instead of the I-131
iodohippurate (lower decomposition rate during the storage).
Other radiochemical impurities are mentioned only scarcely
(iodobenzoate in iodohippurate may contain only 1% of the
total activity).

c) Solutions of simple inorganic ions. The description is
simple for stable, nonhydrolyzable ions like Na-24 ion, K-42
ion, Se-75 selenite, Tc-99m pertechnetate. The identity can be
verified by radiochromatography. Protective substances must be
added to the solutions of those ions which are unstable at
very low concentrations (thiosulphate in I-131 solution).

Ionic state of hydrolyzable cation (Fe, Ga, In) depends on
the pH of the solution and on the concentration of the present
anions. Sometimes the solution contains several partially

hydrolyzed ions in an equillibrium. Determination of the "true" state requests some special methods which do not change the equillibrium between hydroxo-, chloro-, or aquo-complexes (2). On the other hand, a good reproducibility of the ionic state (even in the case of mixture) will be achieved if the anion concentration and pH of the injection remain constant.

2.1.2. <u>Radionuclide substitutes an atom of some other element in the molecule</u>. The labelling process results in a new chemical compound with the properties similar but never identical with the original compound. The differences in chemical properties increase with decreasing molecular mass.

Various radioiodinated protein will conserve their basic behaviour as macromolecules with respect to membranes, electric field, etc. Albumin iodinated to low extent (less than one iodine atom per one molecule of albumin) cannot be separated from noniodinated albumin by means of gel chromatography, electrophoresis, etc. Structural changes cannot be proved by physical and chemical studies. The iodination process also results in indirect changes in the molecule - mercapto groups are oxidized and formation of -S-S- bridges can combine either different parts of one molecule or even two molecules. Even the most careful iodination denaturates the protein and the biological behaviour of iodinated protein is always a little different from that of nonlabelled one.

Such opinion that careful iodination does not change the properties of the original molecule is still deep in our mind and it disappears very slowly. As an example the case of "Bromsulphalein labelled with I-131 iodine" will be mentioned. This RPh was introduced by Tubis et al.(3). The authors as well as some other investigators (4-6) tried to find such conditions of iodination which would yield the product of identical biological properties with those of bromsulphalein (BSP). In that period it had been recognized that iodination of BSP leads up to the formation of monoiodo-BSP and diiodo-BSP (7-9). In our country we have studied in detail the properties of iodinated BSP in connection with introduction of this RPh into routine production. We have found that the

iodination results in a mixture of unchanged BSP, its mono-
iododerivative and diiododerivative. The spectra of these
compounds apparently differ (Fig. 1) and different are also
the pH values at which the colourless form of phthalein
dissociates into the coloured anion (Fig. 2) (10).

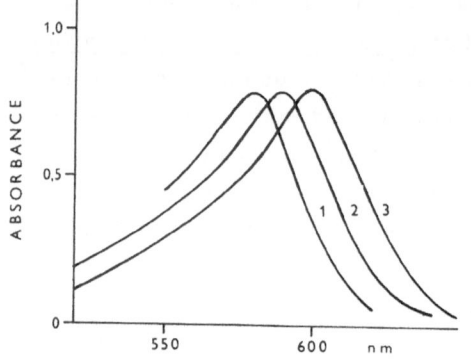 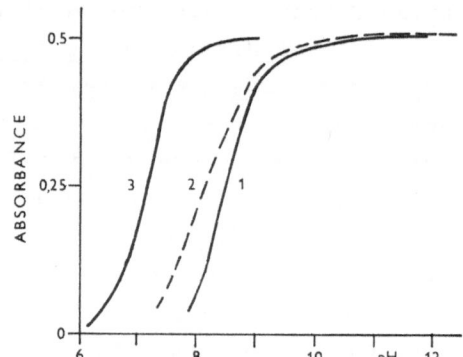

FIGURE 1. Visible spectra of
BSP (1), monoiodo-BSP (2) and
diiodo-BSP (3).

FIGURE 2. The change of absor-
bance as a function of pH. For
curves shown in Fig. 1.

There is also difference in the biological properties of both
iodinated derivatives and the biological behaviour of BSP.
Albumin molecule does not release diiodo-BSP after addition of
alcaline solution to plasma, while in the case of BSP this
effect is being used for its spectrophotometrical
determination. The blood clearance (Fig. 3) and the
hepatobiliary transit (Fig. 4) of diiodo-BSP are slower than
those of monoiodo-BSP and they depend also on the administered
dose (11). These results explain differences in clinical
behaviour of iodinated BSP from various producers. It is
evident that the impurity limits should be given not only on
the content of iodide but also on that of diiodo-BSP. In
addition, the chemical content of BSP must be kept on a steady
level due to the biological competition of BSP and
iododerivatives. Hence,the description of an injection should
be as follows: BSP solution with approximately 0.5 - 1.0% of
iodinated molecules, 90 - 95% of the activity in the form of
monoiodo-BSP, 2 - 5% in diiodo-BSP and 1 - 3% as inorganic
iodide. Other iodinated compounds may not be present.

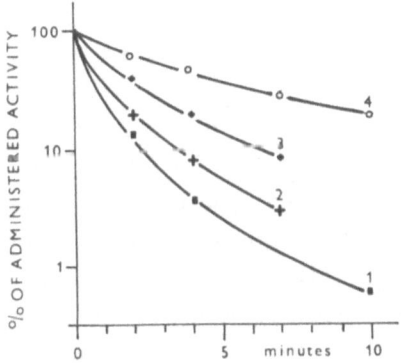

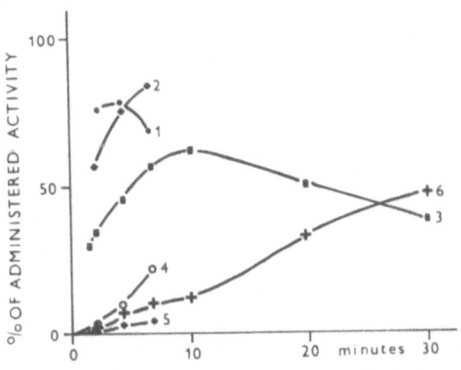

FIGURE 3. Blood clearance in rats. BSP, 5 mg/kg (1); monoiodo-BSP, 0.29 mg/kg (2); diiodo-BSP, 0.33 mg/kg (3) and 6.5 mg/kg (4).

FIGURE 4. The activity in liver (1-3) and intestine (4-6) of rats. Monoiodo-BSP, 0,29 mg/kg (1,4); diiodo-BSP, 0.33 mg/kg (2.5) and 6.5 mg/kg (3,6).

2.1.3. <u>Radionuclide is bound to the molecule by means of chelating groups</u>. The reaction creates completely new compound, a chelate, properties of which differ from those of the chelating compound as well as from those of the radionuclide ion.

All RPhs in this group can be characterized with the two fundamental properties - a) the radionuclide is present at a very low (trace) concentration, b) the chelate can dissociate. The trace concentration makes inapplicable all the detection methods with the exception of the methods of radiochemistry. The dissociation complicates radiochemical separation. Chelate with low stability constant dissociates even by simple dilution. Different mobility of the chelate and the chelating agent causes decrease of the chelating agent concentration in the chelate band during chromatography or electrophoresis. In consequence, the chelate dissociates during the separation and this process is responsible for the peak tailing and formation of artifact peaks. The dissociation can be diminished by addition of the chelating agent into the solvent or electrolyte (12-14). This procedure sometimes changes the separation ability of the system, sometimes it leads up to false positive conclusions and therefore it is inconvenient in the quality control. Similar effect occurs in the case of dilution of the sample with chelating agent. For example, dilution of a sample with 0.2% sodium citrate according to the USP monograph on gallium Ga-67 citrate injection (15) can substantially "improve" the result of radiochemical analysis. We have found that the solution of Ga-67 gallium chloride when diluted with 0.2% sodium citrate can be interpreted as Ga-67 gallium citrate. This injection is now clinically tested in CSSR. Since the "Ga-67 gallium citrate" is in fact a mixture of various chelates in equillibrium and its exact composition is not known, we decided to describe the solution. The citrate (0.078 M) and the chloride (0.004 M) concentrations as well as the pH (kept close to pH 5.6) are checked in each batch. The radiochemical purity determination has been considered only as a qualitative test and it is carried out for completeness. It must be emphasized that equillibrium of gallium citrate chelates is being conserved only until the administration. Then the citrate concentration rapidly decreases, the pH increases and the binding of gallium-67 to transferrin improves. This conclusion follows from in vitro experiments (Table 1). Our results are in agreement with the final part of Hnatowich et al.'s paper (17). Because of low binding forces of Ga-67 to plasma proteins (18), the salting out method was used in our study.

Chelates with high stability constants (DTPA or EDTA chelates of In or Ga isotopes) can be described much easily since they are stable in vivo (their chelates are excreted unchanged) as well as in the course of analysis. The majority of the chelates now applied in the injections were formerly studied at normal cation concentrations for the purpose of analytical chemistry. Therefore, the composition of these chelates at trace concentrations can be calculated in a high degree of approximation to the real state. On the other hand, the majority of chelates containing technetium-99m were used first as RPhs and then their physical and chemical properties have been explored. Technetium forms chelates only at lower oxidation state and therefore the reaction mixture contains Tc-99m chelating substance and reducing agent. The RPhs containing Tc-99m were developed and still are developed empirically. The description of individual RPhs is based mainly on the description of a) biological behaviour, b) the composition of the reaction mixture, and c) the consequences of addition of individual reagents into the mixture.

Within the last ten years several laboratories started with systematic study of technetium chemistry with respect to RPhs. The oxidation state of Tc in various chelates was determined

Table I. The effect of citrate ion concentration on in vitro binding of gallium-67 to globulin fraction of heparinized human plasma (16).

molarity of citrates in original solution	plasma	% of bound Ga-67
0.104	9.5×10^{-3}	6.4
0.094	8.6×10^{-3}	8.7
0.063	5.7×10^{-3}	13.6
0.033	3.0×10^{-3}	29.4
0.033	1.6×10^{-3}	41.9
0.033	8.0×10^{-4}	44.8
0.033	4.7×10^{-4}	47.6
0.104	2.1×10^{-4}	42.6 + 6.3[a]

a) The mean (with 95% fiducial limits) of 13 detn., in other cases the mean of 3 detn. Bloodsamples are from different persons.

with the aid of long-lived Tc-99. It has been found that the chelates of Tc (V) state, Tc (IV) state and even Tc (III) state (19, 20) are formed. The extrapolation of the results of model experiment to a trace concentration is sometimes quenstionable. The role of stannous chelate, as a catalyst

52

only, was also mentioned (21). The final oxidation state of
Tc-99m depends both on the total amount of divalent tin in the
reaction mixture and on the redox potential given by the ratio
of Sn (II)-chelate to Sn (IV)-chelate (19). It has been
recognized that tin does not participate in the chelate
molecule, however the recent paper shows the tin as a
constituent of the Tc-chelates with EHDP (22). Technetium is
even able to form several chelates with one chelating agent.
In these chelates technetium is present in various oxidation
states and these chelates are different in their structure and
in their biological behaviour (23, 24). Model experiments are
seriously complicated due to the presence of stannous and
stannic chelates. Nevertheless, many methods now being used
for the study of the chelates, i.e. spectrophotometry
(including molar ratio method), redox titrations, NMR spectra,
ligand exchange method, etc. contribute to better knowledge of
Tc-chelates (25-35).

In general, the clinical testing of new technetium-99m
containing RPhs is being permitted without perfect description
of the respective RPh. However, the time interval between the
first administration and consequently improved description
shortens. Thus in the case of hepatobiliary radiopharma-

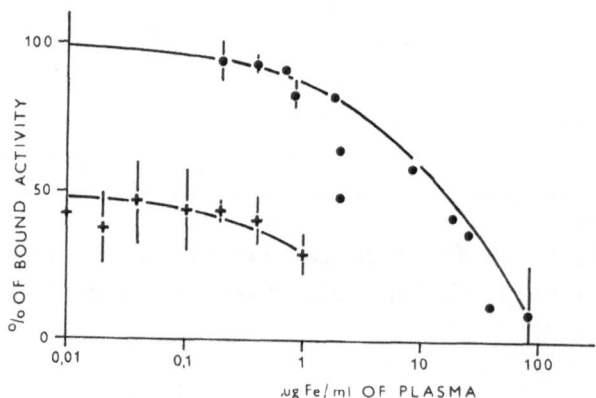

FIGURE 5. The effect of iron (III) on the binding of Ga-67 and
In-113m to transferrin (16).

ceuticals of HIDA-type the results of model experiments were published within two-three year sequence past the first paper (36-39) had appeared and in the case of new renal RPhs the results were published even in "right" sequence (40-42).

As there is no general guide, the level of chemical impurities in RPhs containing chelates must be estimated individually. We have tried to estimate the maximum permissible iron (III) content in gallium Ga-67 citrate injection by means of in vitro experiments. Is was found that an iron (III) content less than 0.2 µg per ml of plasma had no effect on the binding of Ga-67 to transferrin (Fig 5). It can be calculated using this result that the content of approximately 0.1 mg Fe per ml of injection is acceptable. However, the content of Fe can be kept below 2 µg per ml and we have adopted this low value as limit. So, there is a safety factor of approximately 50.

2.2. Injections containing particles

Description of the injection should include the soluble substances as well as the particles. RPhs can be classified with respect to the particle size.

2.2.1. Colloidal particles. The injection of colloidal radiogold is a good example of well described RPh. The particle size and the number of particles can be determined by electron microscopy. Since the particles are homogeneously space labelled, it is possible to calculate the total mass (and hence the activity) of particles in the respective range of diameter. The relations between the particle size distribution and the activity distribution are presented in well known figures in the Catalogue of RCC Amersham (43). In the body the particles of larger diameter are preferably detected. Biological behaviour of radiogold colloids depends also on the type and the concentration of the protective colloid (44). The impurity, i.e. the activity in ionic gold fraction is determined chromatographically. Sometimes a false high activity appears in the spot of ionic gold. The impurity is simulated by very small colloidal particles, which in the presence of high concentrations of the protective colloid move on with the solvent front (45).

From several colloids containing Tc-99m applications of Tc-99m sulphur colloid prevailed for at least ten years. Sulphur particles are prepared by decomposition of thiosulphate in the presence of Tc-99m pertechnetate. The first papers mentioned only the reaction conditions for complete incorporation of the activity into the particles and conditions of improving the stability of colloidal solution. The properties of particles have been studied later. Electron microscopy cannot be directly used due to the volatility of sulphur. The particles can be sized by means of filters with defined pore diameter. In this procedure either some special material (etched polycarbonate) must be used (46, 47) or the analysed solution must be diluted with surface active agent (0.1% benzalkonium chloride) (48), to prevent adsorption of the particles on the filter. This technique, however, does not give any information on the number of particles in the particular fraction. It has been found (sedimentation technique in centrifuge) that the activity of Tc-99m is proportional to the sulphur mass in the fraction, i.e. the particles are labelled homogeneously (49); similar results have been obtained recently by another method (50). It can be concluded that in the solution approximately 90 - 95% of the particles exist with the diameter less than 0.1 μ, but this fraction contains only 5 - 20% of the total Tc-99m activity. The activity distribution depends on several factors. Figure 6 shows the effect of thiosulphate concentration on the particle size with maximum activity (49). Table 2 summarizes the effect of the protective colloid on the activity distribution in the particles and on the biological distribution in rats (49, 51); all the colloids were prepared at a constant thiosulphate concentration in the reaction mixture. The results show serious discrepancies in particle sizing by some of the methods. Nevertheless, the results explain considerable difference between the colloids used in nuclear medicine.

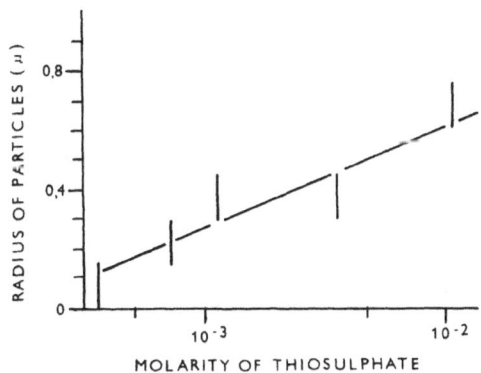

FIGURE 6. The effect of thiosulphate concentration in the reaction mixture on the particle size with the maximum of Tc-99m activity.

Table 2. The effect of protective colloid on the particle size with the maximum of Tc-99m activity and on the biological distribution (49, 51).

protective colloid	radius of sulphur sedimentation	particles filtration	% of activity in liver	spleen
none	0.6 – 0.8	(0.11-0.37)[a]	93.6±1.5	4.0±1.3
mannitol	0.35– 0.5	(0.23-0.37)[a]	92.3±1.4	3.4±0.7
CMC[b]	–	0.11-0.23	90.7±0.5	3.3±1.0
dextran	0.4 – 0.55	(0.23-0.37)[a]	90.6±1.7	3.7±1.6
gelatin	0.15– 0.30	0.05-0.11	88.7±0.7	3.0±0.8
rheodextran	–	(0.23-0.37)[a]	87.7±4.0	4.7±1.8
PVP	0.15– 0.30	0.11-0.22	87.4±1.1	4.8±0.4
Haemaccel	–	0.05-0.23	84.7±1.4	4.9±0.9

a) Unreliable results due to extremely high adsorption of particles on filters. b) Carboxymethylcellulose.

As far as the radiochemical purity is being concerned unbound Tc-99m is not always present as pertechnetate (52). The control methods based on the USP (53) can therefore not neither describe unambiguously the individual colloid, nor distinguish the bad colloid and colloid with small particles (radiochemical purity at least 92% and at least 80% of activity in liver of mice are required).

Tc-99m antimony sulphide colloid will be the second example to show, how carefully the methods of the radiochemical purity control must be selected. It was observed that during the labelling process Tc-99m forms an intermediate product, i.e. a chelate with tartrate ions (54). This chelate is excreted rapidly into urine and therefore kidneys can be sometimes visualized. Special radiochemical system was developed for separation of labelled particles, pertechnetate and Tc-99m chelate with tartrate ions (49).

2.2.2.Suspensions of macroaggregates. Today's RPhs of this type are prepared presumably from preformed particles so the radionuclide binds to their surface. This is the reason why the biological behaviour of the activity does not correspond to the biological fate of the particles.In vivo metabolism of the particles depends on the nature of the particles and on the process used for their formation (coagulation), but at every respect it starts from the surface. Optical microscopy is quite suitable for the determination of the particle size distribution.

3. KITS FOR INJECTIONS

The sense of introduction of the preparation kits is to facilitate the daily preparation of short-lived RPhs and to improve the reproducibility of their properties. Kits may consist of one or more solutions, freeze-dried solids or in-house prepared solutions stored in a frozen state. The kit is usually described by a recipe, i.e. only the masses of initial reagents (per ml or per vial) are being stated. The chemical reactions involved in the kit preparation (formation of stannous chelate and sodium chloride, etc.) are not mentioned.

3.1. Kits for the preparation of RPhs containing Tc-99m

The majority of the kits contains the chelating agent and

some reducing agent usually a stannous compound. In the kit the content of divalent tin can be determined with the aid of iodometry or polarography. Chelating agent can be identified by infrared spectrometry. Its content can be determined by chelatometric titration provided the point of equivalence has not been disturbed by stannous or stannic chelates. In addition, the injection prepared from the kit must comply with all the demands on the respective RPh, i.e. radiochemical purity, pH, biological behaviour (if necessary), etc.

From the toxicological point of view certain amount of divalent tin and its compounds, which is present in RPhs, is being considered safe. However, even micrograms of tin per kg of body mass can alter metabolic pathways in red blood cells (55, 56). On the other hand some divalent tin must be present in the kit. It must be present in a considerable molar excess with respect to Tc-99m, to ensure its complete reduction and subsequent stability. This excess must be sufficient to reduce all Tc-99 carrier possibly present (first eluate) (57) and all other oxidizing substances in the eluates including the dissolved oxygen in the eluant. Sometimes the transfer of Tc-99m into the desired chelate is also influenced by the concentration of divalent tin in the reaction mixture. This is the case of HIDA-type radiopharmaceuticals. It has been found that in the reaction mixture there are two Tc-99m chelates formed successively (58). The biological behaviour of both the chelates has been considered almost identical, however, reaction period of 15-30 minutes is being recommended for the kits by several manufacturers. We have observed formation of two different chelates in reaction mixtures of more than 10 radiopharmaceuticals of this type. The biological behaviour of the two chelates is not identical (Table 3). Figure 7 shows the effect of stannous chelate concentration on the transformation rate of chelate 1 to chelate 2. It is evident, that the transformation rate depends on the volume of the eluate added into the kit vial. In addition, the transformation rate also increases with increasing temperature of the reaction mixture. The results explain some

Table 3. The effect of the solution composition on the biological distribution of the activity in rats, 5 hours after i.v. administration of two hepatobiliary radiopharmaceuticals (59).

organ or sample	% of administrered activity			
	Diethyl-HIDA		Trimethyl-HIDA	
	a	b	a	b
Total blood	1.08+0.23	0.29+0.06	1.04+0.29	0.20+0.08
Liver	1.94+0.28	0.83+0.11	0.88+0.23	0.31+0.05
Interstine	77.0 +5.1	93.2 +3.4	75.5 +3.5	92.6 +2.3
Kidneys	5.4 +0.72	1.19+0.17	4.4 +0.82	0.68+0.11
Urine	8.9 +4.2	3.4 +3.4	14.4 +4.4	4.9 +2.1

a) solution contained 60-70% of chelate 1 and 30-40% of chelate 2. b) solutions contained 98-99% of chelate 2.

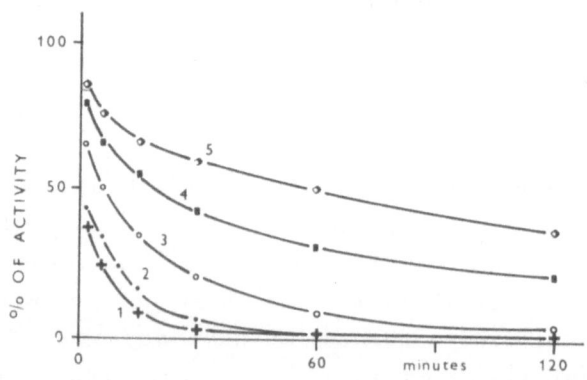

FIGURE 7. Decrease of the percentage of the chelate 1 in the reaction mixture as a function of the time (room temperature). Trimethyl-HIDA concentration $6.5 \times 10^{-3}M$, divalent tin concentrations $8.8 \times 10^{-4}M$ (1), $4.4 \times 10^{-4}M$ (2), $1.8 \times 10^{-4}M$ (3), $8.8 \times 10^{-5}M$ (4), and $4.4 \times 10^{-5}M$ (5).

discrepancies in the literature and give a guide to an improved diagnostics - either to use higher divalent tin content or to heat the reaction mixture. It can be concluded that the kit description must also include exact description of preparation procedure with respect to the volume of the eluate added, reaction time and temperature.

The content of divalent tin in freeze-dried kits slowly decreases within the shelf-life. Any water residue accelerates this decrease. Thus, the water content represents an unwanted impurity and should be kept at a certain level (for example below 2% of the total mass of the residue).

3.2. Kits   for   the   preparation   of   radioiodinated
      radiopharmaceuticals

The preparation of RPhs containing iodine-123 requires rapid and reliable methods. It has been found that the isotopic-exchange reaction can be catalyzed by traces of ions like Cu^+, Cu^{2+}, Pd^{2+}, etc. The kits for the preparation of o-iodohippurate were recently developed and are now used in several laboratories (60-64). All the substances in the kit can be determined by usual chemical methods and radiochemical methods are quite sufficient for the description of the final injection (see 2.1.1.). The exact chemical form of the catalyst is sometimes questionable.

4. GENERATORS

A generator is a device for repetitive separation of shortlived daughter radionuclide from its long-lived parent. The daughter radionuclide must be easily transformable into the solution which comply with all the demands on the injections. Although the generator is a device, the licensing proceedings are similar to those for the RPhs. Both the device and the product must be described. The description of the device must include the separation efficiency. The quality of the generator is evaluated indirectly from the quality of the product.

Chromatographic generators of Tc-99m are the most widely used generators. Manufacturers ensure the high quality of the eluate and I refer to recent papers (65-67) for the details.

The solution of daughter radionuclide is either administered directly or it is used for the preparation of other RPhs. Hence, the product must be evaluated also from this point of view. Partial dissolution of the adsorbent material in chromatographic generators is the main source of chemical contamination of the product. These chemical impurities usually do not disturb in the primary injection, however, they can influence the properties of RPhs prepared from the eluate. The effect of aluminium on the quality of Tc-99m RPhs is well known (68). We have studied the effect of silica on the quality of In-113m RPhs. Silica is always present in the eluates from In-113m generators of the silica-gel type. The total content of silica in the eluate (0.5 - 1.0 mg) depends on the time interval between sequential

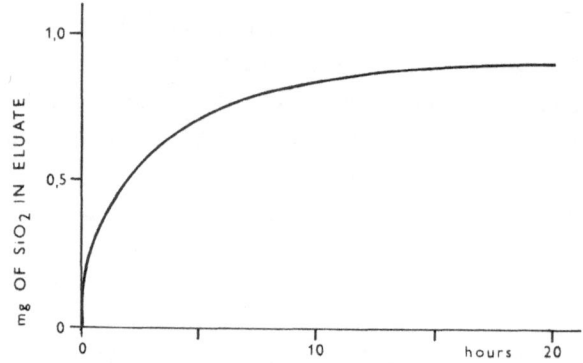

FIGURE 8. The total content of silica in the eluate as a function of the time interval between sequential elutions (69).

elutions (Fig. 8), on the bed size, on the temperature and on the previous treatment of the silica-gel bed(69). In the presence of other chemical impurities like zinc, the voluminous precipitate of the corresponding silicate is formed after the neutralization (zinc is leached from rubber closures during autoclaving of vials containing eluant). Model experiments on rats verified that silica does not alter the essential diagnostic behaviour of In-113m RPhs (70). However, significantly higher excretion of In-113m into urine and lower activity in liver were found in the presence of silica after the administration of diluted eluate and EDTA-chelate. The presence of silica improves the formation of colloids and higher uptake of the activity in liver was found for colloid prepared without added carrier as well as for colloid prepared with added ferric chloride as a carrier. The citrate added to the eluate prevents formation of the silicate precipitate; no differences has been found between the solution with and without silica.

It can be concluded that the compatibility of the generator product and the procedure for preparation of RPhs should be verified experimentally. The recipes and all the details of the procedure for the preparation of the respective RPhs should be adjusted, if necessary. The description of the generator product should include the content of trace chemical impurities and any additives.

REFERENCES
1. WHO Expert Committee on Specifications for Pharmaceutical Preparations, 25th Report Techn Rep Ser 567, Geneva;: WHO, 1975:62.
2. Penkoske P, Potchen EJ, Welch MJ, Welch TJ. Clinical chemistry of the tin-indium generator. J Nucl Med 1969; 10: 646-650.
3. Tubis M, Nordyke RA, Posnick E, Bladh WH. The preparation and use of I-131 labelled sulfobromophthalein in liver function testing. J Nucl Med 1961; 2: 282-288.
4. Mani RS, Prabhu TP. Trace labelling of bromsulphalein/BSP /with radioiodine. Isotopenpraxis 1969; 5: 277-282.
5. Suarez AF de, Gomez SJ, Mitta AEA. Rapid method for preparation of iodine-131 labelled bromsulfalein. Radiochim Acta 1969; 12: 172.
6. Iya VK, Mani RS, Desai CN. Preparation of labelled molecules. In: Radioisitope Production and Quality control, IAEA Techn Rep Ser 125, Vienna, I.A.E.A., 1971; 823-860.
7. Kato S, Kurata K. Radioactive mono and diiodo sulfobromphthalein. US Patent No 3,743,713; June 22, 1971.
8. Kato S, Kurata K, Wakebeyashi T. Structure of iodine-131-labelled 3,3'-/tetrabromophthalidylidene/bis/6-hydroxybenzene sulfonic acid. Chem Pharm Bull 1972; 20: 581-583.
9. Saguansri P, Songkhla SN, Suwanik R, Plechachinda R, Intarusput C. Simplified method of preparation of iodine-131 labelled BSP/bromsulphalein/ and identification of its major component as iodine-131-labelled BSP monoiodide. Siriraj Hosp Gaz 1973; 25: 1877-1889, Chem Abstr 81: 10681j

10. Angelis B, Cifka J. Quality control of bromsulphalein-I-131 injections. 2nd CMEA Symposium on Radiopharmaceuticals, Poland, Kazimierz Dolny, 1977, 7 pp
11. Cifkova I, Cifka J. Biological behaviour of individual fractions of I-131 labelled bromsulphalein. 2nd CMEA Symposium on Radiopharmaceuticals, Poland, Kazimierz Dolny, 1977, 6 pp
12. Eckelman WC, Reba RC, Kubota H. Tc-99m Pyrophosphate for bone imaging. J Nucl Med 1974; 15: 279-283.
13. Brand JAGM van den, Dekker GB, Ligny Cl de. A comparative investigation of various Sephadex G-types and Biogel P-10 in the gel chromatographic analysis of Tc-99m labelled ethane-1-hydroxy-1,1-disodium diphosphonate. Int J Appl Radiation Isotopes 1979; 30: 129.
14. Darte L. A Comparative investigation of the gel chromatography column scanning method for quality control of Tc-99m-methylenediphosphonate. Nucl Med 1981; 20: 51-63.
15. Gallium citrate (Ga-67) injection. The Pharmacopoeia of the United States of America, XXth Rev., Addendum a to Supplement I, 1980: 127.
16. Kopecky P, Polackova E, Cifka J et al. Progress report on gallium-67 preparation. Nucl Res Inst Rez, Report UJV 5546 1980: 36 pp.
17. Hnatowich DJ, Kulprathipanja S, Beh B. The effect of preparation quality on biodistribution for Ga-67 citrate. J Labell Comp Radiopharm 1977; 13: 180.
18. Vallabhajosula SR, Harwig JF, Siemsen JK, Wolf W. Behavior of gallium-67 in the blood. The role of transferrin. J Labell Comp Radiopharm 1979; 16: 112-114.
19. Steigman J, Meinken G, Richards P. The reduction of pertechnetate-99 by stannous chloride 1. The stoichiometry of the reaction in HCl, in a citrate buffer and in a DTPA buffer. Int J Appl Radiat Isotopes 1975; 26: 601-609.
20. Eckelman WC, Meinken G, Richards P. The chemical state of Tc-99m in biomedical products. 2, The Chelation of reduced technetium with DTPA. J Nucl Med 1972; 13: 577-581.
21. Billinghurst MW, Rempel S, Williams S. Reduction Requirements of technetium-99m pertechnetate for the formation of technetium radiopharmaceuticals. J Labell Comp Radiopharm 1979; 16: 185-187.
22. Brand JAGM van den, Dekker BG, DAS HA, Ligny CL de. Gel chromatographic separation and identification of Tc/Sn/EHDP complexes using the radiotracers P-32, Tc-99m, and Sn-113. Int J Appl Radiat Isotopes 1981; 32: 637.
23. Johannsen B, Syhre R, Spies H, Münze R. Chemical and biological characterization of different Tc complexes of cysteine and cysteine detivatives. J Nucl Med 1978; 19: 816-24.
24. Johannsen B, Spies H. Chemie und Radiopharmakologie von Technetiumkomplexen. ZfK Rossendorf Bericht 1981;213 pp
25. Marzilli LG, Worley P, Burns HD. A new electrophoretic method for determining ligand: technetium stoichiometry in carrier free Tc-99m radiopharmaceuticals. J Nucl Med 1979; 20: 871-876.

26. Russell CD, Crittenden RC, Cash Ag. Determination of net ionic charge on Tc-99m DTPA and Tc-99m EDTA by a column ion-exchange method. J Nucl Med 1980; 21: 354-360.
27. Kievet W de. Technetium radiopharmaceuticals: chemical characterization and tissue distribution of Tc-gluco-heptonate using Tc-99m and carrier Tc-99. J Nucl Med 1981; 22: 703-9.
28. Mulder G, Oldenburg SJ, Oort WJ van, Hartigh J den. Valence state of technetium in technetium methylene diphosphonate at tracer concentrations, measured by amperometry. Int J Appl Radiat Isotopes 1981; 32: 675-677.
29. Vanlic-Razumenic N, Petrovic J. Preparation of technetium-99-DMS renal complex in solution and its chemical and biological characterization. Int J Appl Radiat Isotopes 1982; 33: 277-284.
30. Johannsen B. Reaction of Tc-99m diphosphonate with N-donor ligands. Int J Appl Radiat Isotopes 1982; 33: 429-432.
31. Garcia R, Galvez J, Moreno JL. Stoichiometric and kinetic study of the Tc-99 DMSA complex obtained with stannous excess: a possible model for the physico-chemical behaviour of the radiopharmaceutical Tc-99m DMSA. Int J Appl Radiat Isotopes 1982; 33: 521-524.
32. Johannsen B, Syhre R. Untersuchungen zur Komplexierung von Tc-99 mit Gluconat. Radiochem Radioanal Letters 1978; 36: 107-110.
33. Russel CD, Cash AG. Oxidation state of technetium in bone scanning agents as determined at carrier concentration by amperometric titration. Int J Appl Radiat Isotopes 1979; 30: 485-488.
34. Burns HD, Sowa DT, Worley P, Vaum R, Marzilli LG. Electrophoretic determination of charge on carrier-free Tc-99m labelled complexes. J Pharm Sci 1981; 70: 436-439.
35. Jones AG, Davison A, La Tegola MR et al. Chemical and in vivo studies of the anion oxo /N, N,-ethylenbis/2-mercap-toacetimido//technetate/V/. J Nucl Med 1982;23: 801-809.
36. Loberg MD, Cooper M, Harvey E, Callery P, Faith W. Development of new radiopharmaceuticals based on N-substitition of imidodiacetic acid. J Nucl Med 1976; 17: 633-638.
37. Callery PS, Faith WC, Loberg MD, Fields AT, Harvey EB, Cooper MD. Tissue distribution of technetium-99m and carbon-14 labelled N-/2, 6-dimethylphenylcarbamoylmethyl /iminodiacetic acid. J Med Chem 1976; 19: 962-964.
38. Ryan J, Cooper M, Loberg M Harvey E, Sikorski S. Technetium-99m-labelled N-/2, 6-dimethylphenylcarbanoyl-methyl/iminodiacetic acid /Tc-99m HIDA/: A new radiophar-maceutical for hepatobiliary imaging studies. J Nucl Med 1977; 18: 997-1004.
39. Loberg MD, Fields At. Chemical structure of technetium -99m-labelled N-/2, 6-dimethylphenylcarbamoylmethyl/ iminodiacetic acid /Tc-HIDA/. Int J Appl Radiat Isotopes 1978; 29: 167-173.
40. Davison A, Jones A, Orvig C, et al. A new class of oxotechnetium/+5/ chelate complexes containing a TcON$_2$S$_2$core. Inorg Chem 1981; 20: 1629-1632.

64

41. Fritzberg AR, Klingensmith WC, Whitney WP, et al. Chemical and biological studies of Tc-99m N,N‚bis/ mercaptoacetamido/ethylenediamine: a potential replacement for I-131 iodohippurate. J Nucl Med 1981; 22: 258-263.

42. Fritzberg AR, Kuni CC, Klingensmith WC, Stevens J, Whitney WP. Synthesis and biological evaluation of Tc-99m N, N‚bis/mercaptoacetyl/-2, 3-diaminopropanoate: a potential replacement for I-131 o-iodohippurate. J Nucl Med 1982; 23: 592-598.

43. Medical Products 1976/7 (Catalogue). The Radiochemical Centre Amersham: 42-43.

44. Caro RA, Ciscato VA, Radicella R. Kinetics of the phagocytosis of radiogold colloids by the reticuloendothelial system in the rat. Int J Appl Radiat Isotopes 1970; 21: 405-8.

45. Spevacek V, Vesely P, Cifka J. Cromatographic determination of the radiochemical purity of colloidal radiogold Au-198 Nucl Res Inst Rez, Report, 1968, 96 pp; see: Analytical Control of Radiopharmaceuticals. Proc. Panel, Vienna 1969. I.A.E.A., Vienna 1970; 171-175.

46. Davis MA, Jones AG, Trindade H. A rapid and accurate method for sizing radiocolloids. J Nucl Med 1974; 15: 923-928.

47. Pedersen B, Kristensen K. Evaluation of methods for sizing of colloidal radiopharmaceuticals. Eur J Nucl Med 1981; 6: 521-526.

48. Krogsgaard OW. Technetium-99m-Sulfur Colloid. Eur J Nucl Med 1976; 1: 31-35.

49. Cifka J. Methods for the quality control of macroaggregates and colloids labelled with technetium-99m or indium-113m. Part of a joint coordinated research programme on radiopharmaceuticals. Final Report. I.A.E.A. Research contract IAEA-R-1021. 1975, 48 pp.

50. Frier M, Griffiths P, Ramsey A. The physical and chemical characteristics of sulphur colloids. Eur J Nucl Med 1981; 6: 255-260.

51. Cifka J, Rajman I, Cabalfin E, Cifkova I. The activity and particle size distribution in sulphur colloid S-Tc-99m of various origin. 3rd European Congress Nucl Med, Karlovy Vary, May 1979.

52. Cifka J, Vesely P. Non-pertechnetate radiochemical impurity in sulphur colloid labelled with Tc-99m. In: Radiopharmaceuticals and labelled compounds. Proc Symp Copenhagen, March 1973. Vienna, I.A.E.A., 1973; Vol. 1: 53-62.

53. Technetium Tc-99m Sulfur Colloid Injection. The Pharmacopoeia of the United States of America, XIXth Rev 1975; 489.

54. Morcellet JL, Rousset C, Le Mignant A. Sulfure d'antimoine et de technetium, agent scintigraphique de la rate et du foie. J Biol Med Nucl 1972; 7: 33-39.

55. Khentigan A, Garrett M, Lum D, Winchell HS. Effects of prior administration of Sn/II/ complexes on in vivo distribution of Tc-99m pertechnetate. J Nucl Med 1976; 17: 380-4.

56. Holt JT, Spitalnik SL, Wilson G. Inhibition of chromium-51 RBC labelling by stannous pyrophosphate. J Nucl Med 1982; 23: 934-935.
57. Srivastava SC, Meinken G, Richards P. The chemistry of Tc-99m labelling kits. J Labell Comp Radiopharm 1977; 13: 158.
58. Fonda U, Pedersen B. Tc-99m Diethyl-HIDA. A contribution to the study of its structure. Eur J Nucl Med 1978; 3: 87-89.
59. Angelis B, Cifka J, Cifkova I. The preparation of liver diagnostic containing Tc-99m and its characteristic. Radioisotopy 1981; 22: 633-648.
60. Kronrad L, Hradilek P. Brousil J, Svihovcova P. Kits for preparation of radiopharmaceuticals labelled with iodine isotopes. 3rd European Congress Nucl Med, Karlovy Vary, May 1979.
61. Hradilek P, Kronrad L, Kopicka K. Method of preparing radioactive iodinated derivatives of hippuric acid. Czechoslovak Pat Docum 188692/B/, July 15, 1981.
62. Hinkle GH, Basmadjian GP, Kirschner AS, Ice RD. Kit preparation of radioiodinated o-iodohippuran. J Pharm Sci 1981; 70: 312-316.
63. Jeyasingh K, Jewkes RF. Simplified kit preparation and use of I-123 hippuran. In: Proc. 19th Internal Annual Meeting Geselschaft fuer Nuklearmedizin, Bern 1981. 1982; 314-317.
64. Hawking L, Elliot A, Shields R, et al. A rapid quantitative method for the preparation of I-123 iodohippuric acid. Eur J Nucl Med 1982;7: 58-61.
65. Boyd RE. Molybdenum-99: Technetium-99m Generator. Radiochim Acta 1982; 30: 123-145.
66. Molter M. The current status of Tc-99m generators. Nucl Med 1981; 20: 7-10.
67. Technetium-99m. Generators, Chemistry and Preparation of Radiopharmaceuticals. Eckelman W.C., Coursey B.M., eds. Special Issue. Int J Appl Radiat Isotopes 1982; 33: No 10.
68. Hesselwood SR. Quality control procedures for Tc-99m complexes. Nucl Med 1981; 20: 3-6.
69. Cifka J, Rokos A. The silicium content in eluates from indium-113m In generators. Ceskoslov farm. 1979; 28: 399-403.
70. Cifka J, Rokos A, Cifkova I. The silicium content in the eluates from In-113m generators and its effect on radiopharmaceuticals. 3rd European Congress Nucl Med, Karlovy Vary, May 1979.

3.   ANALYTICAL QUALITY CONTROL

GERTRUDE PFEIFFER

1. INTRODUCTION

Quality control is the sum of all arrangements made to ensure that a product will be safe and suitable for the intended use. But as Kristensen pointed out (1) "Quality is not an absolute term. When setting up recommendations for preparation and quality control, consideration must be given to economy and time available". First of all governmental regulations have to be met, but there is a lack of official directions concerning radiopharmaceuticals in many countries and the pharmacopoeias are often not up to date. So decisions concerning the degree of quality control required and the setting of limits for impurities, especially in the case of new radiopharmaceuticals must be made by the manufacturers. They are always looking for fast, precise and simple methods for quality control, so that the given specifications can be tested before the product reaches the patient. Another question is responsibility. It is obvious that the responsibility of the manufacturer ends with the delivery of his products to the hospital. All further manipulations, including dispensing of radiopharmaceuticals and the preparation of Technetium-99m compounds from generator and kits is the responsibility of the hospital pharmacy or the nuclear medicine department, wherever this work will be done.

2. THE QUALITY OF RADIOPHARMACEUTICAL PRODUCTION

2.1 Quality control of primary products

Nearly all chemicals used for the production of radiopharmaceuticals (raw materials) are listed in the pharmacopoeas and in these cases tests for identity and quality control can be found there. For new products, however, tests must be worked out. This also applies to target material. For identification, simple chemical tests, melting points, IR- or UV-spectra are most commonly used. If material of "analytical grade" (e.g. pro analysii) is used, quality tests can often be replaced by the certificate of the manufacturer.

Some years ago we had problems with our Hippuran. Suddenly the amount of labelled o-I-benzoic acid increased. We first thought of an increased rate of decomposition, because at this time the labelling activity was increased, but afterwards we found, that the new batch of hippuric acid, which was used for the production of Hippuran, contained more o-I-benzoic acid than before. This observation was in agreement with a later publication by Kaspersen (2).

2.2. Process control

The continuous supervision of the production process is absolutely necessary in radiopharmaceutical production, because some of the test results, e.g. the sterility test, are not known before application to the patient. Therefore an effective quality assurance system must be established, covering raw materials, instruments, production process, air control and quality control of the endproducts. The regulations are given by GMP and GRP-manuals (1) and will be discussed in chapter 6.

3. TOTAL RADIOACTIVITY

Standardization of radionuclides should be based on national or international standards. The dose calibrator used should be submitted to a quality assurance programme. Some of the critical points are: - calibration of the instrument used
- tests for function/geometry/linearity/volume should be performed for all radionuclides and preparations
- precision of the instrument
- environment: is the calibrator close to a collection of radionuclides?
- response to impurities
A few remarks on the last point: High gamma emitting

radionuclides can falsify the result of the activity measurements in the dose calibrator to a great extent, e.g.:1 μCi I-132 is equivalent to 13 μCi Mo-99 (3), 0.5 % I-126 in I-125 : error more than 5%, I-124 in I-123 : error 20-30%. (3,4)

4. RADIONUCLIDIC PURITY

4.1 Definition

The ratio, expressed as a percentage, of the radioactivity of the radionuclide concerned to the total radioactivity of the source. Radioactive daughter products do not fall under this limitation (5).

The source of radionuclidic impurities can be systematic or non-systematic:

systematic: - side reactions e.g.: Te-124 (p,2n) I-123 and Te-124 (p,n) I-124 or I-127 (p,5n) Xe-123-I-123 and I-127 (p,3n) Xe-125 - I-125.
 - reactions with the target material: Co, Fe, Cu, Cd, Al radioisotopes

Non-
systematic: - leakage of mother nuclide in a generator: Mo-99-break-through
 - contamination during processing

Side reactions are very common in the field of cyclotron isotopes. They cannot be absolutely avoided, only reduced by choosing the optimal bombarding conditions (excitation functions, energy etc).

4.2 Principles

In producing a new radionuclide all possible radioactive impurities should be listed (side reactions, target reactions). This enables a first choice of the necessary tests to be made, but a complete assay must be performed too. As these complete assays are very time consuming and therefore expensive, for routine purposes the tests will be reduced to the assay of radionuclidic impurities which introduce a risk to the patient, such as particle emitters or radionuclides with a long half life. But from time to time in routine production, too, a complete analysis should be performed. The

same rule should apply to the certificates of the
manufacturers (e.g. fission-Mo) which should also be
controlled.

4.3 Methods

Rhodes and Hoppes (6) reviewed methods and instrumentation
for detecting γ-emitters, including the pitfalls of the
evaluation of spectra such as: double peaks, escape peaks etc.
Nearly all radionuclides emit a series of γ-rays of different
energies and many of these energies are the same for different
radionuclides. So it is nearly impossible to analyze a complex
γ-spectrum by hand using radionuclide tables (7,8). Looking at
the gamma spectrum is sufficient for identity tests and a
rough purity check, but for quantitative determination of
impurities a computed system is absolutely necessary.

In our Institute we are very satisfied in using the well
equipped analytical section of our department of radiation
protection. They possess very sensitive instruments with a
full automatic evaluation, which they use for all low level
tests, including urine analysis for α-emitters.

For the determination of α or β-emitting radionuclides
chemical separation must often be performed. This procedure
can only be done in specially equipped laboratory.

4.4 Technetium-99m

Reviewing the recent literature only Tc-99m is studied. Of
course, Tc-99m is the radionuclide most often used in nuclear
medicine, but the other radionuclides should not be forgotten
completely. In this paper only recent publications will be
discussed (9, 10, 11, 12, 13): the method used for the
detection of γ-emitting radionuclides was the same in all
cases. Everybody used a Ge-Li-system, but the identified
radionuclides in the eluates of technetium or in old
generators are different, though there are only very few
sources of Mo-99 (fission-Mo) in the world.

Vlcek (12):   Co-60, Ru-103, I-131, Cs-134, Ba-140, La-140,
               Re-188
Vinberg (10): Co-60, Ru-103, I-131, Cs-134, Nb-92m, Nb-95,
               Rb-86

Väyrynen (13): Co-60, Nb-92m, Sb-124, Sc-46, Cr-51, Nb-95

The problem in the determination of α and β -emitting radionuclides is the sensitivity of the detection method: the concentration of α and β -s in a Tc-99m-eluate fall within the range of the detection limit, which lies for alphas between 0.1-3 pCi per sample (10, 11, 14). Therefore it is useful to accumulate the eluates from one week before the assay. This we did some years ago and compared loaded and unloaded generators. Our detection limit was for urine analysis: 0.2pCi ± 0.2pCi/l and our results:

loaded: A)   0.12 ± 0.14 pCi   B)   0.12 ± 0.09 pCi
unloaded: 0.10 ± 0.02 pCi   0.12 ± 0.08 pCi

But independent of the methods used, all values for alpha- and beta-emitting radionuclides are far below the limits of the pharmacopeias.

An unexpected result was published by Johansson (15). He found an "enormous" amount of Plutonium in the eluate of a non-fission generator, but we can hope, that this was a unique observation.

Now some critical remarks on the Mo- break-through tests. Because of the high difference in the energy of the emitted gamma-rays between Tc-99m (140 keV) and Mo-99 (740 keV) the determination of Mo-99 in the eluate can easily be done by two activity measurements: with and without a lead shield of about 6mm, which reduces the gamma rays of the Tc-99m by a large amount. Nearly all commercial dose-calibrators are equipped with a "suitable" lead shield and instructions for the calculation of the amount of Mo-99. But Williams (16) found, that of 3 tested systems only one accurately reflected the activity of Mo-99. Therefore it is recommended to check the system with pure solutions of Mo-99 and Tc-99m.

4.5 Iodine-131

Though I-131 has been used for many years there is no data about its radionuclidic purity, neither in the pharmacopeas, nor in other papers. We have produced I-131 for many year and therefore we started a study to estimate the content of the possible radionuclidic impurities,

Tellurium-and Antimony isotopes (17). We waited 30-90 days before analysis and found nothing. This result could be interpreted as a radionuclide purity of more than 99.99%. But this value is not an absolute one. It can only be related to defined impurities, because very low γ-s (e.g. I-125), low β-s or α-s could not be found with this test.

4.6 Iodine-123

The limits for the radionuclidic impurities, set up by the USP are very low: 93%, and 85%. This fact shows, that practical considerations play an important role in setting the limits. In Europe, where I-123 is produced by different reactions with a high radionuclidic purity (only 1-2% of I-125) the pharmacopoea limits will be different. We have produced I-123 since 1976. On account of the compton spectrum of I-123 the low gammas of I-125 can only be detected after decay of I-123. We use a Si-Li detector or a special Na-I-detector for counting I-125 in I-123. If I-123 is contaminated with I-124 it is possible to determine the radionuclidic purity at once in the gamma-spectrum, since I-124 emits high energy gammas.

4.7 Summary

- In general the detection and determination of the radionuclidic purity is limited to specially equipped laboratories (except Mo-99 essay in Tc-99m).
- The exact quantitative determination of α or β-emitters is very often impossible, because the count-rates are in the range of the detection limits.
- The limits are often given by the production process: side reactions can not be excluded only reduced.
- No stated values are absolute, they are related to defined impurities.

5. RADIOCHEMICAL PURITY

5.1 Definition

The ratio, expressed as a percentage of the radioactivity of the radionuclide concerned which is present in the chemical form declared, to the total radioactivity of that radionuclide present (5).

Sources of radiochemical impurities:

- remainings of the labelling agent (I^-, $TcO_4...$)
- intermediate products (TcO_2, mono-labelled products)
- products from a side reaction (*I-benzoic acid in Hipppuran)
- decomposition products (instability, radiation effect)

The term "declared chemical form" in the definition of the Pharmacopoea is not clear. If we look at Rose Bengale e.g. nobody knows which iodine atom will be replaced by radioiodine and what is the exact chemical form. Therefore, organ distribution and blood clearance will be the most important criteria for radiochemical purity (18). With labelled proteins the case is similar. Here, too, the behaviour in a specified manner under given conditions will be the limiting factor (19).

A new problem appeared with better analytical techniques for Technetium-compounds. Especially in the HPLC analysis more than one peak was detected: some have a different biological behaviour, some not, but in general we can find an equilibrium between 2 or 3 chemical forms. As our knowledge in Technetium chemistry is just in its infancy, we can only guess, that some of these peaks belong to the same substance, but to a different molecular size, probably monomer, dimers or similar. So these newer techniques will probably lead us to a new definition of the term "radiochemical purity".

5.2 <u>Methods and evaluation of the results</u>

Methods, commonly used for the determination of the radiochemical purity are:

- chromatography: paper chrom. (PC) / thin layer chrom. (TLC)/ gel chrom. (GCS scanning/ instant-thin layer chrom. (ITLC)/ high performance liquid chrom (HPLC).
- electrophoresis
- filtration and precipitation

In practice the rapidity of an analysis is the most important criterium: Therefore in the hospital laboratory ITLC-mini-chromatograms are preferred and in the quality control departments of the manufacturer HPLC methods.

The main problem of the determination of the radiochemical purity consists in the correct calculation of the impurities from the scanned chromatogram. There are some factors which influence the level of uncertainty:

- counting equipment and scanner characteristics: slit width, scan speed, statistics
- influence of background from environment and on the scanned material
- tailing of the peaks: difficulty in separation of the peaks.

In the paper of Mellish (20) all these problems in the evaluation of chromatograms are discussed in detail. In practice everybody has to find the best compromise between precision, accuracy and time available for the test.

5.3 Review of literature

Cohen reviews the literature up to 1973 (21). Later, summaries of methods for radiochemical quality have been published by Eckelman (22), Pauwels (23), Kristensen (1), Phan The Tran (24), the Canadian Department of Health and Welfare (25), Strehlau (26) and Heide (27). Especially the work of the German group belonging to the office of health (27) can be regarded as a complete list of all publications up until 1980. For instance there are 29 methods listed for Hippuran and 27 for Tc-99m EHDP. In this review only some newer aspects and pitfalls will be discussed in detail.

5.4 Tc-99m compounds

Most of the published specifications deal with the quality control of Tc-radiopharmaceuticals. Looking at the labelling kinetics of Tc-DTPA using Tc-99 and paper chromatography we found that pertechnetate disappears very quickly, but the Tc-DTPA-complex is not formed at once: there are some intermediates, which disappear later on. The same observation was made by Srivastava with MDP (28) and Fritzberg with HIDAs, using HPLC (29). But today we know very little about the chemical structure of the intermediates.

Especially for the routine control of Tc-99m kits in the hospital the Mini-chromatograms (size ca 1 x 6 cm) were developed (30, 31). Mainly ITLC-strips (fa Gelman), with cellulose or silicagel are used. The solvents mentioned are 70-85% methanol, acetone / methylethylketon, NaCl-solutions, (0.9%-20%), acetate buffer, (1M /2M) 15% Phosphoric acid with

and without pretreating with NaOH (32), acetone plus saline
(33).

All these methods only work if they are very carefully
performed. There are some factors which can interfere with the
separation process, as probe volume, spot size (34), pencil
marks (35), drying or not before running, temperature, air or
nitrogen atmosphere, chromatographic medium (36, 37), cutting
line (38, 39).

Technetium complexes with a low stability constant will be
decomposed by silicagel or sephadex. Phosphor containing
radiopharmaceuticals may react with the calcium in
chromatographic papers. The cutting line is a very critical
point: using saline or other hydrous solutions the start peak
will show a tail. It is therefore necessary to find the
optimal line for cutting the strip for any chromatographic
system used.

The gelchromatography in the form of GCS (gel
chromatography scanning), developed by Persson (40) seems to
be a method which can be used by the manufacturer and by the
hospital staff as well. It is quite simple and the scanning
can be done by using the gamma-camera. The analysis of Tc-bone
scanning agents works very well (41, 42), but the method can
also be used for the analysis of macroaggregates (43) and a
lot of other Tc-compounds (44): -HSA, -Bleomycin etc. One
critical point is the interaction of weak complexes with
sephadex. Therefore Biogel is preferred now. Another point
under discussion is the choice of the correct solvent: saline
or the ligand with or without tin are in discussion. The
result of gelchromatography can be disturbed by Tc-labelled
additives in the kit, e.g. citrate in a HSA-kit (45). One
group prefers the combination of different columns, filled
with sephadex and resins (46) and call the system "Sorbgel".

The determination of the radiochemical purity of
Tc-labelled macroaggregates or HSA by filtration or
precipitation of the protein are well established methods.
Especially in the case of labelled HSA the blood clearance is
the most sensitive test for quality until now (47). Some
confusion arose in the quality control of macroaggregates with

added HSA, but this problem is now solved (48).

In recent years HPLC has been used for analysis of Tc-99m radiopharmaceuticals. As mentioned before, the very good separation of HPLC showed some unexpected results: too many, unidentified peaks. Starting with the analysis of HIDAo (29), methods for the quality control of MDP (28), HSA (49) and other substances were published (50, 51). Though this method is very sensitive and precise, it is not suited for the routine control in the hospital.

5.5 Iodine labelled radiopharmaceuticals

All radioiodinated radiopharmaceuticals contain a certain amount of radioiodide: remainings from the labelling agent or labelling efficiency less than 100% or decomposition. In the last years some rapid methods for the determination of radioiodide have been published using:
- ITLC-SG and the solvents 2N HCl and 5% KI (52)
- PC in 33% Ammoniumsulphate (53)
- PC plus electrophoresis in Dimethylformamide-ammonia (54)
For the analysis of hippuran the pharmacopoea prescribes paper or thin layer chromatography. The separation of hippuran, radioiodide and o-iodobenzoic acid is good, but it takes very long. Too long in the case of I-123 Hippuran, if one wants the result before delivering the product. Even the HPLC-method described by BOEGL (55) takes too long. So we had to modify the technique using a reverse phase system and 15% acetic acid or 30% methanol as solvents (56). The precision of HPLC is very good, it is easy to repeat an analytic run, and the correlation with the "classic" chromatogram is very good in the case of o-iodobenzoic acid (r = 0.9474) and quite good in the case of radioiodide (r = 0.4850). The variation seen when analysing I-123 Hippuran is very low (2-4%), for I-131 Hippuran it is a bit higher (5-8%). Both values are in the range well known for analytic procedures in clinical chemistry.

5.6 Others

Besides the chromatographic methods, electrophoresis is used too for the determination of the radiochemical purity in radiopharmaceuticals. The group of Jovanovic uses this method for the quality control of Tc-99m labelled HSA and macroparticles (57) and for Hg-labelled chlormerodrin (58).

For radiopharmaceuticals labelled with short lived cyclotron radionuclides (C-11, F-18, etc) HPLC is the chosen method (59).

6. CHEMICAL PURITY

6.1 Definition and general remarks

The ratio expressed as a percentage, of the mass of substance present in the declared chemical form to the total mass contained in the source disregarding any excipients or solvents (5). The results of the analysis of the raw materials, including toxicity tests, prove that the material is safe. In general the injected amount of a radiopharmaceutical is so low that there will be no risk by toxicity. With the increasing use of cyclotronproduced radionuclides metallic impurities from the target material may appear. Their concentration is in general far below the toxic range, but there may be a competition between these metals and the radionuclide in the binding reaction with a ligand: Indium-111 always contains traces of iron, cadmium and copper. One must consider this fact when calculating the necessary DTPA-concentration for preparing In-111 DTPA. Though the problem of toxicity through chemical impurities can be neglected, they can play an important role on the biodistribution of radiopharmaceuticals. Even bacteriostatics, if not added at the correct level may disturb the kinetics of a radiopharmaceutical (60).

6.2 Methods

All methods known in analytical chemistry can be used for detecting chemical impurities. For practical reasons, simple and quick methods are preferred, such as spot tests, atomic absorption, UV-, IR- and emission spectroscopy, activation analysis, chromatography, especially HPLC.
Two systems, one classic, one new, will be discussed in details.

6.3 Aluminium

Aluminium in the Tc-99m pertechnetate disturbs the

labelling of blood cells and influences the biodistribution of pertechnetate, sulphur colloids (61) and bone-kits (62). A test to check the aluminium content of pertechnetate is described in all pharmacopoeias. Recently some work was published to quantify the aluminium content. In general this was done with a two-step test: after localization of the aluminium with a spot-test the exact amount was determined by atomic absorption (61, 63) and/or by activation analysis (63).

6.4 Tin (II)

For the labelling of many kits the technetium of the pertechnetate (Tc-VII) must be reduced to a lower valence state. For this purpose tin (II) salts are very often added to the ligand. But tin (II) is very easily oxidized to tin (IV), so that the actual amount of tin (II) in the kit may be reduced to a critical value, where the amount is insufficient for a complete reduction of pertechnetate. Therefore, in the last years a lot of papers have been published which gave more or less simple recipes for the determination of tin (II) in kits:

- Spot tests: .4-N-methyl-pyridyl-porphine-tosylate (64)
                  . 4-methyl-pyridyl-porphyrine (65)
                  disappearance time measured
                  .phosphor molybdate impregnated paper (66)
                  .N-bromo succinimide with methyl-red
                  indicator (67)
- Polarography: .differential pulse polarography (68)
                  .polarometry, a very sensitive method (69)
                  .polarography (70)
- Iodometric titration (70)
- Potentiometry in HCl using KIO_3 (71)

The manufacturer should use a very sensitive and precise method for tin (II) determination. For the user in the hospital a good spot test should be sufficient.

6.5 Quality of saline

The quality of saline for generator elution and for the dilution of the generator eluate before kit-labelling is very important. Sometimes the labelling efficiency may decrease due to

- pH higher than 6.5 (Technetium-colloid will be formed)
- bacteriostatics (72)
- addition of EDTA

6.6 Others

Most work in this area is done on technetium and kits. A few other examples can be mentioned. The determination of Thallium in Tl-201 with a fluorometric technique using Rhodamine B (73) and the influence of different amounts of citrate on the radiochemical purity and on the biodistribution of Galliumcitrate Ga-67 (74).

6.7 The quality of "quantity"

The quantity, the mass of the substance injected, should always be kept in mind: sometime results vary, not due to a lack of "quality", but because very different amounts of the substance may have been injected: variations in the kinetics and in the biodistribution may be the result.

The so-called "Monday-effect" (Tc-99 disturbs the labelling) has been discussed in details during the last years and should be well known now.

Less well known is the effect of high-specific activity or high activity concentrations on the stability of iodine labelled compounds. In the case of Hippuran this effect was described in the 60`s (75), but many customers still ask for the highest possible specific activity and concentration.

7. PARTICLE SIZE

7.1 Macroaggregates and micropheres

The distribution of particle size in a batch of macroaggregates or microspheres can be measured by light microscopy using a hemocytometer. It is easier and less time consuming to use a scanning system on the microscope or a coulter counter. This instrument gives only good results in the analysis of microspheres. Methods and limits are prescribed in the pharmacopeias.

7.2 Colloids

The determination of the particle size of colloids is rather more tedious. Because of the vacuum the electron microscope can not generally be used and it is also a very expensive instrument. Therefore, the most commonly used methods are filtration through filters with a defined pore size, such as Nuclepore (76, 77, 78, 79). Better results gives the separation of the colloids on Biogel (77, 80), but the time needed for a complete analysis is very long. The method of the future will be a coulter counter technique using laser light (Nanosizer), but this instrument is not yet established for routine work (77).

8. PHARMACEUTICAL QUALITY
8.1 Sterility

The disadvantage of the classic sterility test is well known: the results come after application. Therefore the process control in radiopharmaceutical production is very important. Nevertheless, more effort is needed to devise faster sterility tests. After the first attempt, many years ago, using the metabolization of radioactive glucose or other substances through bacteria (BACTEC), sponsored by the IAEA (81, 82, 83), very little has happened. Some experiments with a microbiological contamination of a generator column showed that the column itself is a very good filter. In all cases the pertechnetate was steril (84). So, in practice sterility problems in radiopharmaceuticals are rare, but anyway it would be better to have a result before injecting the substance into a patient.

8.2 Apyrogenicity

Nearly the same thing happened with the Limulus test. It is now mentioned in the USP, but there are no more recent publications which show whether this test really can be used instead of the rabbit test in the pharmaceutical control of radiopharmaceuticals. The reason is probably, that tests for pyrogens are only demanded if more than 10 or 15 ml of a solution are injected, and these volumes will never be injected in nuclear medicine. Therefore no-one feels forced to develop a new method or to undertake systematic experiments on pyrogen tests.

3 Others

The same consideration as mentioned above are true for

"tonicity" and "pH". Of course it is desirable to use solutions with a physiological value in pH and tonicity, but as the injected volumens are very small (less than 2 ml in general) these factors do not play an important role in the analytical quality control of radiopharmaceuticals, though they should be observed and registered.

REFERENCES
1. Kristensen K. Preparation and control of radiopharmaceuticals in hospitals. Technical Reports Series No 194 IAEA Vienna 1979.
2. Kaspersen FM, Westera G. Radioiodinated o-iodo benzoic acid as impurity in hippuran preparations. Int J Appl Radiat Isotop 1980;31:97.
3. Hauser W, Cavallo L. Measurement and quality assurance of the amount of administered tracer. In Rhodes BA, ed. Quality Control in Nuclear Medicine, SV Mosby, 1977:154.
4. Johnston AS et al. Dose calibrator readings due to radionuclide impurities found in radiopharmaceuticals. Nuclearmedizin 1980; XIX:1.
5. Radiopharmaceutical Preparations. European Pharmacopoea, 1975;III:371ff.
6. Hoppes, DD. Radionuclidic Purity. In Rhodes BA ed. Quality Control in Nuclear Medicine; SV Mosby, 1977:164.
7. Perolat JP. Table de radionucleides. Commissariat à l'energie atomique, Saclay, 1977.
8. Erdtmann G, Soyka, W. The gamma rays of the radionuclides. In Lieser KH ed. Topical presentations in nuclear chemistry, Vol. 7. 1979.
9. Vinberg N, Kristensen K. Comparative evaluation of Tc-99m-generators. Eur J Nucl Med 1976;1:219.
10. Vinberg N, Kristensen K. Fission Mo-99/Tc-99m generators - a study of their performance and quality. Eur J Nucl Med 1980;5:435.
11. Braun H et al. Determination of   and pure -emitting impurities in Mo-99/Tc-99m generator eluates. J Radioanalyt Chem 1981;67:215.
12. Vlcek J et al. Results of regular study on radionuclidic purity of Tc-99m obtained from Mo-99/Tc-99m generators. Eur J Nucl Med 1979;4:385.
13. Väyrynen T et al. Residual activity of Tc-generators. Eur J Nucl Med 1981;6:269.
14. Sauter P et al. Alpha-aktivität in Technetiumeluaten von Spaltmolybdängeneratoren. In Oeff K, ed. Nuklearmedizin und Biokybernetik, 14. Internat. Jahrestagung der Gesellschaft für Nuklearmedizin, 1978: 609.
15. Johansson L, Mattsson S. Plutonium in Tc-99m pertechnetate for clinical use. J Nucl Med 1980;21:1091
16. Williams CC et al. The accuracy of 99-Molybdeneum assays in 99m-Technetium solutions. Radiology 1981;138:445.
17. Zehnder P. Bestimmung der Nuklidreinheit von Jod-131 aus der Eigenproduktion IP. EIR-interner vertraulicher Bericht, 1978, K 7701.

18. Krohn KA, Jansholt A. Radiochemical quality control of short lived radiopharmaceuticals. Int J Appl Radiat Isotop 1977;28:213.
19. Bayly RJ. Chemical and radiochemical purity. In Rhodes BA, ed. Quality Control in Nuclear Medicine, SV Mosby, 1977:173.
20. Mellish CE. Limits of accuracy in the determination of purity by thin layer and paper chromatography. In "Analytical control of radiopharmaceuticals", Proceedings of a panel, IAEA, 1970, PL-336/10:115.
21. Cohen Y, Besnard M. Analytical methods of radiopharmaceutical quality control. In Subramanian G, Radiopharmaceuticals, SNM, New York 1975:207.
22. Eckelman WC, Levenson SM. Chromatographic purity of Tc-99m compounds. In Rhodes BA, ed. quality Control in Nuclear Medicine, SV Mosby, 1977:197.
23. Pauwels EKJ, Feitsma RIJ. Radiochemical quality control of Tc-99m labelled radiopharmaceuticals. Eur J Nucl Med 1977;2:97.
24. Phan The Tran, Wasnich R. Practical Nuclear Pharmacy. In "Practical Nuclear Medicine Series", Banyan Enterprises, Honolulu, 1979.
25. Health and Welfare Canada. Results of quality control studies of Tc-99m labelled radiopharmaceuticals prepared from kits (1978, 1979). Canada 1982, 82-EHD-75.
26. Strehlau E, Weiland J. Erfahrungen mit der Qualitätskontrolle kommerzieller and eigenmarkierter Radiopharmazeutika. Radiobiol Radiother 1980;21:376.
27. Heide L et al. Analytik radiochemischer Verunreinigungen in Radiopharmazeutika. Institut für Strahlenhygiene des Bundesgesundheitsamtes, STH-Berichte, Teil I, 1979:15, Teil II, 1980:7, Teil III 1980:9, Teil IV 1981:65.
28. Srivastava SC et al. Characterization of Tc-99m bone agents (MDP, EHDP) by reverse phase and ion exchange HPLC. J Nucl Med 1981;22:P-69.
29. Fritzberg AR, Lewis D. HPLC analysis of Tc-99m iminodiacetate hepatobiliary agents and a question of multiple peaks. J Nucl Med 1980;21:1180.
30. Colombetti LG et al. Rapid determination of oxidation state of unbound Tc-99m and labelling yield in Tc-99m-labelled radiopharmaceuticals. J Nucl Med 1976;17:805.
31. Majewski W et al. Radiochemical evaluation of commercial iminodiacetate hepatobiliary radiopharmaceuticals. J Nucl Med Technol 1981;9:185.
32. Belkas EP, Archimandritis S. Quality control of colloid and particulate Tc-99m labelled radiopharmaceuticals. Eur J Nucl Med 1979;4:375.
33. Cooper PA, Zimmer AM. Radiochemical purity and stability of commercial Tc-99m stannous DTPA kits using a new chromatographic technique. J Nucl Med 1975;3:208.
34. Taukulis RA et al. Technical parameters with miniaturized chromatography system. J Nucl Med Technol 1979;7:19.
35. Williams CC. Radiochemical purity of Tc-99m oxidronate. J Nucl Med 1981;22:1015.
36. Owunwanne A et al. Factors influencing paper

chromatographic analysis of Technetium-99m phosphorous compounds J Nucl Med 1978;19:534.
37. Gasche W et al. Chromatographic investigations of Tc-99m-MDP and Tc-99-pyrophosphate. J Nucl Med All Sci 1982;26:148.
38. Mock BH et al. Rapid miniaturized chromatographic quality procedures for Tc-99m radiopharmaceuticals. J Nucl Med 1978;19:1086.
39. Zimmer AM et al. Rapid miniaturized chromatography for Tc-99m-IDA-agents: comparison with gel chromatography. Eur J Nucl Med 1982;7:88.
40. Persson BRR. Gel chromatography column scanning: a method for identification and quality control of Tc-99m-radiopharmaceuticals. In Subramanian G. ed. Radiopharmaceuticals, SNM, New York, 1975:228.
41. Darte I. A comparative investigation of the gel chromatography column scanning method for quality control of Tc-99m-methylene disphosphonate. Nuclearmedizin 1981;20:51.
42. Van den Brand JAGM et al. A comparative investigation of various Sephadex-G types and Biogel P-10 in the gelchromatographic analysis of Tc-99m labelled l-hydroxy-ethylidene-1, 1-diphosphonate. Int J Appl Radiat Isotop 1979;:30:129.
43. Darte I et al. Quality control and testing of Tc-99m macroaggregated albumin. Nuclearmedizin 1976;15:80.
44. Johansen B. Gelchromatographische Qualitätskontrolle von Tc-99m-Radiopharmazeutika. Radiobiol Radiother 1976;17:91.
45. Pszona A, Sakowicz A. The influence of citrate ions on the radiochemical purity of Tc-99m human serum albumin. Int J Appl Radiat Isotop 1981;32:349.
46. Vilcek S et al. Analysis of Tc-99m labelled compounds using sorb gel method. Radiochem Radioanalyt Lett 1982;52:55.
47. Millar AM et al. An evaluation of 6 kits of Technetium-99m-human serum albumin injection for cardiac blood pool imaging. Eur J Nucl Med 1979;4:91.
48. McLean JR et al. Quality control procedures for Tc-99m-MAA. Int J Nucl Med Biol 1979;6:142.
49. Vallabhajosula S et al. Radiochemical analysis of Tc-99m human serum albumin with high pressure liquid chromatography. J Nucl Med 1982;23:326.
50. Russell CD, Majerik JE. Determination of pertechnetate in radiopharmaceuticals by high pressure liquid, thin layer and paper chromatography. Int J Appl Radiat Isotop 1979;30:753.
51. Wong SH et al. Quality control studies of Tc-99m labelled radiopharmaceuticals by high performance liquid chromotography. Int J Appl Radiat Isotop 1981;32:185.
52. Rosenberg A, Teare FW. A novel rapid thin layer chromatographic monitoring system for the radioiodination of protein and polypeptides. Analyt Biochem 1977;77:289.
53. Siuda A, Lucka, B. Determination of inorganic radioiodine in solutions of I-125-labelled proteins. J Lab comp and radiopharm 1980;18:915.

54. Dreyer I et al. Untersuchungen zur Elektrophorese und Papierchromatographie radioaktiv markierter anorganischer Halogenverbindungen im System Dimethylformamid-Ammoniak. Radiochem Radioanalyt Lett 1978;33:281.
55. Bögl W, Stockhausen K. Hochdruckflüssigkeitschromatographische Qualitätskontrolle einiger auf dem Markt befindlicher J-123/J-125/J-131 ortho-jod-Hippurane. Nuclearmedizin 1978;17:283.
56. Beranek I, Pfeiffer G. Anwendung der Hochleistungsflüssigchromotographie (HPLC) zur Qualitätskontrolle von Radiopharmaka. EIR-interner Bericht, 1982, TM-52-82-05.
57. Jovanovic V et al. Radiochemical quality control of Tc-99m-labelled radiopharmaceuticals J Radioanalyt Chem 1980;59:239.
58. Jovanovic V et al. Determination of radiochemical purity of chlormerodrin-Hg-203 by electrophoretic method. J Radioanalyt Chem 1977;35:383.
59. Machulla HJ et al. Radioanalytical quality control of C-11, F-18 and I-123 labelled compounds and radiopharmaceuticals. J Radioanalyt Chem 1976;32:381.
60. Bayly RJ. Chemical and radiochemical purity. In Rhodes BA, ed. Quality Control in Nuclear Medicine, Sv Mosby 1977:173.
61. Shukla SK et al. Effect of aluminium impurities in the generator produced pertechnetate-99m ion on thyroid scintigrams. Eur J Nucl Med 1977;2:137.
62. Zimmer AM, Pavel DG. Experimental investigations on the possible cause of liver appearance during bone scanning. Radiology 1978;126:813.
63. Müller T, Steinnes E. On the purity of eluates from Tc-99m-generators. Scand J clin lab invest 1971;28:213.
64. Hambright P et al. Rapid spot test for stannous tin levels in Tc-99m kits. J Nucl med Technol 1977;5:88.
65. Zimmer AM, Spies SM. The paper spot test: a rapid method for quantitaing stannous concentrations in radiopharmaceutical kits. J Nucl Med 1981;22:465.
66. Lin TH et al. Instant spot test for SN (II) in Tc-99m radiopharmaceuticals and kit reagents. J Nucl Med 1981;22:P-72.
67. Study KT. Determination of stannous ion content on radiopharmaceutical kits using N-bromosuccinimide. J Nucl Med Technol 1982;10:161.
68. McBride MHD et al. Stannous ion quantitation in pyrophosphate and polyphosphate radiopharmaceutical kits using differential pulse polarography. J Pharmaceut Science 1977;66:870.
69. Liebscher I et al. Sn (II) Bestimmung in Tc-99m-Sn-DMSA. Radiochem Radioanalyt Lett 1979;37:313.
70. Colombetti LE, Barnes WE. Effect of chemical and radiochemical impurities from eluants on Tc-99m labelling efficiency. Nuclearmedizin 1977;16:271.
71. Chervu LR et al. Stannous ion quantitation in Tc-99m radiopharmaceutical kits. Eur J Nucl Med 1982;7:291.
72. Study KT et al. The effect of bacteriostatic saline on Tc-99m labelled radiopharmaceuticals. J Nucl Med Technol 1981;9:115.

73. Study KT et al. Acceptance testing of Thallium-201. J Nucl Med 1979;20:684.
74. Waxman AD et al. Are all Gallium citrate preparations the same? Radiology 1975;117:647.
75. Bremer KH. Herstellung und in vitro Stabilität der Testsubstanzen für Nierenuntersuchungen. In Höfer R, ed. Nierenclearance, Hoechst, 1968/69.
76. Krogsgaard OW. Technetium-99m sulfur colloid. Eur J Nucl Med 1976;1:31.
77. Pedersen B, Kristensen K. Evaluation of methods for sizing of colloidal radiopharmaceuticals. Eur J Nucl Med 1981;6:521.
78. Warbick A et al. An evaluation of radiocolloid sizing techniques. J Nucl Med 1977;18:827.
79. Billinghurst MW, Jette D. Colloidal particle size determination by gel filtration. J Nucl Med 1979;20:133.
80. Persson BRR et al. Radioanalytical studies of Tc-99m labelled colloids and macromolecules with gel chromatography column scanning technique. J Radioanalyt Chem 1978;43:275.
81. Servian JL. Report of an international atomic energy agency meeting on quality control of radiopharmaceuticals. Int J Appl Radiat Isotop 1977;28:653.
82. Gopal NGS et al. Radiometric sterility test for radiopharmaceuticals. Isotopenpraxis 1976;12:257.
83. Rhodes BA. Radiometric sterility testing. In Rhodes BA, ed. Quality Control in Nuclear Medicine, CV Mosby, 1977:226.
84. Sørensen K et al. Microbial contamination of radionuclide generators. Eur J Nucl Med 1977;2:105.

4.   PHARMACEUTICAL FORM - PACKAGING

PER O. BREMER

1. INTRODUCTION

Radiopharmaceuticals may be divided into three categories
according to use: Diagnostic radiopharmaceuticals, therapeutic
radiopharmaceuticals,   research radiopharmaceuticals.

At a first glance radiopharmaceuticals look like a very
homogeneous group of products, as the majority of the products
are supplied as injectables in standard glass vials. However,
a closer look at the preparations in current use will show a
wide variety of dosage forms, and the radiopharmacist will
encounter several dosage forms that are rarely found among
non-radioactive drugs. The most common dosage forms to-day
are:

1. Oral solutions
2. Injectable solutions
3. Colloidal solutions for injection
4. Suspensions of labelled particles for injection
5. Capsules
6. Gases for inhalation
7. Gases for injection
8. Preparations from radionuclide generators
9. Preparations from kits used with radionuclide generators

The production of radiopharmaceuticals introduces new
problems that are unknown in the manufacture of conventional
drugs. The radioactive nature of these products makes it just
as important to protect the personnel against the product
during the production as it is to protect the product against
the influence of the personnel. Special precautions must
therefore be taken for each of the dosage forms to ensure a
satisfactory quality of the final product. A quality assurance
programme designed for the individual product must cover all
aspects of the production from the starting materials to the

final labels and package inserts.

2. ORAL SOLUTIONS

This group of relatively simple radiopharmaceuticals should not be expected to give many problems in manufacture or routine use, as most products are aqueous solutions of radioactive compounds dispensed in standard single-dose or multi-dose vials. However, it is already in this group we start to meet the problems that make radiopharmaceuticals so special compared to non-radioactive drugs: the problems that are related to the radioactive nature and the chemical composition of the product. Most of the problems are connected to the stability of the products and are due to the low physical concentration of the active molecules of the product. Irradiation in cyclotrons and reactors transforms only fractions of the target material to the desired radionuclide. When dilutions are made of the stock solutions, the concentration of radioactive material will become so low that the normal macrochemical laws will seem not to be valid for these solutions. The stability problems are often caused by small amounts of chemical impurities in the product that can change the chemical form of the radionuclide by acting as an oxidizing or reducing agent. Such impurities can be introduced in the product in several ways, for example with the raw materials, by the water or other solutions used in the production, and from the glass vials, the rubber stoppers or other packaging materials. Only pure grade chemicals should therefore be used in the preparation of radiopharmaceuticals. The cleansing procedures for glass containers and rubber stoppers are of utmost importance, and these procedures must ensure that all remains of detergents used in the process are removed, as to avoid interaction with the product. Another major source of stability problems is the leaching of additives from the stoppers, as the minute quantities of chemicals that are released into the solutions, are enough to introduce chemical changes and even produce insoluble forms of the radiopharmaceutical. The choice of stoppers must therefore be considered carefully with regard to the quality 'and the materials. The same applies to the glass quality of the vials. Soft soda glass should be avoided, as soluble alkali from the glass may cause pH changes in the solution. It is furthermore important to note that radionuclides in very low concentrations tend to adhere to glass surfaces, thereby making it difficult to withdraw the total amount of radioactivity from a container. A high specific activity and a high radioactive concentration are generally not optimal for the stability of the product, and these factors can lead to self-decomposition by internal radiation effects in the molecule and to the induction of radiolysis in the solution. Some of these effects can be avoided by supplying the radio-pharmaceutical in more dilute solutions. However, dilute solutions can be the origin of new stability problems, as oxidation processes may occur more rapidly at high dilutions if the solvent used for the dilution contains much dissolved oxygen.

To protect and ensure the efficacy of radiopharmaceuticals it is common to use additives in the formulation of these products. Stabilizers can act chemically or physically. Typical examples of chemical stabilizers are antioxidants, such as ascorbic acid and gentisic acid, that are added to technetium-99m preparation kits, and sodium thiosulphate added to iodide solutions to prevent the liberation of fumes of radioactive iodine due to oxidation processes in the solution.

The pH value of a solution is important to the stability of the product, and in radiopharmaceutical solutions radiolysis can produce such pH changes. Adjustment of the pH by a proper buffer solution is therefore often advantageous. The buffer must not react unfavourably with the product, and it must be kept in mind that the buffer can also be affected by radiolysis.

Certain compounds improve the stability of radiopharma-ceuticals by protecting against radiolysis, as they act as scavengers for the free radicals produced by the radiation in the solution. One of the most common preservatives used to prevent microbial contamination, benzyl alcohol, exerts this effect, and is therefore extensively used in radiopharmaceuticals.

3. INJECTABLE SOLUTIONS

Radiopharmaceutical preparations for parenteral administration must be prepared using precautions to exclude microbial contamination and to ensure sterility, thereby meeting the same requirements as to standard parenteral solutions. The composition of these products do not differ much from the oral solutions, it is the means of production and presentation that make them different. In addition to the problems described for the oral solutions, several new aspects must be taken into consideration for the injectable solutions. The methods of production are limited compared to the preparation of conventional parenteral products. Most products are sterilized in the final container by autoclaving, but some must be prepared using aseptic working techniques. For such products membrane filtration is applied less frequently, as this technique often will give high radiation doses to the operators. Many of the products cannot undergo membrane-filtration as they contain particles or colloids that will clog the filter.

Antimicrobial preservatives are added to many of the parenteral solutions, but the European Pharmacopoeia states that this is not obligatory for such radiopharmaceuticals in multi-dose vials, unless this is prescribed in the individual monograph. Only for certain preparations a pyrogen test is prescribed, but to avoid pyrogens in the final product it is advisable that the manufacturer verifies the absence of pyrogens in the starting materials.

The parenteral solutions may be supplied in single- or multi-dose vials or in single-dose syringes. The presentation form will not cause any major problems if the packaging material has been chosen with care. Surface treatment of glass vials and especially of the plastic surfaces of syringes may lead to interaction with the solution.

4. COLLOIDAL SOLUTIONS FOR INJECTION

The products in this group generally have a particle size

distribution between 10 nm and 1 µm, and only products with a
mean particle size in the lower range can be defined as true
colloids. The homogeneous phase, the solvent, is most often
aqueous with the addition of stabilizing agents. The particles
are usually electrically charged, and some of the additives
act as stabilizers by forming a protective colloid on the
primary particles and thereby preventing aggregation in the
system.

The classical radiopharmaceutical in this group is the
colloidal solution of gold-198, in which a lyophobic sol of
gold particles is made thermodynamically stable by the
formation of a lyophilic layer of a protective gelatine
colloid. Technetium-99m tin colloid and technetium-99m sulphur
colloid belong also to this group.

The main problem of this dosage form is the aging effects
of the colloids that tend to give an increase in the particle
size with time. This tendency for particles to grow larger may
be stopped by additives such as protective colloids. If this
growth is not controlled, a radiopharmaceutical colloid that
was suitable for liver and spleen studies at the time of
labelling due to uptake in the reticuloendothelial system, may
a few hours later contain such large particles that a high
uptake in the capillary bed in the lungs will be the result,
and thereby give a very unsatisfactory examination.

5. SUSPENSIONS OF LABELLED PARTICLES FOR INJECTION

These products can be divided further into Macroaggregated
particles and Microspheres. These products contain generally
particles with a mean particle size larger than 10 µm. The
size can be determined under a light microscope using a
hemocytometer. It is not an exact division in particle size
distribution between the products with large colloidal
particles and the suspensions with small particles, but it is
this difference in particle size that decides the quality of
the product and the diagnostic use of the product. In theory
any particles of suitable size might be used in
radiopharmaceutical suspensions if they could be labelled with
radioactivity. However, in human medicine the choice is

limited to non-toxic, non-antigenic, biodegradable materials. Human serum albumin is the material used most frequently today. Ferrous hydroxide labelled with technetium-99m was used previously, but this product is not used today because of adverse reactions. The most common method for the production of aggregates is to denature a solution of human serum albumin chemically or by heating. The mean particle size will depend on the conditions of the production process, such as temperature, rate of stirring, composition of the liquid medium, etc. The first aggregated particles were supplied to the hospitals ready labelled with iodine-131. Today the radio-pharmaceutical is supplied as a freeze-dried preparation kit containing prefabricated albumin particles. In addition the kit contains a reducing agent, which will take part in the formation of the complex of albumin particles and technetium-99m, when an eluate from a technetium-99m generator is added to the vial. The number of particles injected should be so low that only a minor fraction of the smallest blood vessels are blocked. The study will not endanger the patient when only a small part of the total number is closed. As the particles are biodegradable, they are metabolized by the body within a few hours, and normal blood-flow will be restored to the lung tissue. It is of great importance that the particles are within the correct range. If the particles are smaller than 10 m, they will also be taken up in the RES system, and it will be difficult to interpret the study. If the particles are too large, they will block some of the greater blood vessels, alter the perfusion patterns and cause pulmonary hypertension.

The main disadvantage with macroaggregated albumin is that the particle size and shape are not well defined. The spread around the mean diameter may vary, and the mean particle size is different from producer to producer. The international pharmacopoeias set strict limits for the size range of the particles allowed in such products. The search for a physical stable, uniformly sized biodegradable particle lead to the development of the microspheres. As the name indicates, they are small, spherical particles, and they are also made for medical purposes by denaturing albumin. They can be made with a very narrow particle size distribution, as their greater mechanical resistance allows sorting according to size by sieving after production. One batch can therefore be divided into fractions with different mean particle size. The microspheres may be supplied in suspensions or in freeze-dried form, both for labelling with technetium-99m before use. One disadvantage with this product is a slower metabolism than for macroaggregated albumin, which prolongs the time to restore normal blood flow. The rate of biodegradation is determined by the amount of heat used to prepare the microspheres.

For medical research purposes another type of microspheres can be applied. They are called tracer microspheres and are made of an organic matrix which contains a solution of the radionuclide. After carbonization of the organic material the solution is sealed inside the microsphere. Tracer microspheres can be produced in a wide range of particle sizes and with many different radionuclides. They are not readily metabolized.

Sedimentation is the most common problem in the routine use of radiopharmaceutical suspensions. Sedimentation will take place in the vial after labelling and in pre-dispensed syringes. To ensure that the patient receives the correct number of particles, the dose should be drawn from the vial immediately before use. The vial should be inverted several times to ensure that the dose is drawn from a homogeneous preparation. Adsorption of particles to the walls of vials and syringes has also been observed, making it difficult to administer the correct dose to the patient. The adsorption problem can be made less by treating the walls with a surfactant agent.

6. CAPSULES

Radiopharmaceuticals in liquid form for oral use are sometimes administered in capsules. This is primarily done to reduce the risk of spilling and contamination. The solution is dispensed in ordinary, hard gelatine capsules, filled with a carrier substance such as sodium phosphate. The volume of radioactive solution in each capsule is normally so small that there is no danger of the capsule wall dissolving because of the liquid present.

Capsules are also used to supply radioactive solutions as standards for diagnostic purposes. For these capsules special emphasis must be laid on content uniformity and the release of the radioactive material from the capsule.

7. GASES FOR INHALATION

The gases used most frequently are radioactive noble gases, such as xenon-133, xenon-127, krypton-85 and krypton-81m. They are usually presented as precalibrated doses in a definite volume. The gases are often diluted with air. The various manufacturers have developed different systems for the delivery of acurate doses of gas from the pre-calibrated vials, ampoules or metal cylinders. A multi-dose container has been introduced for xenon-133, where the gas is supplied in a shielded, collapsible bag, that allows samples with known radioactive concentration to be drawn from the bag with a syringe. Radioactive gases for inhalation may also be supplied from radionuclide generator systems, where the patient is breathing a gas that comes directly from the generator. An example is krypton-81m, that is eluted from a column containing rubidium-81 by passing humid air or nitrogen through the column and with subsequent mixing with air in a special breathing mask.

8. GASES FOR INJECTION

The same radioactive gases for inhalation may also be applied in perfusion studies, when the gases are available in sterile, isotonic solutions in single-dose or multi-dose containers. For ultra short-lived isotopes, such as krypton-81m with a half-life of 13 seconds, it has been necessary to design generator systems that allow continuous infusion to the patient direct from the generator. This system demands a very high standard in design, production and use, and special emphasis must be laid on the aseptic aspects of the procedure.

9. RADIONUCLIDE GENERATORS

The radionuclides with short physical half-lives allow the administration of larger doses without increase in the radiation exposure above the accepted levels. With high photon fluxes better images can be obtained in a shorter time. Economic limitations and transport difficulties would generally make it impossible to supply these nuclides to medical centres that are distant from the site of production. However, for some of these nuclides the problems have been solved by the development of radionuclide generator systems. The generators are based on the principle of decay/growth relationship between a long-lived parent radionuclide and a short-lived daughter radionuclide. Upon formation the daughter nuclide is separated from the parent nuclide and used for the preparation of radiopharmaceuticals. In nuclear medicine several generator systems are used routinely today.

The ideal radionuclide generator for parenteral solutions should have the following properties:

a. The system supplies a sterile, apyrogenic solution
b. 0,9% saline solution can be used as eluent
c. The generator may be stored without special precautions at room temperature
d. The daughter nuclide has suitable radiation characteristics and half-life
e. The chemical separation gives minimal content of parent nuclide in the eluate
f. The parent nuclide must have a relatively short half-life, so the "in-growth" of the daughter nuclide is not too long.
   However, the half-life should be long enough to make possible a convenient transport system from the manufacturer to the hospitals.
g. The eluate contains the daughter nuclide in a chemical form that makes it suitable for the formation of complexes with other agents to produce various radio-pharmaceuticals.

The Mo99/Tc99m generator, the most important system in use, fulfills most of these criteria. The principle of the generator is the same as when it was first introduced in 1957, but as it is the single most important product in nuclear medicine today and an important economic factor for the producers of radiopharmaceuticals, much work has been done in the development and design of this generator system. The modern generators are reliable and easy to use as they allow automatic elution, and they are designed as closed systems to prevent contamination by microorganisms. Both vacuum and pressure systems are employed in the elution process. Some systems have one large eluent reservoir in a glass bottle or plastic bag, and the column is kept wet permanently. In other systems the eluent is supplied in individual portions for each elution, and the column is kept dry between each elution. Following the manufacturer's instructions the present generator systems will supply a sterile eluate when aseptic working techniques are applied. Still a couple of problems remain that may upset the routine work in the nuclear medicine department: No yield of activity upon elution of the generator or reduced yield upon elution.

When no yield at all is obtained, this can be due to large, internal damages of the bed during transport, which makes it impossible to pass the saline solution through the column, or the needles of the canulas may be clogged with particles from the rubber stoppers of the vials. In systems based on evacuated vials, a leak in these vials will also make it impossible to elute the generator. Reduced yields have two main causes. The presence of reducing agents on the column may lead to the reduction of pertechnetate to ionic species of other oxidation states that will bind to the column material. This can be due to the presence of reducing substances in the eluent or the column material, or induced by the strong local radiation at the upper part of the column. Reduced vacuum in the vials may give only a partial elution and thereby reduced yield. Low yields are also obtained when the eluent only reaches a fraction of the surface of the column material on which the parent nuclide is bound. This can be caused by use of poor quality column material, improper initial packing of the powder bed or disturbance in the bed during transport.

10. PREPARATION KITS FOR USE WITH RADIONUCLIDE GENERATORS

The introduction of preparation kits for use with radionuclide generators has made the production of short-lived radiopharmaceuticals in hospitals much easier. The radiopharmaceutical is prepared by addition of eluate from a radionuclide generator to vials with pre-dispensed, sterile materials in lyophilized form or solution. The preparation kits are very simple to use, as most modern kits require only a one-step procedure. The kits have a long shelf-life and can therefore be kept in stock in the hospitals. As the labelling procedure is performed in a closed system and the final preparation is used within one working day, it is not necessary to take too many precautions when planning the preparation area for these products. The finished preparation should be inspected behind lead glass shielding to make sure that a complete solution or suspension has been obtained.

11. LABELS AND PACKAGE INSERTS

Labels and package inserts are an important factor in the presentation of a radiopharmaceutical. The labelling should comply with the relevant national legislation and international agreements. The radioactive nature of the products makes it undesirable to read all the relevant information from the label of the container, as this will give unnecessary radiation doses to the eyes and the fingers. The information has therefore been divided between the label on the container and the package inserts.

On the label of the container should be stated:
a. The name of the preparation
b. The name of the manufacturer
c. The total radioactivity in the container at a stated date and, if necessary, hour. For liquid preparations just a statement of the radioactive concentration may be given
d. An identification code that makes it possible to trace the manufacture and distribution history of the product.

Additional information should be given on a package insert or on a label on the package. Such information should include:
a. The period of validity or the expiry date
b. The route of administration
c. The name and the concentration of any added antimicrobial preservative
d. Any special storage conditions
e. Any special information on the product or that particular batch, including warnings and special precautions.

The package inserts for preparation kits are often very elaborate. They contain detailed instructions for how the labelling procedure should be performed. Furthermore there is information on the indications for clinical use, contraindications, adverse reactions, radiation dosimetry, toxicology etc. The manufacturer´s instructions for use must be carried out carefully, and changes in these recommendations must only be made on the basis of quality evaluations. It should be noted that the responsibility for the quality of the final preparation is shared between the manufacturer of the kit and the personnel responsible for the preparation in the hospital.

The expressions "period of validity" and "expiry" have special significance for radiopharmaceuticals. For non-radioactive medicinal products these definitions indicate the period of time the manufacturer guarantee the product for use with regards to quality and "potency". For radiopharmaceuticals the "potency" is given by the amount of radioactivity present in the product, and thereby related to the time of calibration. The choice of calibration date may be made on various backgrounds, such as the day of production, the day of dispatch or according to the demands of the customer. In addition, the special nature of radiopharmaceuticals make it necessary to give an expiry date, that is depending both on the chemical and radiochemical stability of the product. After the expiry date the product may also contain an insufficient amount of radioactivity for the intended use because of decay. The radionuclidic purity of the product may change considerably as the amount of longlived radionuclidic impurities increase with time in preparations of short-lived radionuclides. It should therefore be noted that the manufacturer´s specification for a product should be valid for the whole period of use.

The various principles applied to fix the calibration time have lead to a certain confusion. Earlier it was common to ship radiopharmaceuticals with activity precalibration to the day the customer would receive the product. Lately, however, extended periods of precalibration have been used as a marketing tool, especially in the sales promotion of technetium-99m generators. There is now a tendency to restrict such extreme use of precalibration. The Isotope-Pharmacy in Denmark does not allow a precalibration longer than half of the half-life of the radionuclide in question. For radionuclides with a half-life shorter than 4 days, a precalibration of maximum 4 days is allowed.

Apart from labelling according to pharmaceutical legislation, shipments of radiopharmaceuticals are also subject to special national and international regulations with regard to the packaging and the labels on the outside of the packages. The internationally accepted regulations for transport of radioisotopes have been drawn up by IAEA. Special regulations have been issued by the relevant authorities for transport by air (IATA), sea (IMCO), rail (RID) and road (ADR), and these are all based on the IAEA regulations. The requirements for packaging of radioisotopes take into consideration both the safe containment of the radioactive material and the protection of the personnel that will handle the package during transport. The radiopharmaceutical is generally first enclosed in a leak-proof and securely sealed container, and then enclosed in a secondary shielding container. The shielding should be adequate to prevent external dose rates in excess of certain limits, and the material and thickness of the shielding are therefore determined by the radionuclide and the amount of radioactivity. The inner containers are enclosed in a sealed can to further ensure a leak-proof package. For liquid products it is specified that sufficient absorbent material is provided to absorb twice the volume of the liquid in event of leakage. The shipping carton must withstand certain tests to ensure that it will not be damaged by weather conditions or handling during transport. The outside of each package shall be provided with a seal that is not readily breakable and which, while intact, will prove that the package has not been opened. According to the external radiation dose on the surface of the cartons, the packages are divided into 3 categories, and this is clearly indicated by corresponding labels on the surface. These labels shall state the radionuclide(s) in the package, the total amount of radioactivity and the transport index, which is the highest dose rate measured at one meter from any point on the surface of the package. It is important to note that both transport index and amount of total radioactivity should be given with reference to the date of dispatch.

REFERENCES
1. Basics of Radiopharmacy. Rhodes B A, Croft B Y, C.V. Mosby, St. Louis, 1978.
2. Fundamentals of Nuclear Pharmacy. Saha G B. New York, Springer Verlag, 1979.
3. The Preparation and Control of Radiopharmaceuticals in Hospitals. Kristensen K, Vienna, International Atomic Energy Agency, 1979.
4. Radiopharmacy. Tubis M and Wolf W. New York, John Wiley and Sons Inc. 1976.
5. European Pharmacopoiea, Second Edition 1981.
6. Radioisotope Production and Quality Control. Vienna, International Atomic Energy Agency, 1971.
7. 25. report WHO Expert Committee on specifications for Pharmaceutical Preparations. Geneva, World Health Organization, 1975.
8. Regulations for the Safe Transport of Radioactive Materials. 1973 Revised Edition (As amended). Safety Series No. 6. Vienna, International Atomic Energy Agency, 1979.
9. IATA Dangerous Goods Regulations. 24 Edition International Air Transport Association. Montreal, 1982.

5. STABILITY OF RADIOPHARMACEUTICALS
CHARLES FALLAIS, FRANCIS SMAL

1. INTRODUCTION

The concept of the stability for a radiopharmaceutical is not different from that of a common drug. As in the pharmaceutical industry, stability problems are routinely classified into three types: physical, chemical and microbiological (1,2).

The degradation of a radiopharmaceutical can produce the following effects:
- change in its biological behaviour (physiological distribution);
- increase of side effects (organ and whole body dosimetry);
- changes in content uniformity (colloids);
- changes in the pharmaceutical aspects (colored solutions);
- formation of impurities (free radioisotopes in labelled compounds);
- interaction with the container (absorption-adsorption);
- presence of micro-organisms (non-sterile radiopharmaceuticals, pyrogenic effects).

The specific characteristics of a radiopharmaceutical product may have an influence on the stability studies. Of particular importance are: Its radioactive content (physical half-life, nature and energy of radiation), its use after a short time after its preparation, the small quantity of active product, the limited number of different galenic forms and its use in a small and selected population of patients by specialised medical users.

Stability studies are commonly undertaken during two stages in new drug research. During development, such studies are used to evaluate different formulations and to determine the conditions of storage and the shelf-life of the product. Later stability studies on different batches in the final package are undertaken to guarantee that the results are reproducible. In terms of duration, the first step of stability studies is particularly important for the radiopharmaceuticals. The second one is particularly considered with regard to the effective shelf-life of the product which is generally in terms of days or weeks with radioisotopes of short or mean physical shelf-life. Some examples can illustrate these aspects.

2. PHYSICAL STABILITY

2.1. For inorganic radioisotopes, the adsorption on glass or absorption into rubber closures must be determined. For radiopharmaceuticals with shelf-life of months like Sr-85, Fe-59, P-32, it has been proposed to siliconize glass vials and rubber closures. But by using neutral glass and chloro- or bromo-butyl rubber, the losses in activity are less than 5% for ferric (Fe-59) citrate and P-32 phosphate at expiry date.

2.2. More important is the absorption of Xenon-133 in rubber closures. When the use of cartridges was proposed to avoid the presence of gas and solution phases in vials, this major problem was recorded (Fig. 1).

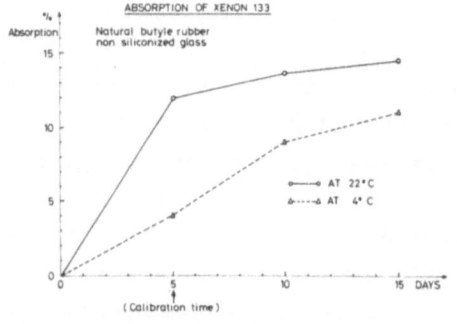

Figure 1

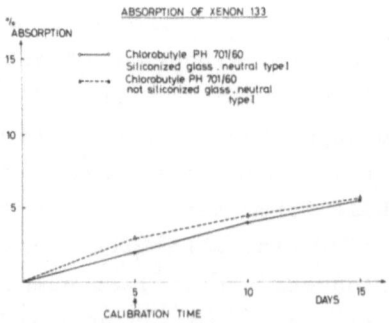

Figure 2

To ensure a usable activity in the solution, the manufacturer was obliged to overdose the activity at production time. The effect of storage temperature is not negligible so that the real activity which is taken by injection can be different from time to time. To solve this problem, stability studies were undertaken with different rubber closures and siliconized glass to reduce this effect as much as possible (Fig. 2).

2.3. It is wellknown that the pH has an important effect on the adsorption of In-111 chelates. When In-111 oxine is prepared in Tris-buffer, the radioactive product is catched in a few hours by the glass walls of the vial. So In-111 chelates are generally prepared in an acidic solution and the buffer is supplied in separate vials.

2.4. Colloids and suspensions are particularly sensitive to dilution and pH changes and less to room temperature. The pH can be fixed by the production method and the use of suspension agent like dextran or gelatine to increase the viscosity of the preparation is generally adopted. It is however very important to avoid dilution or to inject immediately any even slightly diluted suspension of colloid.

3. CHEMICAL STABILITY
3.1. To check this type of stability, all the chemical methods such as polarography, electrophoresis, paper-, TL-, HPL-chromatography, UV-, visible-, IR-spectrophotometry, etc. are useful. The biological behaviour in man of the radiopharmaceutical can be estimated by the biodistribution in animals. By assays at different times after the labelling, it is possible to evaluate the stability in vivo and protocols of assays must report the accepted percentage of organ uptake.Table 1 and 2 give examples.

TABLE 1 - DMSA - Biological distribution

Rats are sacrified one hour after injection

	Time of injection after reconstitution of the vials	
	15-45 min.	210-270 min.
% injected activity in kidneys	⩾ 41%	⩾ 41%
% injected activity in liver	⩽ 5%	⩽ 5%
Activity in kidneys / Activity in liver	⩾ 10%	⩾ 8%
% injected activity in stomach	⩽ 1%	⩽ 1%
% free Tc-99m	⩽ 2%	⩽ 2%
Recovered activity / Injected activity	⩾ 83%	⩾ 83%
% injected activity in whole blood	⩽ 15%	⩽ 15%

TABLE 2 - MDP - Biological distribution

Rats are sacrified 2 hours after injection

	Time of injection after reconstitution of the vials
	20-45 min. and not less than 6 hours
Recovered activity minus activity in whole skeleton	⩽ 9%
% injected activity in kidneys	⩽2.5%
% injected activity in liver	⩽ 1%
% injected activity in stomach	⩽ 1%
% injected activity in whole blood	⩽1.2%
Activity in femur / Activity in liver	⩾ 1%

Note -Skeleton uptake of MDP-Tc-99m is dependent on the age
of the rats. Uptake is higher with young rats. Usually,
overall bone uptake is higher than 4o% of the injected
activity and any batch with bone uptake less than 3o%
will be discarded.
-If the biodistribution in one rat appears to be
abnormal (very different from the 5 others), the
decision to take into account will be taken case by
case by the pharmacist in charge of Quality Control.

3.2. Stability of radio-labelled o-iodo-hippuric acid

The impurities levels, free iodide and ortho-iodo-benzoic acid (OIB) represent the sum of the amount initially present at preparation time and the amount produced by decomposition. (3,4,5).

It has been described that I-131-iodohippurate decomposition is mostly due to absorbed radiation. By chromatographic procedures this degradation was followed during 28 days at different temperatures (Table 3).

TABLE 3 - Stability study - Ortho-iodo-hippuric acid (I-131)

Method: TL-chromatography. Eur.Pharm.Vol.III, 1977, Method b.
Radioactive concentration: 0,5 mCi/ml at day 0.
Specific activity: 50 μCi/mg.

Time elapsed after preparation (days)	Iodide			O I B			O I H		
	4°C	22°C	42°C	4°C	22°C	42°C	4°C	22°C	42°C
0	0.8	0.8	0.8	0.7	0.7	0.7	98.4	98.4	98.4
6	1.1	1.1	1.0	1.2	1.1	1.1	97.2	97.3	97.3
12	1.9	2.0	1.7	1.8	2.0	1.6	96.0	95.9	96.2
18	2.2	2.1	2.0	2.2	2.1	2.3	95.1	95.1	95.3
22	3.6	3.2	2.8	2.3	2.7	2.6	93.8	93.7	94.0
28	5.2	5.0	-	5.4	4.2	4.3	91.6	91.1	91.8

The percentage of IOB and iodide are increasing during the time of the study. The influence of the temperature cannot be proved (Fig. 3, 4, 5). Taking this study into account for I-123-o-iodo-hippurate shelf-life evaluation, it is expected that the content of iodide and OIB-level will remain the same during storage as the initial percentage determined at production time.

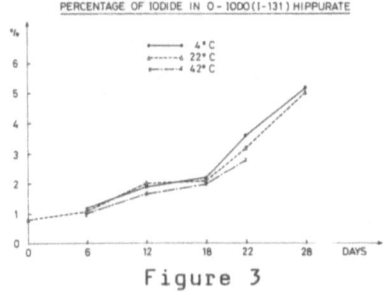

Figure 3

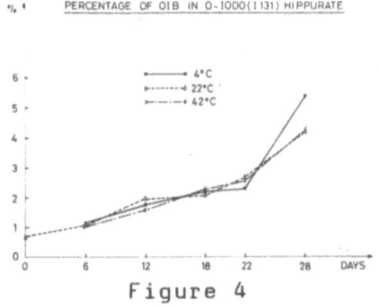

Figure 4

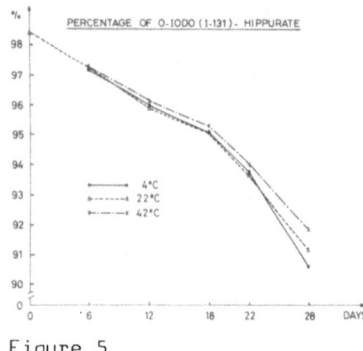

Figure 5

The most important precaution must therefore be to use a very pure o-iodo-hippurate with very low (0.2-0.3%) content of OIB and to make sure that the exchange reaction is as complete as possible (98-99%). To control this quality, a rapid HPLC-procedure is particularly useful and reported by Millar (6).

The comparison between TLC and HPLC shows a significant difference between the results obtained by the two techniques. The higher resolution of HPLC can explain the better percentage (99,1% ± 0,2 Standard deviation, against 98,3% ± 0,2 for TLC).

3.3. Tc99m-compounds

Many papers and communications are available concerning this large field of radiopharmaceuticals. They must be consulted for each particular product. During the development of the IDA derivatives, the structure activity relationship (SAR) has been studied and reported (7). It is a demonstration of the importance of stability studies at this development stage of a radiopharmaceutical (8,9).

Many molecules are proposed in kit forms. A stability program must be developed before marketing and a stability survey during marketing must be carried out. This program is particularly important to detect unexpected changes of the product when the kit is produced routinely. The assays are based on the radiochemical assay of the product (described in its specifications) and on the biological distribution. The program is only applicable on accepted batches (Table 4).

TABLE 4 - Stability Program

Number of batches	0-5	6-10	11-15
At 1/3 of the validity period: physical assay	Each batch	Max. 4 batches (8 different samplings)	
At 2/3 of the validity period: physical assay radiochemical assay biological assay	Each batch	Max. 4 batches (8 different samplings	
At expiry date (plus up to one month): acceptance procedure	One batch	two batches	three batches

The sampling is made after the acceptance of the batch. The vials are labelled with the estimated date of the assay. All the results are recorded on an analytical sheet and are a part of the Q.C. documents. On-going stability program can be used to extend the expiry date. Therefore all the batches must be fully checked at the proposed date and 3 months later. If in one year none of the batches shows a defect product at the proposed date it can be accepted and the adapted on-going stability program can be re-adjusted.

4. STABILIZING AGENTS

Some agents are proposed to stabilize the radiopharma-ceutical. The use of benzylic alcohol as antimicrobial preservative, the buffering of solutions are reported as well by the manufacturer's formulation as by pharmacopoeia's monographs. For technetium kits, ascorbic acid and gentisic acid are generally proposed to stabilize and protect the oxydo-reduction agent during storage. It is important to know the stability of these stabilizers. An example can be given by ascorbic acid.(10). Under aerobic conditions the ascorbic acid is oxidized to dehydroascorbic acid followed by hydrolysis and oxidation to give diketogulonic acid and oxalic acid. Under anaerobic conditions, it undergoes dehydration and hydrolysis to give furfural and carbon dioxide. The pH at maximum stability is pH 6. In the case of freeze-dried kits with absence of oxygen (air), dried form and low concentration ascorbic acid is under the best condition for keeping its integrity. But it is certain that an identical formulation for a solution will show an important degradation of the ascorbic acid.

REFERENCES
1. Rhodes C T. Drug Product Stability and Shelf-life. The Center for Professional Advancement, Amsterdam, 15-17 Nov. 1982.
2. Glenn H J, Kidwell R E. Radioactive Pharmaceuticals and the concept of stability: Radioactive Pharmaceuticals. Conf. USAEC 65IIII 1966: 171-174.
3. Hotte C E, Ice R D. In vitro Stability of I-131 o-iodohippurate. J Nucl Med 1979;20:441-447.
4. Smal F. I-123 hippuran: Preparation, Quality Control and Clinical applications. Fourth European Congress of Nuclear Medicine, May 20-23, 1980, from Eur J Nucl Med 1980;5:A34.
5. Kappersen F M, Westera G. Radioiodinated o-Iodobenzoic acid as impurity in Hippuran Preparations. Int J Appl Rad Isotop 1980;31:97-99.
6. Millar A M. High performance liquid chromatographic method for determination of the radiochemical purity of iodohippuric acid (I-123) injection. J Pharm Pharmacol 1982;34:14-17.
7. Cox P H. Development in Nuclear Medicine, Vol.I, Cholescintigraphy, 1981. Nijhof, Amsterdam.
8. Loberg M D, et al. Development of new radiopharmaceuticals based on N-substitution of Iminodiacetic acid. J Nucl Med 1976;17:633-38.
9. Loberg M D, Fields A T. Chemical structure of Tc99m labelled N-(2.6-Dimethylphenylcarbamoylmethyl)-iminodia-cetic acid (Tc-HIDA). Int J Appl Rad Isotop 1978;29:167-73.
10. Blaug S M, Hajratwata B. Kinetics of aerobic oxidation of ascorbic acid. J Pharm Sci 1972;61:556-62.

6.   PRODUCTION DESIGN - G.M.P. INDUSTRY
MAURIZIO VILLA

1. INTRODUCTION

A pharmaceutical manufacturer has to comply with a number of regulations and/or guidelines which, by law, regulate the approval of a pharmaceutical. Examples are "Medicines Act", "Product Licence", etc., which are rules generally in force in many countries and which have to be fulfilled by the manufacturer. Within these "regulations and/or guidelines" the Good Manufacturing Practice, also known as G.M.P., plays a fundamental role. G.M.P. could be unofficially referred to as a collection of rules either established by law, or proposed as a guide, or self-fixed by the manufacturer to be followed in order to guarantee consistency, safety, identity and strength of a pharmaceutical. Radiopharmaceuticals for diagnostic as well as for therapeutic use are a "sort of pharmaceuticals" containing radionuclides with specific characteristics and performances. The manufacturer of Radio-pharmaceuticals has to fulfill the "regulations and/or guidelines", and therefore also the G.M.P., regulating the approval of Radiopharmaceuticals. Because of the specific characteristics of these products, these "regulations" may be specific to Radiopharmaceuticals. However, pharmaceutical G.M.P. are also usually adopted for the production of Radio-pharmaceuticals. Once importance and role of G.M.P. are established, the definition of "manufacturer" helps to identify the entity who must follow such rules. The term "manufacturer" normally means production of Radio-pharmaceuticals most often for sale and therefore is referred to as the industry. Nevertheless, the production of Radio-pharmaceuticals in hospitals, even if not for sale or profit purposes, should be characterized by the same guarantee of consistency, safety, identity and strength and therefore it should follow the G.M.P.

2. G.M.P. DEFINITION

G.M.P. is defined by the British "Guide to Good Pharmaceutical Manufacturing Practice" as that "part of quality assurance aimed at ensuring that products are consistently manufactured to a quality appropriate to their intended use". It is thus concerned with both Manufacturing and Quality Control. (1).

The legal status and therefore the application of G.M.P. may vary considerably from country to country. The G.M.P.s drafted by the European Free Trade Association - E.F.T.A. -and followed in many European Countries are legally to be considered as guidelines which "do not have any statutory force, but indicate the main areas of interest and expectations of the various Inspectorates in the performances of their duties in respect of manufacturers".(2). On the other side, the American Authorities, F.D.A., give a legal status of code to the G.M.P. in force in the U.S.A., being defined as "the minimum G.M.P. for methods to be used for the manufacture (......) of a drug to assure that such drug meets the requirements of the act as to safety, and has the identity and strength and meets the quality and purity characteristics that it purports or is represented to posses. The failure to comply with any regulations renders such drug to be adulterated (......) and such drug should be subject to regulatory action". (3).

The force, the definition and interpretation of G.M.P. may substantially vary from country to country and therefore the "manufacturer" must deeply consider and evaluate the legal status, force and interpretation given to G.M.P. by National Authorities.

3. HISTORICAL AND GEOGRAPHICAL CONSIDERATIONS

This section intends to report the most significant steps

of the G.M.P. history during the recent years, and it will discuss the actual interpretation given to G.M.P. in some countries.

In 1972 the "European Free Trade Association" (E.F.T.A.) under the "Convention for the Mutual Recognition of Inspections in respect of the Manufacture of Pharmaceutical Products" first established the "Basic Standards of G.M.P. for Pharmaceutical Products": annexes to this general G.M.P. guidelines were then published by E.F.T.A. in 1973, 1976 and 1981. (4-7). The E.F.T.A. G.M.P.s are followed as originally drafted in Germany, Italy and Norway, or have been slightly modified and detailed to be adapted to local situations as in France and U.K.

The E.F.T.A. guidelines still represent a suitable working tool for manufacturers and Inspectors and are well balanced within the four main aspects of the production design: Facilities and Personnel, Manufacturing Procedures, Quality Control and Post-Marketing Follow-up.

The E.F.T.A. guidelines are quite general. They do not pay particular attention to how to document and record the main steps of production design and, of course, they do not refer specifically to Radiopharmaceuticals.

In 1977 the Danish authorities published a "Promulgation order on production, control, stockkeeping and sale of medicinal products". (8). This G.M.P. is the first and to our knowledge the only one to refer specifically to "radioactive medicinal products". The Danish G.M.P. is largely derived from the E.F.T.A. guidelines, but some aspects neglected or absent in the original document are particularly considered here, such as: Production documentation, Raw materials and Sale and distribution. In general the Danish G.M.P.s are more detailed and specific and particular attention is given to the bureaucratic system of production documentation such as records, files, etc.

Also in 1977, the British Authorities published the "Guide for Good Pharmaceutical Manufacturing Practice". (1). This guide was under revision in 1982, and a new version should be

available within 1983. The existing guide was also considered
the tool and the instructions routinely used by the British
Authorities (D.H.S.S.), to inspect facilities and production
procedures of manufacturers. This guide is in some respects
very similar to the Danish Promulgation order and gives
particular care to: Personnel and Training, Premises and
Equipment. The policy followed in drafting this guide and
therefore in inspecting facilities to control the adherence of
manufacture to such guide is based on the assumption that the
"quality of a pharmaceutical" is mostly assured by a good
design (layout) of facilities and their maintenance; quality
and training of the personnel; proper use of equipment, their
maintenance and routine control; design of the manufacture
procedure. On this basis, the quality control of the final
pharmaceutical is substantially the confirmation of the
intended product characteristics.

In contrast, the G.M.P.s from the Food and Drug
Administration are mostly based on the assumption that the
most strict "in-process" and final Quality Controls would
guarantee rejection of all "unsatisfactory" batches. A heavy
paper work documents all steps during production, quality
control, distribution, and post-marketing follow-up.

Table 1 lists the actual situation in some European countries.

TABLE 1

BELGIUM	No G.M.P. guidelines
DENMARK	"Promulgation order on Production, Control, Stockkeeping and Sale of medicinal Products" - No. 496, Sept. 1977
FRANCE	"Pratiques de bonne Fabrication Commission Nationale de Pharmacopee" - Oct. 1978 (12)
GERMANY	At present, no G.M.P. guidelines: in preparation on the basis of W.H.O. - E.F.T.A.
ITALY	The same as GERMANY
NORWAY	"Basic Standards of G.M.P. for Pharmaceutical Products" E.F.T.A.
U.K.	"Guide to Pharmaceutical G.M.P." -Oct. 1977 (Under revision)

This review, far from being a detailed analysis of all
national policies and legal aspects related to G.M.P., should
put in evidence the wide range of interpretations which may be

given to a "G.M.P." by Authorities, Inspectors and Manufacturers. It is interesting to note that specific G.M.P.s for Radiopharmaceuticals have not been drafted or published so far by legal Authorities. In 1971 a paper entitled "Good Practices in the Manufacture of Radiopharmaceuticals:A Proposal put forward by a Group of Pharmacists from the Nordic Countries" was the first attempt to set up, even if unofficially, specific G.M.P. for Radiopharmaceuticals (9). More recent reviews on G.M.P. for Radiopharmaceuticals represent in fact a list of protocols and specification for Q.C. on final products. (10,11).

4. SORIN G.M.P.
4.1. Introduction

The differences between the G.M.P.s in force in various countries and the wide range of interpretations and policies of regulatory affairs oblige an international manufacturer to follow and respect in some ways the regulations established in the countries where its products are distributed. Industry general policy is to draft and adopt an "in-house" G.M.P. combining the most strict points and the parts characteristics to each national G.M.P. Moreover the Radiopharmaceutical manufacturer includes in its G.M.P.s all specific rules for good manufacturing practice of specific pharmaceutics as Radiopharmaceuticals. For these reasons at Sorin Biomedica we drafted and adopted the "Sorin G.M.P.". The most important and peculiar items of "Sorin G.M.P." are here discussed. "Sorin G.M.P." can be described in detail using the five main documents reflecting the company's organization and policy.

4.2. Quality Assurance Master File

It reports all legal documents and information on the company, describes organizations, personnel (chart, education, responsibility and training), facilities, main equipment, items like components and composition, production and in-process controls and laboratory quality controls. The Master File establishes the general and main rules and regulations of all aspects referring to Radiopharmaceuticals.

References to the other four main documents of the G.M.P. are continuously and frequently made. This document has been mainly drafted on the basis of the F.D.A. requirements.

4.3. S.O.P. File

This file lists and reports all "Standard Operating Procedure" regulating all production and Q.C. activities. It turns out that S.O.P. is the internal official channel to transmit to the personnel specific rules and instructions for each single operation. Each S.O.P. describes the purposes and responsibilities of the S.O.P., instructions for use (in case of equipment or facility), validation process, calibration of equipment, method and responsibility for data and results recording, maintenance. Of course, particular attention is given to the records and their forms. For the production of about 25 different radiopharmaceuticals more than 100 S.O.P. files are used.

4.4. Raw Material File

This document lists and describes the monographs for test and release of raw materials used in production.
The term Raw Materials indicates chemical reagents, glassware, equipments (e.g.: filters, pipettes, etc.), containers, closures and packaging materials as labels, instructions for use, etc.

Most monographs derive from the European or/and the U.S. Pharmacopoeias. When European or U.S. Pharmacopoeias do not report such items, they are alternatively searched for, in accordance with the following sequence: National Pharmacopoeias (as B.P., France, Italy, etc.), National Formulary or American Chemical Society.

Routine procedures and specification are maintained as in the original: in some cases specification might be more strict in order to meet final product specification. For special raw materials where no official references are available from the above mentioned documents, an "in-house" monograph is drafted, on the basis of our experience.

4.5. Master Formula (M.F.) and Batch Sheet (B.S.)

Each production run (both of semimanufactured or final

products) is characterized by its M.F. and B.S. The M.F. reports a fully detailed description of the material to be produced and statements on any calculated excess of ingredients, theoretical yield, manufacturing and control instructions, procedures, specification, special notes and precautions.

The B.S. consists of:

a record of each significant step in the manufacture, processing, packaging, labelling, testing and controlling of the batch including:

a) dates, individual major equipment and lines employed,

b) specific identification of each batch of components used,

c) quantities of components and products used in the course of processing,

d) in-process and laboratory control results,

e) identification of the individuals performing and checking each significant step in the operation,

a batch (lot) number identifying all production and control documents and run numbers associated with the batch,

a record of any investigation made on the batch.

When appropriate, M.F. and B.S. refer to the Quality Assurance Master File or to a specific S.O.P. M.F. and B.S. were drafted by Sorin mostly following the F.D.A. requirements.

4.6. Quality Control

The Sorin Q.C. Department is routinely taking care of: Validation, Facility, Equipment and Environmental Q.C., Raw Materials, In-process Q.C., Final Product Q.C. and G.M.P. Some of these aspects have already previously been described. In order to satisfy different national requirement, procedures and specification for general tests and assays, like sterility, pyrogenicity, etc., Sorin drafted and follows "in-house" procedures and specification resulting from the combination of the European and U.S. Pharmacopoeias. As previously said for Raw Material Q.C., monographs for final product testing are usually derived from the European Pharmacopoeia or, if not applicable, from either the British or U.S. or Japanese Pharmacopoeias. In fact they are actually reporting the largest number of monographs for Radiopharmaceuticals. Batches of final products to be distributed within the U.S.A. are tested on the basis of the U.S. Pharmacopoeia or on the basis of the protocols given in the IND/NDA (Applications for approval). From what has been described it can be concluded that "Sorin G.M.P." is equivalent or similar to a Pharmaceutical G.M.P.

5. RADIOPHARMACEUTICAL G.M.P.

Because of peculiar characteristics of some Radiopharmaceuticals, like the short validity period due to the short radioisotope half-life, these products must be distributed and commercialized before completion of certain Q.C. tests. In fact sterility, general safety and radionuclide purity tests must begin before dispatch, but results to assure quality of the product will be known only several days later. Therefore some special precautions reflecting the peculiar characteristics of Radiopharmaceuticals were kept in mind during "Sorin G.M.P." drafting:

-sterility of the ambient air in shielded cells and laminar flow hoods are almost continuously monitored

-particular attention is paid to sterilization and sterility test of glassware and equipment to be used in direct contact with the Radiopharmaceutical

-particular care is generally given to all operations performed in sterile units

-layout and equipment of sterile rooms for radioactive materials are specifically designed to reduce to a minimum the risk of bacteriological contamination, though still meeting the specific requirements of radioactive manipulation for a "negative pressure" environment

-cross-contamination is avoided by using a cell for each product, by adopting particular care in reprocessing and controlling glassware or equipment to be used in handling radioactive material and by decontamination of all equipment before its re-use.

Moreover, if at Q.C. completion, results show unsatisfactory quality of a released product, two consequent actions are specifically adopted:

-very strict and efficient recall system for the adulterated lot/batch

-re-validation of the production process before a new lot/batch is released.

6. CONCLUSIONS

G.M.P.s for Radiopharmaceuticals are not just law-prone procedures, but are a really necessary tool intended to minimize the importance of the final Q.C. and the potential risk connected to distribution of not completely tested Pharmaceutical (see sterility, general safety, etc.).

Moreover what appears an expensive exercise to be avoided only relying on final Q.C., proves to reduce volume and number of rejected materials. Therefore it turns out that G.M.P. finally works also to optimize all activities of a Radiopharmaceutical manufacturer. The most important rule of the G.M.P. is that there is always room for improvements and that any complaint or report, even if apparently dummy, from the users must be carefully and immediately evaluated and checked. Actions to eliminate discrepancies, failures or breaches to the actual G.M.P. must be immediately taken. Therefore G.M.P. must be daily used, daily revised and daily improved.

Acknowledgements.
The author is indebted to Dr. F. Palmucci for valuable assistance.

REFERENCES

1. Guide to Good Pharmaceutical Manufacturing Practice 1977, London, HMSO.
2. Basic Standards of Good Manufacturing Practice for Pharmaceutical Products - PH 1/72 - E.F.T.A. Sept. 1972.

116

3. Code of Federal Regulations: 21 Parts 200 to 299. Washington - April 1982.
4. Guide to the Preparation of Information requested under Article 2 of the Convention for the Mutual Recognition of Inspections in Respect of the Manufacture of Pharmaceutical Products. PH 2/72 - E.F.T.A. Dec. 1972.
5. Guidelines for the Handling of Starting Materials. PH 2/73 - E.F.T.A. March 1973.
6. Guidelines for Manufacture and Analysis under Contract PH 3/76 - E.F.T.A. May 1976.
7. Guidelines for the Manufacture of Sterile Products. PH 1/81 - E.F.F.A. May 1981.
8. Promulgation order on Production, Control, Stockkeeping and Sale of Medicinal Products. National Health Service of Denmark No. 496 - Sept. 1977.
9. Good Practices in the Manufacture of Radiopharmaceuticals. Archiv for Pharmaci og Chemi, 1971;78:1002-1009.
10. Radiopharmaceuticals and Good Radiopharmacy Practice. M.G.Woldring - Pharmaceutisch Weekblad - Scientific Edition, 1981;3:1285-1301.
11. Quality Assurance of Radiopharmaceuticals: A Guide to Hospital Practice Nuclear Medicine Communications (special issue) 1981.
12. Pratiques de bonne Fabrication Oct. 1978, France, Maisonneuve S.A.
13. Fabrication des Medicaments: arrete royal relatif a la fabrication, a la preparation et a la distribution en gros des medicaments et a leur dispensation, Belgique, 6 Juin 1960.
14. Arrête royal portant reglement general de la protection de la population et des travailleurs contre le danger des radiations ionisantes: Belgique 28 Fevrier 1963.
15. Order concerning Radiopharmaceuticals Ministry of the Interior. Denmark July 1978.

7. PRECLINICAL STUDIES - RADIOPHARMACOLOGY AND TOXICOLOGY

PETER H. COX

1. INTRODUCTION

Radiopharmaceuticals exert no pharmacological action on the tissues of the host organism not even in the case of therapeutic agents where the therapeutic effect is achieved as the result of radiation induced damage. Diagnostic reagents tend to follow well defined metabolic pathways in the body or they are passively transported unchanged as the result of physiological activity and the movement of body fluids. In either case the biodistribution reflects physiological activity and a divergence from normal distribution patterns will indicate the presence of pathophysiological processes. This assumption forms the whole basis of in vivo nuclear medical diagnosis.

It is self evident that a radiopharmaceutical must be a stable preparation with a reproducible biodistribution. The purpose of radiopharmacology studies is to select the potentially most suitable reagent and establish criteria for safety and performance prior to the commencement of an evaluation in human subjects. This implies a study of bio-distribution in both normal animals and in animals with induced pathology. The development of animal models which are representative of human disease states can be difficult to realise in practice. The design of animal studies and the choice of species will be considered in chapter 8 and therefore we will concern ourselves with the evaluation of such studies and the extrapolation of the results obtained to humans.

2. IN VITRO OR IN VIVO?

The present climate of increased social awareness has resulted in more stringent legislation concerning the use of experimental animals. This in turn has resulted in an expansion of the use of in vitro techniques to select optimal formulations prior to carrying out in vivo studies thus reducing the incidence of indiscriminate use of animals.

An evaluation of the physicochemical characteristics of labelled compounds can serve to predict their biodistribution and hence reduce the need for man screening of derivatives. An example of this is the work of Subramanian (1) on IDA-derivatives in which it was demonstrated that by altering the structural formula the lipophilicity could be increased and as a result of this the degree of excretion in the bile could be raised whilst the renal excretion was lowered.

The recent work of Kung and Blau (2,3) on the synthesis of Se-75 labelled tertiary diamines as scintigraphic agents is another classic example of this approach. A series of selenium-75 labelled tertiary diamines were prepared and the effect of pH shift on lipid solubility was measured in vitro by measuring the octanol/buffer distribution co-efficient. A derivative was developed which had a neutral charge and which was lipid soluble at normal blood pH values (3). This compound diffuses readily across the cell membrane in vivo including into the brain. Within the cell where the pH is relatively low the complex aquires hydrogen ions and becomes charged whereupon the lipid solubility decreases thus fixing the complex within the cell (4).

2.1. Computer Models

The use of computer models to predict the biodistribution of labelled compounds is a potentially useful method of complementing animal studies for screening purposes. It is necessary to develop a compartmental model, representing the various organs, tissues and body fluids, on the basis of in vivo biodistribution studies. Data concerning the structure, solubility, ionic charge, lipophilicity and other physical chemical characteristics of new compounds can then be used to obtain a prediction concerning biodistribution.

Such models can be used to analyse biodistribution data and test the validity of clinical suppositions concerning radiopharmaceuticals in use. Charkes and Philips model (4) for F-18 fluoride kinetics is an excellent example of this approach being used to put anomalous clinical data into perspective.

A further use of computers which has been used in the pharmaceutical industry is the construction of mathematical models representing drug receptor sites and then fitting molecular models to them to identify potentially active compounds. This requires considerable computer capacity and sophisticated software and has not yet been applied to radio-pharmaceuticals.

2.2. Cell Culture

In vitro cell cultures of both normal and malignant tissues have provided useful information concerning the mechanisms of uptake and retention of radiopharmaceuticals, in particular with respect to the evaluation of tumour seeking compounds. Such studies have served to identify transport mechanisms and intracellular binding sites (5,6) but when compared with in vivo studies in animals carrying the same tumour type they may only serve to emphasize the dominating role of other factors such as vascularity (7).

3. IN VIVO STUDIES

It is self evident that while in vitro experimentation can provide prognostic information concerning in vivo behaviour, in vivo studies in the intact animal are an absolute necessity prior to the commencement of human investigations. The extrapolation of animal biodistribution data to humans is necessary to identify potential target organs and allow the calculation of radiation doses. This data can then be used to calculate clinically safe injectable dose levels in man.

3.1. Inter Species Differences

Basically biodistribution studies are required in both normal animals and where possible, in animals with induced pathology which resembles human disease states. Animal studies should not, however, be restricted to one species as considerable inter species differences in biodistribution may occur. Figure 1 shows an example of this phenomenon. A technetium stannous citrate complex was formulated by the author as a potential reagent for skeletal scintigraphy on the basis of the rationale that technetium-tin complexes as such were known to be inherently bone seeking (8) and the citrate carrier molecule is an essential component of the human skeleton, 49% of all citrate present being present in bone.

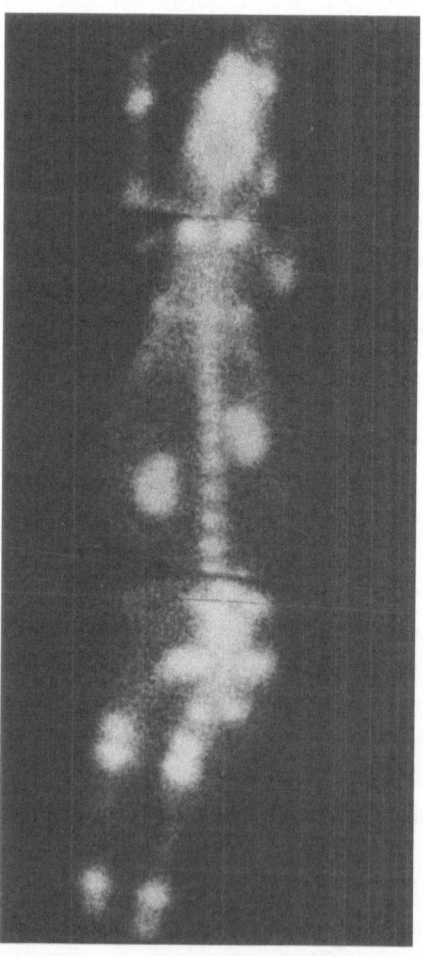
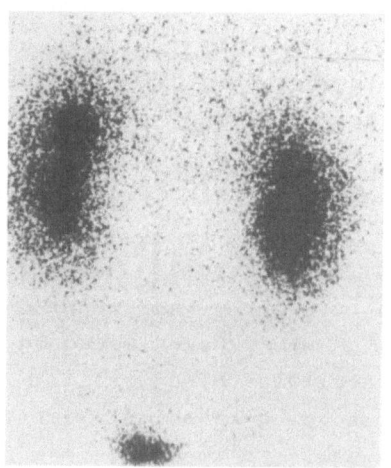

Fig.1. Left: Technetium citrate uptake in the rabbit skeleton after intravenous injection.
Right: The same compound in the human kidney two hours post injection.
There is no skeletal accumulation in the human, a clear interspecies difference exists.

Animal studies in rats and rabbits (8) showed an excellent skeletal localisation with a very low tissue background in both species. Figure 1 left shows a typical scintigram in the rabbit. In humans, however, no skeletal uptake at all can be observed the injected activity being rapidly scavenged by the kidneys and excreted via glomerular filtration, figure 1 right. It is clearly desirable that studies be carried out in more than one species of which only one should be a rodent. This inevitably imposes a limit on the possibility to fully develop new radiopharmaceuticals within the economic framework of a hospital or university environment.

Even in the event that extreme interspecies differences in biodistribution are not evident care should be taken when extrapolating kinetic data from animals to humans. Most animals have different metabolic rates to each other and to humans. Nevertheless comparable biodistribution patterns are usually observed.

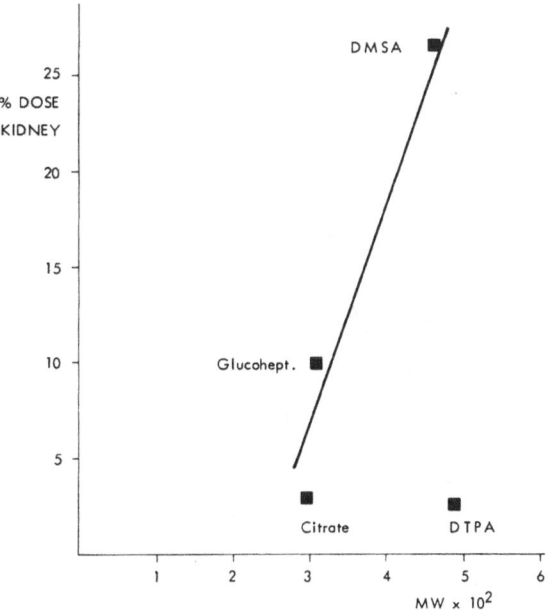

Fig. 2. Kidney uptake in the rat compared with the molecular weight of technetium complexes.

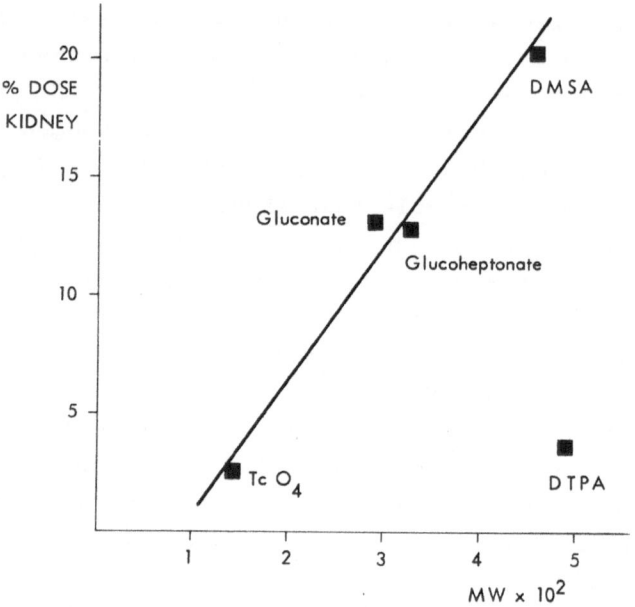

Fig.3. Kidney uptake in the rabbit compared with the molecular weight of
technetium complexes.

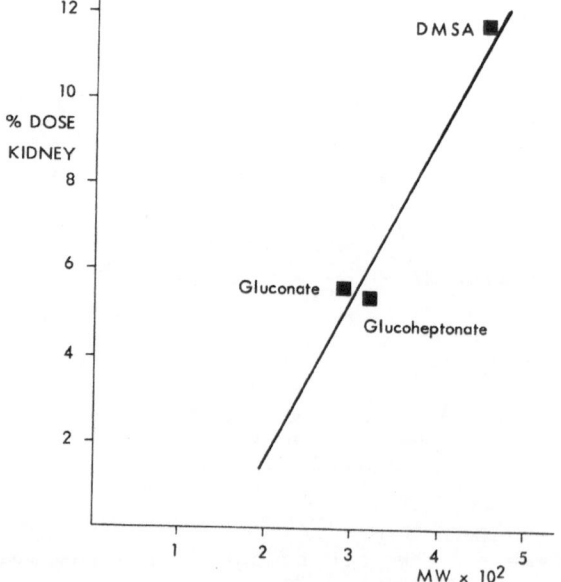

HUMAN KIDNEY UPTAKE

Fig.4. Kidney uptake in humans compared with the molecular weight of
technetium complexes.

For example the percentage uptake of intravenously administered technetium complexes in the kidney shows similar patterns in the rat, rabbit and in man although there are clear differences in the percentage uptake, of the administered dose, between the species (9). Figures 2, 3 and 4 show the appropriate data. In all three species there is a clear tendency for the larger molecular weight complexes to accumulate in the renal cortex to a higher degree. This is also a simple illustration of how biodistribution studies can be used to identify a structure activity relationship, in this case molecular size, between apparently dissimilar chemial compounds and as such serves to introduce the following topic which we should consider namely the presentation and interpretation of biodistribution data.

3.2. The Presentation and Evaluation of Biodistribution Data

The desirability of standardising methods of presenting biodistribution data has been discussed by Subramanian in chapter one and will not be considered further here despite the obvious importance of this topic for the extrapolation of data from animals to humans.

A point which is worthy of fuller consideration is the need to evaluate the biodistribution data relating to the target organ, i.e. the organ which is to be examined scintigraphically or functionally, with regard to other tissues in order to retain optimum objectivity other wise false conclusions may be drawn. To illustrate this let us reconsider the uptake of technetium complexes in the kidney. From the data in figures 2, 3 and 4 it could be concluded that the DMSA complex shows the highest concentration in the renal parenchyma. A study of renal parenchyma uptake in relation to time post injection in rats confirms this, table 1.

Table 1. Renal uptake in the rat in relation to time post injection. % injected dose per organ (9).

Reagent	time hrs post injection		
	0.5	1.0	2.0
DMSA	17.0	20.0	27.0
GLUCOHEPTONATE	8.8	9.1	8.7
DTPA	1.1	0.66	0.46

On the basis of this fact it has long been propounded that DMSA should be the reagent of choice for kidney imaging. Let us, however, now turn our attention to two of the most important tissues related to the kidney with respect to background activity, the bloodpool and the liver. Table 2 shows the kidney to blood ratios of the reagents with respect to time and table 3 the corresponding kidney to liver ratios.

Table 2. Kidney/blood ratios in the rat in relation to time post injection (% dose/g wet tissue)

Reagent	time hrs post injection		
	0.5	1.0	2.0
DMSA	17.0	27.0	47.0
GLUCOHEPTONATE	44.0	93.0	160.0
DTPA	4.8	8.1	44.0

Table 3. Kidney/liver ratios in the rat in relation to time post injection (% dose/g wet tissue)

Reagent	time hrs post injection		
	0.5	1.0	2.0
DMSA	8.7	17.0	28.0
GLUCOHEPTONATE	64.0	76.0	100.0
DTPA	13.0	13.0	12.0

A study of these figures raises some immediate questions with regard to DMSA. From table 2 we can see that the kidney/blood ratios observed with Glucoheptonate are a factor 3 higher than DMSA and this is also reflected in the kidney/liver ratio. It is possible to draw the following conclusions: Although the absolute concentrations of glucoheptonate in the kidney is lower than that of DMSA its blood clearance is more rapid and complete which results in a much higher kidney/background contrast for glucoheptonate.

The differences in blood clearance rates is also reflected in the kidney/liver ratios shown in table 3. These ratios are lower than the blood values which indicates that some accumulations is taking place in the liver. Here once again the data is favourable to glucoheptonate. The final conclusion is obvious : despite the fact that DMSA shows the highest specificity for kidney parenchyma the actual reagent of choice is glucoheptonate because its total biodistribution pattern yields better kidney to background ratios favourable to scintigraphy. When we discuss toxicity we will also observe the influence of these factors on radiation dose.

3.3. The choice of pathophysiological animal models

We have touched upon biodistribution studies in the normal animal and the importance of considering biodistribution parameters other than the degree of accumulation in the target organ. Let us now consider biodistribution as a means of detecting pathophysiology. Normal biodistribution patterns form the basis upon which in vivo nuclear medical studies are evaluated but the prime objective is the detection of pathology and therefore it is desirable to show that pathological changes are detectable before commencing human studies.

An animal model should closely imitate human pathology to be of any value and the development of a suitable model may be quite difficult. In the field of oncology the use of animals with implanted animal tumours has been of considerable value in evaluating the uptake of tumour seeking reagents (10, 11) and with the availability of immuno-deficient strains of animal it is now practicable to implant human tumours without rejection and to examine them under physiological conditions. Nevertheless to date no adequate animal model has been developed for a tumour which develops metastases at a distance and which would only allow the investigation of the problems of early in vivo diagnosis.

A number of alternative models have been tried to attempt to surmount this problem. On the assumption that the tumour uptake of radiopharmaceuticals is related to the rapid cell proliferation associated with repair Hill and Wagner (12) and Hammersley et al (13) used the regenerating rat liver as a model but obtained variable results - compared with each other and with similar work carried out by Orü (14) suggesting that such models are not reproducible.

On the assumption that the uptake of ionic tumour localising radiopharmaceuticals is related to cell metabolic

activity as reflected by cell membrane permeability Cox and
v.d. Pompe (15) investigated the uptake of gallium in the
thymus of the rat and found a definite correlation between age
(metabolic activity) and gallium accumulation. The natural
model appears to work, the pseudopathological not.

A further example of the use of analogue animal models
instead of real pathology can be found in the literature on
skeletal imaging reagents. Subramanian and McAffee (16)
compared a whole series of technetium comlexes for bone and
lesion uptake using a rabbit model in which the lesion was a
burr hole in the tibia induced by a dentists drill. From such
studies it has been concluded that MDP is basically still the
reagent of choice with a high degree of accumulation in normal
bone, a high lesion to bone ratio and rapid blood clearance.
In evaluating these results however it should be borne in mind
that the lesion was regenerating bone following minor trauma.
In the human situation the main use of skeletal scintigraphy
is to detect metastases where there is active bone erosion and
where inflammatory reactions and tumour uptake play a role.

In human studies (17) it has been shown that there is
little difference between these reagents in their ability to
localise in metastases, the tumour to bone ratios being about
1.8 in all cases. This tends to show the fallacy of the use of
pseudopathological models and this should clearly be borne in
mind when designing such experiments.

4. TOXICITY AND SAFETY STUDIES.

The information obtained from the biodistribution studies
in normal animals and pathology models can be used to prepare
a protocol for human studies but there remains one important
aspect to be considered namely toxicity. Radiopharmaceuticals
are in general administered only once to the patient or, in
follow up studies, at the most four or five times over a
period of years. The amount of substance injected is usually
homeopathic in quantity and therefore the use of acute
toxicity testing is not appropriate for the labelled compound.
There is a strong case for special regulations to be applied

to radiopharmaceuticals rather than implementing the general requirements for drugs.

4.1 Radiation Dose

The most likely form of host damage is radiation damage. To minimize the incidence of this the clinically useful diagnostic dose, as calculated from the biodistribution data, has to be related to the radiation dose to the target organ. In this case the target organ is not necessarily the organ to be investigated but the organ which receives the highest radiation dose and in this context one should not forget the bladder and intestines. The variations which can occur are well illustrated by reconsidering the renal agents which we referred to earlier. Table 4 shows the radiation dose to the kidneys of these reagents. It can clearly be seen that whilst glucoheptonate gives the best tissue to background ratio its lower total concentration in the kidney compared with DMSA pays off as a favourable radiation dose.

Table 4. Radiation dose of technetium complexes to the kidney of human subjects.

Reagent	Dose Rad/mCi
DMSA	0.62
GLUCOHEPTONATE	0.17
DTPA	0.042

With reference to this topic the choice of label should not be forgotten when a number of nuclides can be used as label. Table 5 gives calculated values for dose rates, in humanoid phantoms, of several nuclides to illustrate this.

Table 5. Average total $\beta + \gamma$ absorbed dose rates from a concentration of 1 μCi/kg in a 70 kg elipsoid and a 1 kg sphere in mrad/hour.

Radionuclide	Dose (mrad/hr)	
	Elipsoid	Sphere
Gold-198	1.0	0.83
Mercury-197	0.23	0.19
Technetium-99m	0.13	0.07

The choice of nuclide should also be related to the clinical use especially in the case of therapeutic compounds. Gumpel (18) demonstrated that yttrium-9o with a maximum range of 11 mm and an effective range of 5 mm is useful for intra articular therapy of the knee but not for the much finer tissues of a finger joint for which Erbium 169 with a maximum range of 1 mm was more suited. It should also be borne in mind that radiation damage may occur away from the target organs. The leakage of intraarticular preparations such as those mentioned above may cause chromosome aberations in peripheral lymphocytes (19) and it has been suggested that low energy Auger electrons such as emmitted by Thallium-201 may cause more damage to the gonads than has been supposed. (20). Adequate evaluation of the potential of a radiopharmaceutical to cause genetic damage is clearly desirable.

4.2 Sensitisation testing

The second most likely form of side effect of radiopharmaceuticals is the development of an allergic response and this can be tested for by suitable animal tests involving repeat insults. A comprehensive registration of adverse reactions in humans is also important to identify such risks.

4.3 Acute and chronic toxicity testing

The use of the LD 50 and other toxicity tests is of little value in testing radiopharmaceuticals as indeed are chronic toxicity studies particularly since it is virtually impossible to obtain the radiopharmaceutical in a concentrated form. Indeed when this can be done it is doubtful whether the concentrated form will have the same chemical form as the diagnostic complex. Useful studies however are tests for mutagenecity such as the Ames test.

REFERENCES
1. Subramanian G et al. The influence of structural changes on biodistribution of Tc-99m N-substituted Ida derivatives. In: Nuklearmedizin Proceedings 15th Congress Society of Nuclear Medicine (Europe). Ed: Schmidt HAE, and Woldring MG, Groningen.1977
2. Kung HF, Blau M. Synthesis of Se-75 labelled tertiary diamines - New Brain imaging agents. J Med Chem 1980; 23: 1127-1130.

3. Kung HF, Blau M. Regional intracellular pH shift. A proposed new mechanism for radiopharmaceutical uptake in brain and other tissues. J Nucl Med 1980; 21: 147-152.
4. Charkes ND, Philips CM. A new model of F-18 Fluoride Kinetics in Humans: Simulation by analoque computer.IN: Medical Radionuclide Imaging Vol II I.A.E.A. Vienna 1977: 137-144.
5. Larson SM et al., The transferrin Receptor Hypothesis: Mechanism of Tumor uptake of Carrier Free Gallium-67. In: Frontiers in Nuclear Medicine Ed: Horst W, Wagner HN and Buchanan JW, Springer Verlag, Berlin 1980: 134-153.
6. Fernandez - Pol JA. Molecular Basis of the Regulation of Iron-59 and Gallium-67 Transport in normal and Simian Virus 40 transformed cells In: Frontiers in Nuclear Medicine Ed: Horst W, Wagner HN and Buchanan JW, Springer Verlag, Berlin 1980: 162-182.
7. Muranaka A. Accumulation of Radioisotopes with tumour affinity. Acta Med Okayama 1978;32: 407-417.
8. Cox PH, Tc-99m complexes for skeletal scintigraphy Physico-chemical Factors affecting bone and bone marrow uptake, Brit J Radiol 1974;47: 845-850.
9. Cox PH, Technetium Complexes for renal scintigraphy In: Progres in Radiopharmacology 3 Ed Cox PH, Martin Nijhoff The Hague 1982: 31-44.
10. Reinhold HS, Van de Berg, Blox A. Physiology of Tumours-Vascularity and Microcirculation In: Progres in Radio-pharmacology I. Ed: Cox PH, Elsevier North Holland Amsterdam 1979: 13-22.
11. Van der Pompe WB, An ionic model to explain the distribution of metal chelates in normal and pathological tissues In: Progress in Radiopharmacology I. Ed:Cox PH, Elsevier North Holland. Amsterdam 1979: 31-44.
12. Hill JH, Wagner HN. Gallium uptake in regenerating rat liver J Nucl Med 1974;15: 818-820.
13. Hammersley PAG et al. Uptake of Ga in the regenerating rat liver and its relationship to lysosomal activity. Cancer Res 1975;35: 1154-1158.
14. Orü H. Tumor scanning with Gallium and its mechanism studied in rats. Strahlentherapie 1972;144:192-200.
15. Cox PH, Van der Pompe WB. An ionic model to explain the distribution patterns of tumour seeking radiopharma-ceuticals in normal and pathological tissues Proceedings XIII Int Meeting Society of Nuclear Medicine -Copenhagen 1975: 1461-1467.
16. Subramanian G, McAffee TG. New Developments in Radiopharma-ceuticals for Imaging. In Medical Radionuclide Imaging Vol I I.A.E.A. Vienna 1981: 429-452.
17. Cox PH, The Pharmacological Behavior of Technetium in Bone. In: Progress in Radiopharmacology I. Ed: Cox PH Elsevier North Holland Amsterdam 1979: 109-127.
18. Gumpel JM. The role of Radiocolloids in the treatment of Arthritis Rheumatology and Rehabilitation 1974; XIII:1-9.
19. LLoyd DC, Reeder ET. Chromosome aberrations and intraarticular Yttrium-90. Lancet 1978, I: 617.
20. Dandanundi VR et al. Radiotoxicity of Thallium-201 in Mouse Testis. J Nucl Med 1983; 24: 145-153.

8.   ANIMAL MODELS FOR EFFICACY STUDIES - A PRACTICAL
     APPROACH

GERHARD KLOSS

1. INTRODUCTION

Animal tests to determine the suitability of drugs for diagnostic or therapeutic use in humans can be broken down into toxicological and pharmacological studies.

The toxicological investigations include acute, sub-acute (14-days) and chronic toxicity (which runs for up to 2 years) tests and in addition embryo toxicity tests, fertility studies and carcinogenicity studies.

The pharmacological studies encompass the pharmacokinetics, that is uptake in the body, distribution and excretion as well as the biotransformatory processes, the metabolism, that take place during these operations.

In addition there are the most important parameters for the physician and the patient: the functional suitability, that is with therapeutic agents the pharmacodynamics and with diagnostic agents the diagnostic efficacy.

The basic scheme outlined here for the testing of drugs by means of animal studies has now become regarded worldwide as the standard for this aspect of drug safety, but in its comprehensive form it is only used for the therapeutic agents which in practice are always applied over long periods of time.

With diagnostic agents, which as a rule are only used once or only at relatively long intervals, the method can be simplified somewhat. Thus, for instance, the test for chronic toxicity is usually unnecessary.

With radiodiagnostic agents there is the additional factor that one is dealing not only with single administrations but also in most cases with very small amounts of substance, as the chemical compound should not have any pharmacodynamic effect of its own but takes part in physiological or biochemical processes solely as a tracer without affecting them. It must be borne in mind, however, with the final galenical formulation that additives can sometimes have a pharmacodynamic effect. For instance benzylalcohol added as preservative has a vasodilatory effect that must be taken into account during subcutaneous or intramuscular application.

The toxicological effects of radiodiagnostic agents are, unlike conventional drugs, linked to two different basic principles. On the one hand to the chemical toxicity of the compound used but on the other also to the radiotoxicity of the radionuclide used for labelling. Thus with radiopharmaceuticals pharmacokinetics are of central importance both for the determination of functional suitability, which in this case is determined by the pharmacokinetics rather than the pharmacodynamics, as well as for the assessment of the radiation burden.

In the following a basic scheme for pharmacokinetic animal trials will be outlined followed by a discussion of some specific examples.

2. PHARMACOKINETIC TECHNIQUES

First it is important to mention which species of animal are to be regarded as representative for comparison with humans. However, these considerations also include to a large extent questions of economy and trial technique, as well as in some countries also the animal protection legislation and public pressure on the use of animals for experimental work. On the other hand, as in the testing of human albumin, it may of course be that the distribution of human protein in the animal does not need at all to follow its behaviour in humans.

In our laboratories we have selected the rat as the basic animal for distribution studies. Mice seem to us less suitable because of their small size. Other types of animals are too large and, in view of the large number of animal trials that are necessary for statistical reasons, also too expensive. With rats it must be borne in mind, however, that they are less suitable for investigations of the biliary system because they do not have a gall bladder and therefore the kinetics of this system are not directly comparable with those of humans.

The selection of the organs and tissues to be tested during the trial phase is limited at first sight. In addition to the functional target organs the concentration in the major metabolic and excretory organs are of prime importance. With these preliminary trials the amounts and volumes and their galenical constitution are optimized and initial information on stability is obtained. As regards the amounts of substance applied there is in some cases a distribution pattern independent of the dose given, over a range of several factors of ten. With other substances however, there is a marked dependence of the dose given. We have for instance observed this marked dependence with phosphates. As the dose is increased above a critical value there is an increasing and finally very great accumulation in the liver.

The number of animals in the distribution trials is, for statistical reasons, set at six per group, three males, and three females, as the organ concentrations occasionally vary according to the sex of the animal. We have observed this phenomenon for instance with some substances taken up by the kidney, for which females sometimes demonstrate slightly lower concentrations than males.

The test times to be selected depend both on the biological half-life of the compound and on the physical half-life of the labelling nuclide. Thus with technetium-99m compounds it is often unnecessary and, in view of the short half-life, also difficult to investigate the distribution and excretion for longer than 24 hours.

On the other hand it may be advisable to measure the elimination of the substance from the blood or its urinary excretion at very short intervals. Rats are less suitable for this since frequent blood sampling and unavoidable subsequent bleeding leads to a change in the volume of circulating blood which can, at later stages in the study, affect the blood concentrations. We therefore determine the blood elimination curves in dogs. This investigation is usually combined with a

urine collection by means of a catheter and with sequential
scintigraphy of the target organ.

Our investigation technique takes the following form: the
radioactivity contained in a disposable syringe in a volume of
between 0.05 and 0.5 ml is measured in defined geometry. The
preparation is then injected into the exposed thigh vein of a
rat under light ether anaesthesia. The rat is allowed to
recover consciousness and is killed at a predetermined time.
Killing is carried out, by decapitation, under renewed ether
anaesthesia, and the whole blood and serum needed for the
investigation are collected. In the meantime the syringe is
remeasured in identical geometry and, correcting for
radioactive decay, the exact amount of radioactivity injected
is determined. By giving the injection, with visual
monitoring, into the thigh vein rather than the tail it is
possible to ascertain that intravenous administration is
achieved. With injections into the tail veins it is advisable,
after the animal is killed, to remove the tail and determine
whether there are any paravenous deposits of activity. The
amounts of substance applied in our procedure are not directly
related to the bodyweight. We generally use rats of about 200g
which do not vary within the group by more than $\pm$ 10%.
Standardization to a mean bodyweight of 200g is performed
mathematically using the factor by which the actual bodyweight
varies from 200g to correct for each individual organ in order
to arrive at the organ concentrations calculated per g tissue.
This procedure was selected because the use of a dose adjusted
exactly to the bodyweight seems less precise because of the
difficulty of applying these varying volumes exactly.

The measurement of activity in the organs is carried out in
a gamma sample changer where the conversion factor between the
measurement of radioactivity in the syringe and in the organ
in question is found by comparative measurements. Organs with
high activity, such as the liver, lungs or kidneys, are
measured either in the gamma sample changer after a relatively
long period of decay or they are measured in the same geometry
as the syringe. With the rest of the body this is generally
the case although geometric problems can arise. Homogenization

of the tissue can usually be omitted unless, because of the low gamma energy of the labelling nuclide, as with iodine-125, there is a risk of counting losses due to self-absorption.

Recovery of radioactivity in the experiments in relation to the activity applied are calculated by the addition of all the organs measured as well as the amounts excreted and the cage rinsings. Due to some losses of blood or urine 100% recovery is not often attained although for statistical reasons and because of geometric inaccuracies in whole body measurement, the values can occasionally amount to just over 100%. Calculating the recovery by the method of equating the sum of all the samples measured to 100% and then calculating the content of the individual samples proportionally, seems incorrect as it conceals losses of different types. Tissues are measured untreated. In other words reference is not made to the dry mass and no account is taken of the amount of blood in the organ. This can in fact be established quite easily from the available data but is not appropriate for the calculation of the radiation burden. Moreover data on the blood content of organs obtained from the literature might not apply in special cases. The method of removing the blood from the organs by perfusion with physiological solutions has generally been abandoned because uncontrollable amounts of tissue activity are washed out with the perfusate.

3. BONE-SEEKING RADIOPHARMACEUTICALS

In investigations with bone-seeking substances it has been seen how misleading data in the literature can be with regard to the weights of tissue as a percentage of bodyweight. According to the literature, the skeleton forms 10 to 11% of the bodyweight. Using this figure to calculate the amount of technetium pyrophosphate in the skeletal system one arrives at almost 60% of the applied dose. With investigations of MDP up to 80% is obtained and with DPD sometimes even over 100%. However, residual body measurements show only between 35 and 45% activity, although the body of course contains the whole skeleton. In addition, urine excreted in the meantime often contains more than 50% activity so that the values calculated

simply do not fit together. In a study totally skeletonizing
five female and five male 200g rats we found, to our surprise,
that the bone accounted for only a little over 5% bodyweight
in males and slightly less than 6% in females. When these
values are used for the calculation the relationships tally
again and the higher skeletal accumulations described in
earlier publications are not found.(1).

The majority of distribution trials depicted hitherto give
no information as to whether the intact radiopharmaceutical is
measured. In recent years, with the technetium-labelled
compounds in particular, contradictory hypothesis or even
contradictory trial findings have often resulted. These
results are partly due to difficulties in the chemical
analysis of biological materials. Whereas it is still
relatively simple with particle or colloidal preparations to
draw conclusions from the presence of activity in the urine or
the thyroid gland, for instance as to the extent of
decomposition of the preparation, this can be considerably
more difficult with some complex compounds.

Thus it is not always easy to determine whether the intact
technetium chelate complex is accumulated in the target organ
or whether cleavage and deposition of the technetium alone
takes place. Whether the tin which is effective as a reducing
agent is a constituent of the complex is still arguable with
some compounds. Here the results of animal trials can help to
clarify the behaviour of the substances. The question of
whether only the total complex or its unlabelled carrier
substance accumulates in the target organ can be answered by
labelling the various components separately. Thus in the
studies to investigate the biological behaviour of DPD the
distribution pattern obtained with the technetium-labelled
preparation was compared with the distribution of
technetium-and tin-free DPD which was labelled with C-14. No
differences in accumulation in bone over the 24-hour
observation period were detected. Slight differences were
observed in the blood, liver and kidney concentrations which
may be due to the varying modes of excretion of the breakdown
products (Table 1). It was therefore possible to prove that

the intact technetium DPD complex is accumulated in bone.

Table 1. Comparison of Tc-99m DPD and C-14 DPD in rats (% of
        appl. dose; 50 µg/kg)

	45' p.i.		2h p.i.		6h p.i.		24h p.i.	
	Tc-99m	C-14	Tc-99m	C-14	Tc-99m	C-14	Tc-99m	C-14
Skeleton (5% of body weight)	39,8	35,0	42,9	38,5	45,4	42,4	44,5	44,8
Musculature (40% of body weight)	1,6	0,62	0,4	0,6	0,32	0,44	0,24	0,31
Blood (5% of body weight)	1,0	0,54	0,18	0,078?	0,08	0,3	0,04	0,44
Liver	0,33	0,43	0,2	0,34	0,19	0,38	0,19	0,29
Kidneys	0,8	0,56	0,77	0,8	0,57	0,3	0,56	0,22

The extent to which the radioactive material in the urine
retains bone-seeking properties was investigated in another
series of trials. Tc-99m-DPD was injected into rats and the
urine collected for one-and-a-half hours afterwards. Two hours
after the injection these rats were killed and their organ
activity investigated. The urine collected was intravenously
injected into another group of rats, and the 2-hour
distribution measured in these animals. It was found that in
the second group bone storage was only reduced by about
one-tenth compared with the first group, confirming that the
complex excreted in the urine was not broken down. There is
surely no need to stress that in these trials the various
groups of substances all behave in different ways.

4. IDA - RADIOPHARMACEUTICALS

Studies of IDA derivatives carried out by Callery et al (2) have shown that the technetium-IDA complex is in fact concentrated in the bile, but that the corresponding C-14 compound demonotrated completely different behaviour and was excreted via the urine (Table 2).

Table 2. Different Organ-Distribution of an IDA-Derivative labelled with Tc-99m or C-14, respectively after Callery et al. (2)

Mice (%/Organ)	5 min. p.i.		30 min. p.i.		60 min. p.i.	
	Tc-99m	C-14	Tc-99m	C-14	Tc-99m	C-14
Liver	28,2	5,7	10,2	1,3	8,0	0,4
Intestine	38,3	3,8	60,2	1,8	68,3	1,4
Blood	3,3	7,9	1,1	0,5	0,8	0,2
Kidney	1,8	7,5	0,6	1,0	0,8	1,7
Urine		31,9		74,2		74,0

With a number of Tc-99m-labelled IDA derivatives we have studied the metabolic breakdown by injecting, as in the DPD investigations, the urine of rats, which received Tc-99m-IDA by injection, into a second group of rats, or by injecting the bile of the original group into a third group, respectively. By comparing the organ distributions it was possible to show that a more or less marked biotransformation of the complex took place, depending on the chemical constitution (3).

5. TUMOR-SEEKING RADIOPHARMACEUTICALS

A special problem arises when investigating substances used in the visualization of tumors. In this case it is not the images which show the tumor as a negative contrast within an organ, but rather the direct picture of the tumor trapping radioactivity which is of interest. This has been possible for many years as repeatedly shown with experimental animal tumors of which only the Yoshida-Sarcom, the Jensen-Sarcom and the Walker-Carcino-Sarcom of the rat as well as the Ehrlich-Carcinom of the mouse shall be mentioned.(4). Such animal tumors can very often however not be compared with conditions in man. Therefore experimental results with animals cannot be reproduced in man at all or only to a certain extent.

Progress in this respect was made however during the last few years by using nude mice. Nude mice characterize themselves by the fact that they possess no thymus gland and hence no immune resistance (5). Thus human tumors can be transplanted to these animals without a rejection taking place. Recently use was made of these models especially in the investigation of radioactive labelled tumor-specific antibodies. Apart from the difficulties which one faces when working with such small animals the necessity exist to keep these mice in aseptic surrounding to spare them from any infections they might catch (6,7).

6. ANIMAL STUDIES IN QUALITY CONTROL

The trials described hitherto form part of those which can be carried out during the development phase of a radiopharmaceutical to prove its suitability. Of course for the practical collection of evidence, additional trials should be carried out in an identical manner as intended in man. These investigations, which often involve sequential or functional scintigraphy or the determination of organ, blood or urinary excretion is most often carried out in dogs. Sometimes trials with rabbits are advisable such as for instance with IDA derivatives.

As you will have noticed, however, all these animal trials have been described with regard to the new development of a drug, in other words, I have stated how to obtain scientific information which should be available before a radiopharmaceutical is to be used in man. I am not, however, of the opinion that all these studies must be carried out as a basic principle for official approval. I feel that for this the parameters that serve to improve the safety of the patient such as toxicology, radiation burden and functional suitability should be adequate. There are however requirements which, after obtaining official approval for a radiopharmaceutical, must be met by every individual batch. And these requirements are stated in the relevant pharmacopoeias, examples of which may be the European Pharmacopoeia (Ph.Eur.) and the Pharmacopoeia of the United States of America (USP).

For radiopharmaceuticals it has been found that the properties cannot definitely be guaranteed in all cases by chemical, radiochemical or physical test methods, so that with some preparations it is advisable to carry out simple animal trials to confirm their properties. This is especially so with particle and colloidal preparations.

REFERENCES
1. Schwarz A, Kloss G. Beziehungen zwischen chemischer Struktur und Skelettfixierung verschiedener Tc-99m-Phosphonsäuren. In "Nuklearmedizin im interdisziplinären Bezug". Proceed. of the 18th Internat. Annual Meeting of the Soc. of Nucl. Med. -Europe-, Nürnberg, Sept. 1980. Stuttgart, F.K. Schattauer-Verlag, 1981: 120-24.
2. Callery PS, et al. Tissue distribution of technetium-99m and carbon-14 labelled N-(2,6-Dimethylphenylcarbamoylmethyl) iminodiacetic acid J Med Chem 1976; 19: 962-64.
3. Molter M, Kloss G. Neue TC-99m-IDA-Derivate für eine angepasste Leberfunktionsdiagnostik. In "Nuklearmedizin im interdisziplinären Bezug". Proceed. of the 18th Internat. Annual Meeting of the Soc of Nucl. Med.-Europe-, Nürnberg, Sept. 1980. Stuttgart F.K. Schattauer-Verlag 1981: 116-19.
4. Wiebe LI. Small animal tumor models for screening diagnostic radiotracers. In Eckelmann WC, Lambrecht RM eds. (Inpress). Animal Models in Radiotracer Design. New York Springer Verlag 1983.
5. Rygaard J, Povlsen CO. Heterotransplantation of a human malignant Tumour to "Nude" mice. Acta Pathol Microbiol Scand 1969;77: 758-60.
6. Pressman D. et al. The use of paired labelling in the determination of tumorlocalizing antibodies. Canc Res 1957; 17: 845-50.
7. Kloss G, Leven M. Accumulation of radioiodinated tyrosine derivatives in the adrenal medulla and in melanomas. Eur J Nucl Med 1979; 4: 179-86.

9. HUMAN PHARMACOLOGY - PHARMACOKINETICS
YVES COHEN

1. INTRODUCTION

Human Pharmacology and Pharmacokinetics are conducted in services of Nuclear Medicine when new radiopharmaceuticals have passed the experimental step in vitro and on animals. From the results on animals, physicians try to extrapolate to humans, healthy volunteers and patients. They compare the new radiopharmaceuticals to well-known tracers and, in some way, to other diagnostic or therapeutic methods, for instance, new brain radiopharmaceuticals, to pertechnetate, x-ray scanner and nuclear magnetic resonance imaging. The aim of the human assay is to establish the performance of the new radioactive drug, to specify the pathological indications, to delineate the limits of use, to ascertain the reproducibility of the results in different hands, to detect any side-effects and to give data for the calculation of radiation doses. The human assay needs an approval from committees for ethics and safety. Seen from the radiopharmaceuticals producer point of view, human pharmacology and pharmacokinetics of these tracers are a crucial test upon which the future of the drug will depend. Performed in hospitals, independently from the producer research department, the assays of human pharmacology and pharmacokinetics correspond to phases I and II as largely accepted nowadays. In this paper we shall discuss the organization of the assays, we shall explain the main parameters of pharmacokinetics and we shall review the literature of the most important radiopharmaceuticals. We shall also discuss the future of these assays in view of the advancement of new methods.

2. ORGANIZATION OF HUMAN PHARMACOLOGY AND PHARMACOKINETIC ASSAYS

The new radiopharmaceutical is handed to physicians after clinical procedures are established in common agreement between the producer, the committees of ethics and safety and the clinicians. The very first assays of phase I are designed to estimate the radioactive dose to be injected in order to obtain good diagnostic results (images or decrease curves, etc) of the target organs without a too heavy radioactive background. A relationship between doses and images is calculated in different conditions on healthy subjects and on patients. Tolerance to the radiochemical is appreciated in terms of modifications in cardiovascular output, headache, hyperthermia, lung constriction, pain at the site of injection. Indeed, with radiopharmaceuticals, the diagnostic dose has a double component: the radioactive dose (Becquerels or Curies) and the weight (milligrams) of a chemical vector for the radionuclide. In other terms, at phase I the correct specific activity (Becquerels versus milligrams) is adjusted.

At phase II, half-lives are calculated, on healthy volunteers and patients, for the target organ, the blood, the sites of uptake. Excretion rates and clearances are measured. Phase II is largely the pharmacokinetic step of the assay. From the results, mathematical models are conceived, which help to understand the behavior of the radiopharmaceutical in the body. At that stage, metabolic work is performed in order to know whether the radiopharmaceutical is split in two, the radionuclide on one hand, the chemical on the other hand. At that stage, also, first pass effects are appreciated: some organs with-hold the tracer on its way through the blood stream. An intravenous bolus passes the right heart cavities, the lungs, the left heart cavities and, then, the coronaries and the main systemic arteries. Either the myocardium or the pulmonary tissue may retain a significant part of the radiopharmaceutical. At phase II the target organ, known from the preclinical assays on animals or in vitro, is confirmed. Optimal length of time between injection and imaging is looked for. Phase II is reduced to a significant but small number of patients, well chosen regarding their disease and the demonstration of usefulness of the radiodiagnostic.

After phase II, the aim of phase III is to extend to several diagnostic centers the procedure of the clinical assays, to search for other potential applications. At that phase, the radiopharmaceutical has been tested by several groups; the number of patients and the different diagnosis have given enough informations to decide its commercial distribution.

Phase IV brings informations on extensive use, side effects, new diagnostic possibilities and limitations.

During the planning of procedures of phases I and II several decisions are taken on the number of assays and patients, the dose to be injected, the route of injection, the duration of the whole experimentation. Decisions depend upon the character of the radiopharmaceutical. Nowadays new radiopharmaceuticals come from development of radionuclides produced in a cyclotron (positron emitters) or from development of kits easier to us: combining a radionuclide from a generator and a reagent ready to use, mainly on a single step reaction. Recently, new biological radiopharmaceuticals have been proposed: labelled leukocytes, platelets, fibrinogen. Their pharmacokinetics are fundamentally different from other radiopharmaceuticals as they depend mainly on the state of hematological parameters. The use of radioactive liposomes and of radioactive antitumoral antibodies (monoclonal antibodies) brings specific hindrance and asks to overcome the liver first pass effect.

3. PHARMACOKINETIC PARAMETERS

Among several pharmacokinetic parameters we shall select a few which will have an important impact for the understanding of radiopharmaceutical distribution. First, routes of administration are essential to analyze. Second, radiopharmaceutical affinity is the fundament of nuclear medicine. Third, volume of distribution is necessary to understand the limits of the tracer. Fourth, biological half-life is one of the most important parameters. Fifth, it is associated with excretion and clearance. Sixth, area under the curve seems to become a synthetical parameter melting volume of distribution, half-life and clearance. The final point will be the radiopharmaceutical metabolites. All those parameters are useful to calculate the radiation absorbed dose (1).

3.1. Routes of administration of radiopharmaceuticals

Several routes are used for administrating radiopharmaceuticals.Radioactive gases and aerosols are given through the upper airways of the respiratory tract while breathing. The distribution of the radioactive tracers will depend on this peculiarity. Oral administration is preferred for iodide and pertechnetate either in aqueous solution or in capsules. Tracers used to evaluate the function of the digestive tract follow the same route: vitamine B 12, fatty acids or labelled oils. Parenteral injections are made according to the diagnosis: intrathecal, intraarachidian, to look for leakage of the cerebrospinal fluid system; endoserosal injection is proposed for synovia and pleura; subcutaneous injection in a region which is drained by lymphatic vessels is frequent for lymphography; intraarterial injection is chosen for labelled liposomes directed to tumors; finally, the most used administration is intravenous.

3.2. Affinity of the radiopharmaceutical

The labelled drug is designed to show a high ratio in the specific organ versus the rest of the organism. The best known affinity is iodine for thyroid gland, colloids for the reticuloendothelial system in liver, spleen and bone marrow. Nowadays we look for a high specificity of the radioligand to its receptor: acetanilide derivatives for the hepatocyte (IDA derivatives), quinuclidyl derivatives for muscarinic receptors, beta-blockers for adrenergic beta receptors, monoclonal antibodies for tumor marking.

3.3. Volume of distribution

Volume of distribution of a radiopharmaceutical depends on its route of administration, the volume being the lungs volume for aerosol, the cerebrospinal fluid volume for the tracer administered intrathecally, the blood volume for certain plasma proteins such as transferrin.

Volume of distribution is qualified of "apparent volume of distribution" when calculated from the equation:

$$V_d = \frac{Q}{C_0}$$

where V_d = the apparent volume of distribution;

Q = the quantity of radiotracer injected;

C_0 = the concentration of the radiotracer in the considered biological fluid extrapolated at time 0.

In this case, the volume of distribution equals cerebrospinal fluid for labelled serum albumin, injected intrathecally; it equals blood volume, corrected of blood cells volume, for labelled serum albumin, injected intravenously, and for labelled transferrin administered by the same route. Apparent volume of distribution is dependent on affinity when the radioligand is concentrated in some organs. The apparent volume of distribution overpasses blood volume and often body volume. This is the case for labelled derivates of chloroquine which concentrate in melanomas.

3.4. Biological half-life

Biological half-life is important in nuclear medicine as it serves to calculate effective half-life which, in turn, is used in the calculation of the radiation absorbed dose. The biological half-life concerns the whole body, it corresponds to the total excretion; it concerns blood and is, in this case, the sum of different exchanges between blood and organs; it also concerns such organ where the radioligand is concentrated and increases the absorbed radiation dose.

The relation between physical, biological and effective half-life is given below:

$$T\ 1/2\ eff = \frac{T\ 1/2\ phys \times T\ 1/2\ biol}{T\ 1/2\ phys + T\ 1/2\ biol}$$

3.5. Excretion and clearance

The radionuclide is finally excreted, with breathing, for gases, through feces, for some compounds excreted with bile, and through urine for most of radiopharmaceuticals. Excretion is calculated easily by renal clearance of blood:

$$C = U \times V \times \frac{1}{B}$$

where C = clearance, in volume of blood per unit time;

U = urinary concentration of the radiopharmaceutical;

V = volume of urine per unit time;

B = blood concentration of the radiopharmaceutical.

Clearance is also calculated through another way:

$$C = V_D \times k_e$$

where C = clearance;

V_d = apparent volume of distribution;

k_e = excretion constant.

This latter formula may serve for the whole body or for an individual organ.

3.6. Area under the curve

When establishing a curve of concentration of the radiopharmaceutical in blood versus time, this curve has several shapes. When the tracer is given orally, the curve of concentration in blood increases, present a more or less long plateau, then decreases. When given intravenously the curve of concentration in blood shows a decrease. The area under the curve represents the total quantity of the radiopharmaceutical in blood, from time zero to infinite time. Area under the curve serves to compare radiopharmaceuticals of different origin. It depends on volume of distribution, excretion rate, and for radiopharmaceuticals not directly injected in blood, on the rate of absorption and first pass effect (2).

3.7. Radiopharmaceutical metabolites

Radiopharmaceuticals are metabolized in the organism. The radionuclide is split from the labelled molecule. This fact is very current with iodinated radiopharmaceuticals (iodine-131, 125, 123). Technetium coordinates are separated in the body. This fact leads to the difficulty of assuming the chemical identify of the radiotracer which is scanned during diagnosis. The free radionuclide may contract new bonds (with plasma proteins for example) or may be excreted in a different way from the radiopharmaceutical still labelled. On the same sample of biological fluid, one can separate the labelled radiopharmaceutical, the labelled metabolites, the free radionuclide, the radionuclide bound to biological proteins, the unlabelled radiopharmaceutical and the unlabelled metabolites of the radiopharmaceutical.

4. REVIEW OF LITERATURE

The review of literature shows rather few studies on pharmacology per se and on pharmacokinetics. By no means the reports are systematically oriented toward the establishment of clear cut parameters as defined above. We shall classify radiopharmaceuticals according to the target organ under diagnosis and review papers from 1979 to 1982. Before 1979, see Cohen and Besnard(1).

4.1. Brain

Winchell and his colleagues (3,4) have proposed iodoamphetamine I-123 for measuring local cerebral blood flow. This radiopharmaceutical has attracted great interest and several groups are studying it (5, 6). Kuhl et al. (7) showed, in human subjects, after an intravenous injection, a rapid uptake in brain and lungs and a slower uptake in liver. An early washout in lungs has a half-life of about 13 minutes. At 3 hours after injection, the administered dose was distributed among brain 5%, lung 33%, liver 33%, and remainder of the body 29%. A general half-life from all sites was estimated of 66 hours. An important first pass effect is observed in the lungs before the deposition in the brain. The use of glucose by the brain has lead to the development of new radiopharmaceuticals such as F-18 fluoro-2-deoxy-D-glucose in man, adapted from previous work on animals. Deoxyglucose competes with glucose for the membrane transport sites at the capillaries and cell membranes and for hexokinase in its phosphorylation (8). Free fluorodeoxyglucose has a turn-over rate in human cortex of

4.25 $\pm$ 1.8 minutes, while the half time for uptake is 8 minutes in brain (9).

4.2. Heart

A considerable amount of work is devoted to the search for heart radiopharmaceuticals. Among those proposed are indicators of metabolism, such as deoxyglucose, fatty acids, and indicators of blood flow such as analogs of potassium, radioligands of cholinergic and adrenergic receptors such as quinuclidyl benzilate derivatives and iodobenzoyl beta-blockers (10-13). A few of them have passed the animal experimentation stage and have been tried on patients (Syrota et al., (14) for methyl quinuclidyl benzilate labelled with carbon-11).

Real pharmacokinetic work is scarce; Schelbert el al. (15) have used fluorodeoxyglucose intravenously. Regional myocardial glucose utilization rates are derived from selected regions of left ventricular myocardium. According to the authors, the rate constants in myocardium are of similar magnitude as those in the brain. Free fatty acids are extracted from the blood stream by myocardial cells. The exact significance of this fact is not yet fully elucidated. Terminally radioiodinated fatty acids have been prepared with iodine-131, iodine-125, iodine-123. A great interest is seen in the iodine-123 labelled radiopharmaceuticals (16). The initial uptake and distribution in heart parallel those of potassium, but the turn-over rates depend on the healthy regions versus the infarcted ones: about 25 minutes versus 17 minutes (17).

The use of analogs of potassium and their distribution in the heart tissue are of different significance. The initial distribution of radioactivity is proportional to regional blood flow, while the delayed distribution reflects the viability of myocardium (18). Several radionuclides have been tested: N-13-NH$_4^+$, K-43, Rb-81, Cs-129 and Tl-201. Table 1, from Chervu (19), compares blood clearance and myocardial clearance of these radiotracers.

Table 1 - (data from Chervu (19).

Radionuclides	Blood clearance T 1/2 (minutes)	Myocardial clearance T 1/2 (hours)
N-13- NH_4^+	1.0	1.2
K-43	2.0	1.0
Rb-81	2.2	6.0
Cs-129	9.0	5.0
Tl-201	2.9	4.4

On patients with congestive heart failure or cardiogenic and non cardiogenic shock, thallium-201 activity will clear from blood at a slower rate (20). Dipyridamole, a coronary vasodilator, modifies myocardial clearances of thallium-201 (21, 22). That helps prognostics for the assessment of cardiac performance.

4.3. Lung

Regional ventilatory clearance using radioactive gases or radioactive aerosols has given rise to important pharmacokinetic work based on Steward-Hamilton equation already used for 30 years (23). A model has been proposed on patients, with a washin dynamics corresponding to influx of the radioactive gas, a washout dynamics corresponding to the efflux. Passage of the gas into blood circulation is neglected. At equilibrium, which separates washin phase to washout phase, the concentration of radioactive gas is constant in the lungs (figure 1). In chronic obstructive airway disease, area under the washout curve is modified (figure 2; Alderson and Line (24)). The ratio of the height of washin curve at equilibrium to the area under the whole washout curve gives the fractional exchange per unit time.

In the previous example, lungs were estimated as a one compartment model. However Atkins et al. (25); gave a five compartment model for the calculations of radiation absorbed doses from radio Xenons in lung imaging. Instead of radioactive gas, radioaerosol is used. It is made of 5 micron polystyrene particles labelled with Tc-99m. No leakage of Tc-99m is observed from the particles. The radioaerosol is compared to krypton-81m (26).

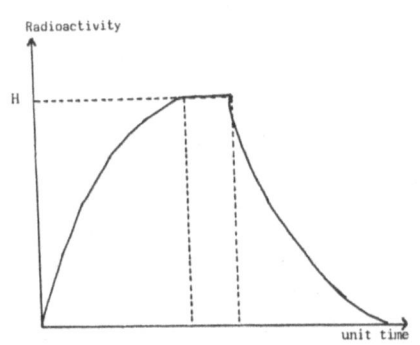

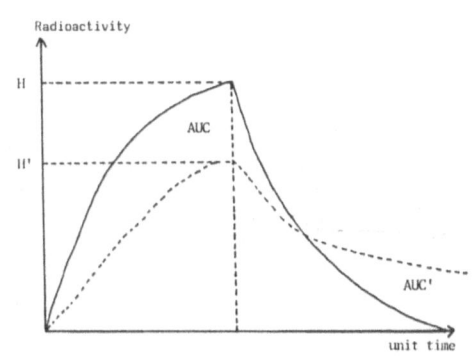

Figure 1
Washin-washout curves of
radioactive gas in lung (24)
H=height at equilibrium.

Figure 2
Modification of the curve (24)
The ratio H/AUC gives the
fractional exchange in normal.
The ratio H`/AUC` gives the
fractional exchange in patient
with obstructive airway disease

4.4. Skeleton
Kinetics of bone seeking tracers have been thoroughly
studied. A five compartment model was proposed by Charkes et
al., back in 1978, for fluoride F-18 (27) and again in 1981,
for methylene diphosphonate labelled with technetium-99m (28).

Figure 3 - Five compartment model for bone seeking
radiopharmaceuticals (Charkes and Makler (28)).

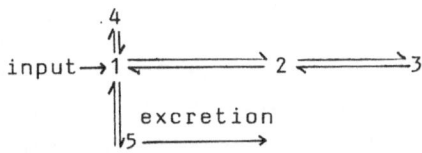

1. blood compartment;
2. bone extracellular fluid compartment;
3. bone compartment;
4. none bone extracellular fluid compartment;
5. tubular urine compartment.

This model takes into account tubular excretion by kidney, distribution in extracellular fluid in and out of the bone. It corresponds to the present concept of skeletal uptake of bone seeking tracers, particularly, diphosphonates (29). Factors involved in skeletal uptake of radiopharmaceuticals are vascularity of the bone, skeletal metabolism, enzymes systems and immature collagen. However, the model of Charkes in figure 3, may be of a good help when comparing different diphosphonates.

Fogelman et al. (30) moved away from these theoritical concepts, and preferred a synthetic approach. They proposed a 24 hours whole body retention technique and used it to compare hydroxymethylene diphosphonate, methylene diphosphonate and hydroxyethylene diphosphonate (table 2).

Table 2 - Whole body retention of diphosphonates in normal volunteers (Fogelman et al. (30)).

	Mean		Lower value	Higher value
Hydroxymethylene diphosphonate	36.5 ±	5.0	25.07	44.23
Methylene diphosphonate	30.3 ±	4.1	23.22	36.40
Hydroxyethylene diphosphonate	18.4 ±	2.9	12.89	22.45

24 hours whole body retention figures are given as a percentage of the 5 minutes after injection counts corrected for the radiactive decay.

It is the first time that, so evidently, a human biological parameter is used to compare the performances of a series of closely related radiopharmaceuticals. The calculated parameters, once established to estimate the activity of osteous cells in normal and in patients, may serve as a tool for clinical pharmacology and pharmacokinetics.

4.5. Kidney

Kidney has been the subject of numerous kinetic works. However pharmacokinetics, per se, is rarely approached. In fact, the problem is complex: several parameters may be studied using different radiopharmaceuticals as shown by Chervu and Blaufox (31). Table 3 summarizes the various use of radiopharmaceuticals to study the kidney functions. A series

of equations relate clearance to renal plasma flow. With
Indium 111-diethylene triamine penta acetic acid (In-111 DTPA)
Ross et al. (32) have calculated the renal clearance (91.1 ±
36.5 ml/min) compared to renal clearance of creatinine (86.0 ±
32.8 ml/min). Houston et al. (33) investigated a simple method
of measuring urinary clearance of In-113m DTPA and
TC-99m-(SN)-DTPA. Although the model cannot be considered as
verified, the results show no difference between the two
radiopharmaceuticals for effective renal clearance from
plasma. A three compartment model is proposed as for
iodohippurate labelled with iodine-131 by Tauxe et al. (34).
These latter authors found an effective renal plasma flow of
318 ± 115 ml/min. They established that in the three
compartment model, one, considered the third, is clearly the
kidneys and post renal pathways, the first must comprise the
plasma volume but the apparent volume of distribution in this
compartment is twice its theoritical size. Regarding
compartment two, it should be extracellular fluid but its
apparent volume of distribution is considerably smaller.

Table 3 - Radiopharmaceuticals for kidney functions

Renal blood flow	Glomerular filtration
Xe-133	inulin C-14
Kr-85	inulin, allyl I-125
HSA, I-131	EDTA, CR-51
HSA, I-125	DTPA, In-113m
	DTPA, Tc-99m
	DTPA, In-111
	iothalamate, I-125

Effective renal plasma flow-

Tubular secretion	Tubular reabsorption
Iodohippurate, I-131	Pertechnetate, Tc-99m
Iodohippurate, I-125	
Iodohippurate, I-123	

Thus, results with radiopharmaceuticals do not adjust with the
theory probably because biological facts such as binding to
proteins are not included in the calculations. This example
shows clearly the limits of pharmacokinetics based on a
limited number of factors, whereas this first approach is
sufficient to characterize radiopharmaceuticals.

4.6. Liver

Radiopharmaceuticals for liver are not only used for scanning, but, more and more, to study the biliary excretion function. In that context, acetanilido-iminodiacetic acid derivatives labelled with technetium-99m, better known as IDA derivatives, will be useful and their pharmacokinetics parameters are well established. The blood radioactivity decreases with three exponentials while radioactivity increases in liver to peak at 20 minutes after intravenous injection to normal subjects (35, 36). Among the derivatives studied, diethyl IDA presents a higher hepatic clearance and a faster biliary excretion rate than parabutyl IDA (37). In patients without hepatobiliary disease, the liver mean transit time is 32 $\pm$ 19 minutes and the mean body disappearance constant is 6.6 $\pm$ 1.1 per cent per minute (38).

All these parameters have been determined to compare patients to healthy people and not to determine the best radiopharmaceutical in the series of the acetanilido iminodiacetic acid. However, Bobba et al. (36) have compared the IDA derivatives labelled with technetium-99m, figured in table 4.

Table 4 - Kinetic parameters of IDA derivatives in normal subjects (Bobba et al. (36)).

IDA derivative	M.W.	Peak hepatic uptake time (minutes after injection)	Mean hepatic excretion T 1/2 (minutes)
HIDA	294	20	48
PIPIDA	306	20	67
DIDA	322	14	37
pBIDA	322	26	153

HIDA   = dimethylacetanilido iminodiacetic acid
PIPIDA = paraisopropylacetanilido iminodiacetic acid
DIDA   = diethylacetanilido iminodiacetic acid
pBIDA = parabutylacetanilido iminodiacetic acid
M.W.   = molecular weight

As may possibly be expected it appears that the heaviest derivative is the longer to reach peak uptake and the longer to be excreted. Nevertheless, molecular weight is not the sole factor, as the dimethylacetanilido derivative is excreted slower than the diethyl acetanilido one.

5. DISCUSSION

The most simple pharmacokinetic work on normal subjects was made with pertechnetate Tc-99m by Prince et al. (39) who showed that the distribution of technetium-99m followed a two compartment model (vascular space and perivascular space) when subjects were given 400 mg potassium perchlorate per os. After distribution between these compartments technetium-99m was excreted (figure 4).

Figure 4 - Two compartment model for pertechnetate distribution (Prince et al. (39)).

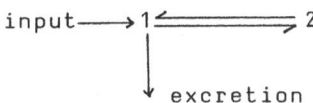

Compartment 1 = blood; Compartment 2 = perivascular space.

In this model, the exponential decrease is solved by the general equation:

$$y = A \cdot e^{-at} + B \cdot e^{-bt}$$

Our review of literature has shown that each of the parameters of pharmacokinetics has been used by the authors, but not all of them in a systematic manner. Half-life is of current use, clearance is expressed with radiopharmaceuticals for kidney, volume of distribution is implemented in compartment models but seldom exploited, area under the curve is not, but once, used. Routes of administration have not deserved a real attention, whereas radiopharmaceutical metabolites are occasionally cited. As good figures of pharmacokinetics are necessary to establish the radiation absorbed dose, we may propose that each radiopharmaceutical be studied, according to one major route of administration. Its blood half-life, excretion clearance, volume of distribution, organ clearance and the associated area under the curve should be established when possible. It might be that these figures are enlisted in the files for drug applications but they are not easily retrieved in scientific literature. In our opinion, sophisticated compartmental models are not of real help for the phases I and II of human pharmacology. An effort of unification of human pharmacokinetic parameters would allow intercomparisons between radiopharmaceuticals and between the results of different scienfific and medical groups. Producers and users would benefit of this endeavour to speak the same language in pharmacokinetics.

6. CONCLUSION

Human pharmacology of radiopharmaceuticals consists in establishing primary side effects due to the chemical counter-part of radiopharmaceuticals and in measuring pharmacokinetic parameters of the radionuclide which is supposed to be linked to the chemical moiety. In that regard, pharmacokinetic of radiopharmaceuticals is of prime importance because it determine the quality of the radiodiagnostic tool and it measures the radiation absorbed dose for the target organ as well as for the rest of the organism. The most used parameters are, in order of frequency, half-life (biological, effective, in blood, in target organs, in whole body), clearance and excretion rate, volume of distribution and area under the curve. The review of literature shows little concern about those parameters as a systematic mean to compare series of radiopharmaceuticals. Only, acetanilido derivatives of iminodiacetic acid, a series of hepatotropic radiopharmaceuticals, have been studied in that way. However, applications for new diagnostic drugs ask, in phases I and II, for an evidence of their qualities objectived by pharmacokinetic studies.

Acknowledgement - We thank Madeleine Besnard for her help and Raymonde Protin for typing the manuscript.

REFERENCES
1. Cohen Y, Besnard M. Radionuclides. Pharmacokinetic. In: Hundeshagen H. (ed) Handbuch der medizinischen Radiologie, Berlin-Heidelberg, Springer Verlag 1980;XV,1:3-76.

2. Ritschel W A. Handbook of basic pharmacokinetics. 2nd edition, Drug Intelligence Publications, Hamilton, 1980.
3. Winchell H S, Baldwin R M, Lin T H. Development of I-123 labelled amines for brain studies: localization of I-123 iodophenylalkyl amines in rat brain. J Nucl Med 1900;21:940-46.
4. Winchell H S, Horst W D, Braun L, Oldendorf W H, Hattner R, Parker H. N isopropyl I-123 p-iodoamphetamine: single pass brain uptake and washout: binding to brain synaptsomes; and localization in dog and monkey brain. J Nucl Med 1980;21:947-52.
5. Carlsen L, Andresen K. I-131 labelled N-isopropyl-p-idoamphetamine. Eur J Nucl Med 1982;7:280-81.
6. Lassen N A, Henriksen L, Holm S, Paulson O B, Vorstrup S, Rapin J, le Poncin-Lafitte M, Moretti J L. Xenon-133 and isopropyl-amphetamine iodine-123 studies of brain blood flow in man by single photon tomography. Proc. IIIrd World congress Nucl Med Biol Paris, Pergamon Press 1982;II:1739-43.
7. Kuhl D E, Barrio J R, Huang S C, Selin C, Ackermann R F, Lear J L, Wu J L, Lin T H, Phelps M E. Quantifying local cerebral blood flow by N-isopropyl-p- (I-123) iodoamphetamine (IMP) tomography. J Nucl Med 1982;23:196-203.
8. Phelps M. Positron computed tomography studies of cerebral glucose metabolism in man: theory and application in nuclear medicine. Semin Nucl Med 1981;II:32-49.
9. Jones S C, Alavi A, Christman D, Montanez I, Wolf A P, Reivich M. The radiation dosimetry of 2 (F-18) fluoro 2 deoxyglucose in man. J Nucl Med 1982;23:613-17.
10. Eckelman W C, Reba R C, Gibson R E, Rzeszotarski W J, Vieras F, Mazaitis J K, Francis B. Receptor binding radiotracers: a class of potential radiopharmaceuticals J Nucl Med 1979;20:350-57.
11. Gibson R E, Eckelman W C, Vieras F, Reba R C. The distribution of the muscarinic acetylcholine receptor antagonist quinuclidylbenzylate and quinnuclidylbenzylate methiodide (both tritiated) in rat, quinea pig and rabbit. J Nucl Med 1979;20:865-70.
12. Hanson R N, Blumberg J B, Poddubiuk Z M, Davis M A, Holman B L. Preparation and biodistribution of a I-125 labelled betaadrenoceptor antagonist bearing a cardioselectivity enhancing N-substituent. Int J Appl Rad Isotop 1981; 32: 429-33.
13. Wieland D M, Brown L E, Rogers W L, Worthington K C, Jiann-Long Wu, Clinthorne N H, Otto C A, Swanson D P, Beierwaltés W H. Myocardial imaging with a radioiodinated norepinephrine storage analogue. J Nucl Med 1981;22:22-31.
14. Syrota A, Maziere M, Crouzel M, Sastre J, Prenant C. Visualization of acetylcholine receptors in the human heart using C-11 methyl QNB and positron emission tomography. Proc IIIrd World Congress Nucl Med Biol Paris, Pergamon Press 1982;III:2503-5.
15. Schelbert H R, Henze E, Phelps M E. Emission tomography of heart. Semin Nucl Med 1980;10:355-73.
16. Poe N D. Rationale and radiopharmaceuticals for myocardial

156

imaging. Semin Nucl Med 1977;7:7-14.
17. Van der Wall E E, den Hollander W, Heindendal G A K Westera G, Majid P A, Roos J P. Dynamic myocardial scintigraphy with I-123 labelled free fatty acids in patients with myocardial infarction. Eur J Nucl Med 1981;6:383-389.
18. Hamilton G W. Myocardial imaging with thallium-201: the controversy over its clinical usefulness in ischemic heart disease. J Nucl Med 1979;20:1201-5.
19. Chervu L R. Radiopharmaceuticals in cardiovascular nuclear medicine. Semin Nucl Med 1979;9:241-56.
20. Pohost G M, Alpert N M, Ingwall J S Strauss H W, Thallium redistribution: mechanism and clinical utility. Semin Nucl Med 1980;10:70-93.
21. Demangeat A, Constantinesco A, Mossard J M, Chambron J, Voegtlin R. Evaluation of myocardial perfusion and left ventricular function by Tl-201 scintigraphy after dipyridamole. Eur J Nucl Med 1981;6:491-503.
22. Harris D, Taylor D, Condon B, Ackery D, Conway N. Myocardial imaging with dipyridamole: comparison of the sensitivity and specificity of Tl-201 versus M U G A. Eur J Nucl Med 1982;7:1-5.
23. Bunow B, Line B R, Horton M R, Weiss G H. Regional ventilatory clearance by xenon scintigraphy: a critical evaluation of two estimation procedures. J Nucl Med 1979;20:703-10.
24. Alderson P O, Line B R. Scintigraphic evaluation of regional pulmonary ventilation. Semin Nucl Med 1980;10:218-42.
25. Atkins H L, Robertson J S, Croft B Y, Tsui B, Susskind H, Ellis K J, Loken M K, Treves S. MIRD dose estimate report n° 9. Estimates of radiation absorbed doses from radioxenons in lung imaging. J Nucl Med 1980;21:459-65.
26. Short M D, Dowsett D J, Heaf P J D, Pavia D, Thomson M L. A comparison between monodisperse Tc-99m labelled aerosol particles and Kr-81 m for assessment of lung function. J Nucl Med 1979;20:194-200.
27. Charkes N D, Makler P T, Philips C. Studies of skeletal tracer kinetics.I.Digital computer solution of a five compartment model of (F-18) fluoride kinetics in humans. J Nucl Med 1978;19:1301-9.
28. Charkes N D, Makler P T. Studies in skeletal tracer kinetics: V. Computer simulated Tc-99m (Sn) MDP bone scan changes in some systemic disorders: concise communication. J Nucl Med 1981;22:601-05.
29. Fogelman I. Skeletal uptake of diphosphonate: a review. Eur J Nucl Med 1980;5:473-6.
30. Fogelman I, Pearson D W, Bessent R G, Tofe A J, Francis M D. A comparison of skeletal uptakes of three diphosphonates by whole body retention: concise communication. J Nucl Med 1981;22:880-3.
31. Chervu L R, Blaufox M D. Renal radiopharmaceuticals. An update. Semin Nucl Med 1982;12:224-45.
32. Roos J C, Koomans H A, Boer P, Oei H Y. Determination of glomerular filtration rate by In-111 DTPA. Eur J Nucl Med 1981;6:551-53.

33. Houston A S, Sampson W F D, Mac Leod M A. A compartimental model for the distribution of In-113m DTPA and Tc-99m (Sn) DTPA in man following intravenous injection. Int J Nucl Med Biol 1979;6:85-95.
34. Tauxe W N, Dubovsky E V, Mantle J A, Dustan H P, Logic J R. Measurement of effective renal plasma flow in congestive heart failure. Eur J Nucl Med 1981;6:555-59.
35. Brown PH, Krishnamurthy G T, Bobba V V R, Kingston E. Radiation dose calculation for Tc-99m HIDA in health and disease. J Nucl Med 1981;22:177-83.
36. Bobba V R, Krishnamurthy G T, Kingston E, Brown P H, Eklem M, Turner F. The comparison of kinetics and image patterns of Tc-99m IDA derivatives in normal subjects. J Nucl Med 1981;22:7.
37. Tarolo G L, Picozzi R, Palagi B, Cammelli F. Comparative quantitative evaluation of hepatic clearance of diethyl IDA and parabutyl IDA in jaundiced and non jaundiced patients. Eur J Nucl Med 1981;6:539-43.
38. Taavitsainen M, Riihimäki E, Tähti E. Body disappearance and liver mean transit time of Tc-99m diethyl IDA. Eur J Nucl Med 1980;5:147-50.
39. Prince J R, Bancroft S, Dukstein W G. Pharmacokinetics of pertechnetate administered after pretreatment with 400mg of potassium perchlorate: concise communication. J Nucl Med 1980;21:763-6.

158

10. RADIATION DOSIMETRY

HANS DETLEV ROEDLER

1. INTRODUCTION

For assessing the safety of a radiopharmaceutical, the radiation exposure of the patient is one of the required parameters. In general, the exposure can only be estimated by initially referring to biokinetic data from investigations in animals and subsequently using available data from man. Mean organ doses are calculated in most instances, but effective doses and local tissue doses may be of considerable importance as well. The quantities needed and methods used for dose calculations are given in this review together with some results. The relevance of these data in assessing the safety of a radiopharmaceutical will be discussed.

2. QUANTITIES DETERMINING THE PATIENT EXPOSURE

The radiation exposure of the patient depends on such factors as the activity administered, the radiopharmaceutical, the pathophysiology and age of patient.

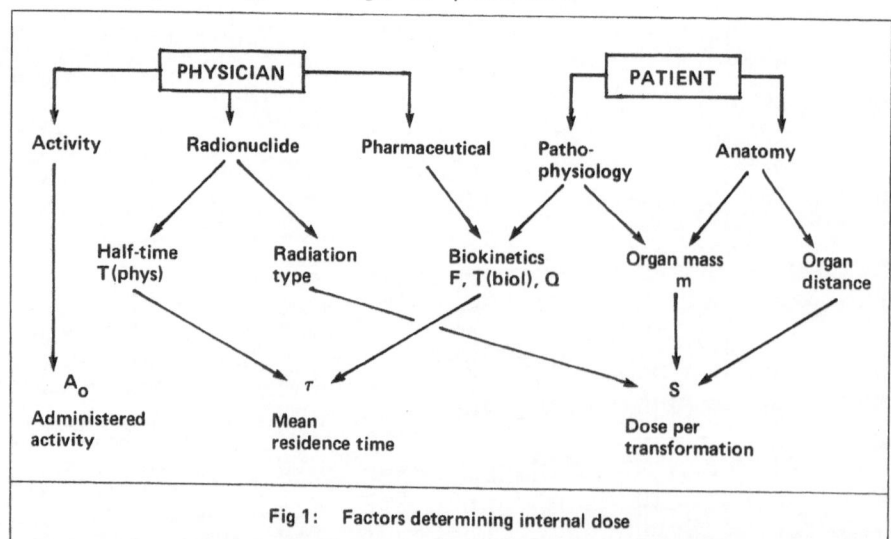

Fig 1: Factors determining internal dose

The term radiopharmaceutical implies not only the radionuclide characteristics of half time and type and energy of radiation emitted per nuclear transformation, but also the basic distribution and elimination pattern which may be described by the mean residence times τ of the radiopharmaceu tical in organs or total body. This pattern may be modified considerably by the pathophysiology of the patient, whereby its diagnosis, in most cases, is the purpose of administering the radiopharmaceutical. Pathophysiology may also refer to the mass of the organ of interest - for instance in cases of struma and splenomegaly - which, however, is primarily age-dependent, as is the mean distance between the organs determining the absorbed fraction of the emitted energy. In the currently used formalism of dose calculation, the above parameters are summarized by three factors:

- administered activity A_o,
- residence time τ ,
- dose S to an organ per transformation.

3. ABSORBED DOSE, EFFECTIVE DOSE EQUIVALENT, LOCAL TISSUE DOSE
3.1. Absorbed dose (1)

The mean absorbed dose $\bar{D}$ in an organ is calculated by

$$(1)$$

where
$$\bar{D} = A_o \times \tau \times S$$

$\bar{D}$ is the mean absorbed dose, that is the energy absorbed in a volume element of unit mass

A_o is the administered activity

τ is the residence time in an organ

S is the mean absorbed dose per transformation.

Considering the contribution from activity in several source organs to the dose in a target organ, equation 1 becomes

$$\bar{D}_k = A_o \times \Sigma_h \tau_h \times S_{k \leftarrow h} \qquad (2)$$

where

$\bar{D}_k$ is the mean absorbed dose in a target organ k (Gy or rd)

τ_h is the residence time (s or h) of activity in the source organ h, i.e. the average time that the administered activity spends in h

$S_{k \leftarrow h}$ is the mean absorbed dose in a target organ k per transformation in a source organ h (Gy or rad $\mu Ci^{-1} h^{-1}$)

3.2 Effective dose equivalent (2)

The effective dose equivalent facilitates the comparison of different dose distributions in the body, based on the individual radiosensitivity of tissues or organs. This concept, which was developed originally for radiation protection purposes of occupationally exposed persons, attributes weighting factors w_k to organs or tissues representing the proportion of the stochastic risk resulting from organ or tissue k to the total risk, when the total body is irradiated uniformly. The effective dose equivalent is then calculated by adding the weighted organ or tissue doses according to

$$H_E = \Sigma_k w_k \times \overline{H}_k \qquad (3)$$

where

H_E is the effective dose equivalent (Sv)

w_k is the weighting factor reflecting the radiation sensitivity of organ or tissue k (gonads 0.25, breast 0.15, red bone marrow and lungs 0.12, thyroid and bone surfaces 0.03, and 0.06 for each of the 5 remaining organs receiving the highest dose)

$\overline{H}_k$ is the mean dose equivalent (Sv or rem) in target organ k; for the radionuclides used in dignostic nuclear medicine its value is identical to that of the mean absorbed dose (Gy or rad), since for these radionuclides the quality factor is 1.

Although the age distribution of patients in nuclear medicine, showing a maximum frequency at approximately age 70 (exception: thyroid patients age 30 - 40), differs considerably from that of occupationally exposed persons and, therefore, the adoption of the weighting factor for the gonadal dose is not justified, this concept is applied here since no decision was made as yet on the use of a more appropriate somatically effective dose equivalent (3, 4, 5) on an international basis.

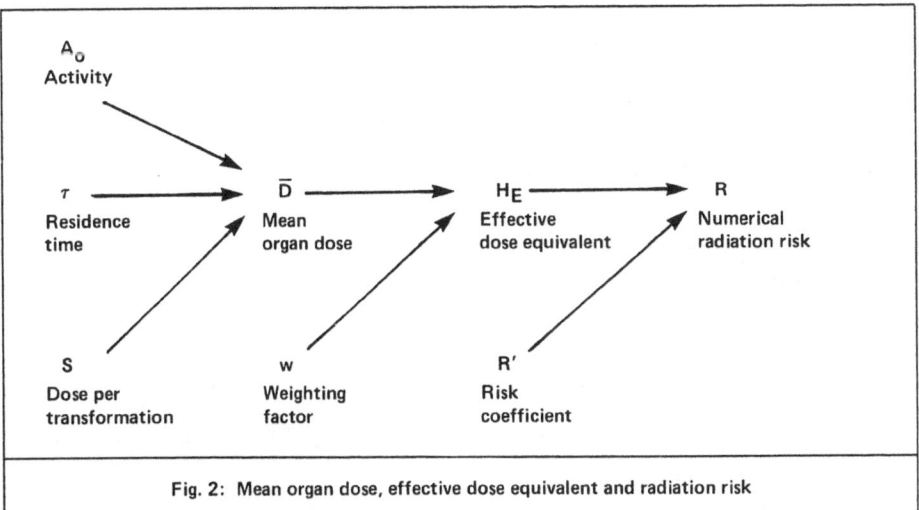

Fig. 2: Mean organ dose, effective dose equivalent and radiation risk

3.3. Local tissue dose

If the distance between activity deposits is equal to or greater than the range of the corpuscular radiation emitted, it is appropriate to consider the distribution of local dose in the vicinity of an activity deposit instead of the dose averaged for an organ or tissue. The local dose $D(x,E_0)$ at a distance x from a point source isotropically emitting electrons of energy E_0 is proportional to the number $\tilde{A}(t)$ of transformations, the energy E_0 and the specific absorbed fraction $\Phi(x,E_0)$:

$$D(x,E_0,t) = \tilde{A}(t) \times E_0 \times \Phi(x,E_0) \tag{4}$$

4. RESIDENCE TIME τ (6, 7)

The residence time τ_h specifies the total number of nuclear transformations in an organ h per unit administered activity. It may be derived from a function describing organ activity versus time which in most cases is given as a sum or a difference of exponential functions. Thus

$$\tau_h = 1{,}443 \times \Sigma_j \alpha_{hj} \times T_{hj} \tag{5a}$$

$$\tau_h = 1{,}443 \times F_h \times \Sigma_j Q_{hj} \times T_{hj} \tag{5b}$$

where

α_{hj} is the fraction of the exponential component j at time t=0 per administered unit activity

T_{hj} is the effective half time of the exponential component j;

$$1/T_{effective} = 1/T_{biologic} + 1/T_{physical}$$

F_h fractional distribution, $F_h = \Sigma_j \alpha_{hj}$ for positive α_{hj}

Q_{hj} intercept of the exponential component j.

The representation according to equation 5b (8 - 11) is advantageous since it reflects the relative distribution of the radiopharmaceutical between different tissues. In summary, the residence times T_h may be calculated for an exponential model from the measured (or estimated) fractional distributions F_h and the effective half times T_{hj} with intercepts Q_{hj}.

4.1. Methods of measurement

4.1.1. Total body retention. The knowledge of the total body residence time is essential for absorbed dose calculations, since the main contribution to the dose in organs not significantly accumulating the radiopharmaceutical, derives from the total body activity outside of the source organs. Appropriate methods are those of total body counting and excretion measurement.

4.1.2. Fractional distribution and retention. The most frequently applied method of determining the fractional distribution and retention of a radiopharmaceutical is the post mortem section of small animals at different times following the administration and subsequent measurement of organ activities. Occasionally, biodistribution data have been derived from human biopsy and autopsy specimens. Non-invasive, external measurements by probes, scanners, gamma-cameras or tomographic systems may be used in humans and larger animals for determining the biodistribution and retention of radiopharmaceuticals. They require, however, careful calibration with appropriate phantoms and special procedures such as conjugate counting methods, peak-to-scatter-methods (12) or advanced attenuation compensation algorithms.

4.2. Evaluation of measurements

4.2.1. Total body retention. The commonly used procedure of evaluation is a least squares fit of a sum, or a difference, of exponential functions with the measured retention data, such as described in (13).

An extrapolation of the biological retention functions beyond the final measurement may be achieved by
a) the exponential component with the longest biological half-time,
b) $T_{biologic}=\infty$ starting from the last measurement
c) basic use of $t_{biologic} = \infty$ as the long-term component of the regression analysis.

From the viewpoint of radiation protection, methods b) or c) are preferable. For the evaluation of published biokinetic data in (14), method c) was used.

4.2.2. Fractional distribution and retention

a) If, from measurements, sufficient results of the retention in the individual source tissues h are available, as is generally the case only from investigations on mice or rats, they may be fitted for each tissue according to the procedures described above for the total body. For instance, this method has been used for pertechnetate (15) as well as for cobalt-, zinc-, and mercury-chloride (16). The advantage of this procedure may be seen in an optimal fit for each investigated tissue h, its disadvantage lies in the purely descriptive nature, which does not require an analysis in the sense of a compartmental model.

b) Scientifically more gratifying is a consistent metabolic model, as used for instance in (17, 18) for iodine and pertechnetate. In these references, the kinetics have been described by four or five half times which characterize the uptake, excretion and translocation of the pharmaceutical for individual tissues, together with respective values of α_{hj} (see equation 5a).

c) A modification of the above model, as used in (19), is the application of reliably known total body half times to the retention functions of organs and the calculation of α_{hj} (see equation 5a) for these half times from available organ retention data by means of a least squares fit. In this procedure, uptake and translocation processes are not taken into account.

d) If the organ retention data are fragmentary, or vary to such a degree that the above mentioned methods are not applicable, a further simplification may be used: the mean (or the only available) value of the fractional distribution in the organ h - if appropriate, after extrapolating back to t=0 - is taken as fractional distribution F_h (see equation 5b). The intercepts Q_{hj} and half-times T_{hj} are assumed to be identical to those of the total body retention function. This is probably the most frequently used procedure not only for radiopharmaceuticals - e.g. for the evaluation of data from literature in (14), or in (20) -, but also for other radioactive compounds, e.g. in (21).

4.3. Extrapolation of animal data to man

Biodistribution and retention data of radiopharmaceuticals are in most cases derived from measurements in animals since measurements in humans, specifically in patients, require considerable cooperation, may exceed tolerable limits or may be questionable for ethical considerations. For extrapolating animal data to man, body weight appears to be of importance, since e.g. life-expectancy, organ weight, cardiac output, kidney clearance or total body retention were interpreted as power functions of body weight (22). For substances undergoing intermediary metabolism, considerable species-related differences of the biodistribution may be expected which prevent an extrapolation to man. For inert tracers, however, an extrapolation may yield reasonably accurate results.

4.3.1. Total body retention. Various procedures have been described in the literature:

a) Extrapolation of the long-term half time of the total body retention function from animal to man by a power function of the body weight: this procedure was proposed e.g. in (23) for Cs-137.

b) Extrapolation of the residence time τ_h from animal to man

by a power function of the body weight:
this procedure was experimentally confirmed e.g. for Zn-65
chloride, Mn-54 chloride, Ag-110m nitrate, Se-75 selenite in
mouse, rat, dog or monkey and man (24 - 27). It could not be
confirmed by the same authors e.g. for Ir-192
hexachloroiridate, Nb-95 oxalate or Ru-106 chloride (28 - 30).
c) Extrapolation of the biological residence time τ_{hb} from
animal to man be the method of "similarity ratios" (31).
d) A more promising approach has been investigated by McAfee
et al. (32) who suggested a normalization of blood and total
body retention by altering the time dimension according to
power functions $W^{0.33}$ of body weight W. For example in a 250
g rat, 9 seconds were considered equivalent to 1 man minute.
This normalization procedure successfully eliminates species
differences for agents which have a predominantly
extracellular distribution and which are excreted chiefly by
glomerular filtration such as DTPA chelates or Tc-99m
pertechnetate. The method failed, however, for agents with a
predominantly intracellular localization or undergoing
extracellular transport such as Tl-201 or I-131 Hippuran.
Nonetheless, this approach is considered as useful for
distinguishing interspecies variability merely due to body
size from interspecies metabolic variations.
e) Tsui et al. (33) extended this concept even further by
transforming not only the time dimension but also the activity
dimension as power functions of body weight. Retention of
Tl-201 in blood was chosen as at test of the theory because
data have been published for several non human species as well
as verifying values for the human.
f) Crawford et al. (34) performed a detailed investigation of
the cumulative probability of correct results when
extrapolating animal data from one or more species to other
species including man. Their results for 10 radionuclides did
not prove a definite relationship between the total body
retention function of different species or an essential
significance of body weight in extrapolating procedures.
 From these results it may be concluded that currently there
is not consistent theory for extrapolating total body

residence times from animal to man.

4.3.2. Fractional activity distribution. In general, the application of animal distribution data as (%/organ) or (%administered activity/% body weight) to man yields different results due to different relative organ weight. For rat and man, both results agree within a factor of 2 - 3 except for the testes where the relative organ weight is greater by a factor of more than 20 in rat than in man.

The quality of biodistribution data measured in humans is generally not sufficient for deciding between these two procedures. The first approach is generally preferred, in particular for organ specific radionuclide accumulation; for the testes, however, the second approach appears to be more appropriate, since otherwise unrealistically high activity concentrations are calculated. In any case the original data should be reported as fractions of administered activity per organ, and 100% of the administered activity should be accounted for, as stated in (35). The reader is referred to this publication which contains useful recommendations for collection and presentation of animal data relating to internally distributed radionuclides.

5. MEAN ABSORBED DOSE PER TRANSFORMATION

For a mathematical phantom of the reference man of 70 kg body weight and 1.75 m body size, as defined in ICRP Publication 23 (36), the mean absorbed doses $S_{k \leftarrow h}$ in a target organ k per transformation in a source organ h were calculated for radionuclides used in nuclear medicine and research, mainly following a Monte-Carlo-method (37). Corresponding values for the newborn, infants and children became recently available that were derived from data for adults by appropriate correction factors (38, 39).

6. RESULTS OF INTERNAL DOSE ESTIMATES: ORGAN DOSES AND EFFECTIVE DOSE EQUIVALENTS

Estimates of organ doses from radiopharmaceuticals have been published elsewhere (40, 41, 42, 43), partially together with the respective biokinetic data for enabling an assessment of the results and a modification for individual circumstances. A revision of ICRP publication 17 (44), summarizing biokinetic data and dose estimates for radiopharmaceuticals, is currently underway. Effective dose equivalents for mean administered activities of frequently used radiopharmaceuticals are summarized in Table 1, based on data given in (45, 46). Selected nuclear medical methods are contained in Table 2 and are arranged in the order of an increasing effective dose equivalent. Approximately 30% of all these investigations have an effective dose equivalent of up to 0.5 mSv, approximately 60% show values between 2 and 5 mSv and approximately 10% (with increasing tendency) result in values from 5 to 7 mSv. The mean annual effective dose equivalent to the population in the Federal Republic of Germany from natural sources is 1.5 mSv (47). The dose limit recommended by ICRP (2) for occupationally exposed persons is 50 mSv. The values in Tables 1 and 2 are referring to the activities listed in Table 1 and the adult reference man, considering physiological biodistribution and retention. The activities administered by the physician in different institutions may be of considerable variance. However, the effective dose equivalent may be easily adjusted because of its direct relationship to the administered activity. It is noted that the rapidly expanding nuclear cardiology is committed to comparatively high effective dose equivalents.

7. DOSE TO BONE SURFACES AND THE BLADDER WALL

According to ICRP Publication 26 (2), a layer of 10 μm thickness on bone surfaces, representing end- and periosteal cells, is considered as radiation sensitive bone tissue. The dose to this layer from a Tc-99m activity distribution on bone surfaces is larger by a factor of 5, when compared to conventional estimates for the total bone volume as a target tissue (48), involving a surface dose of 40 mGy (4 rad) from a 550 MBq (15 mCi) Tc-99m MDP bone scan.

Organ or method	Radiopharmaceutical		Activity A_0 MBq (mCi)	Effective dose equivalent	
				per MBq mSv/MBq	per exami- nation mSv
Thyroid	99mTc	pertechnetate	37 (1.0)	0.011	0.41
	123 I	iodide	3.7 (0.1)	0.12	0.44
	[131 I	iodide	1.9 (0.05)	11	21]
Bone	99mTc	phosphonate	555 (15)	0.0065	3.6
Liver/Spleen	99mTc	colloid	167 (4.5)	0.013	2.2
	[198 Au	colloid	5.6 (0.15)	1.0	5.6]
Kidneys	131 I	Hippuran	1.5 (0.04)	0.16	0.24
	2 % free iodide			11	+ 0.33
					0.57
	99mTc	DTPA	370 (10)	0.010	3.7
	99mTc	glucoheptonate	370 (10)	0.014	5.2
	99mTc	DMSA	111 (3)	0.017	1.9
	[197 Hg	Chlormerodrin	7.4 (0.2)	0.19	1.4]
	[203 Hg	Chlormerodrin	5.6 (0.15)	1.8	10]
Brain	99mTc	DTPA	463 (12.5)	0.010	4.6
	99mTc	pertechnetate	463 (12.5)	0.010	4.6
Myocardium	99mTc	RBC	740 (20)	0.0070	5.2
	201 Tl	chloride	74 (2)	0.0094	7.0
Lungs	99mTc	microspheres	167 (4.5)	0.012	2.0
Schilling-Test	57 Co	cyanocobalamin	0.019 (0.0005)	1.7	0.032
Hepatobiliary	99mTc	HIDA	111 (3)	0.020	2.2
Spleen	99mTc	altered RBC	56 (1.5)	0.053	3.0
Iron kinetics	59 Fe	chloride	0.37 (0.01)	12	4.4

Table 1: Effective dose equivalents (mSv) per MBq administered activity and per examination for some currently and formerly [ ] used radiopharmaceuticals. The values refer to the adult reference man and to physiological biodistribution and retention data.

The dose to the bladder wall from renal radiopharmaceuticals has seldom been adequately considered although it may reach values of e.g. 60 mGy (6 rad) from brain scans with 460 MBq (12.5 mCi) Tc-99m DTPA (46). The radiation sensitivity of the bladder and the appropriate value of the weighting factor w_k are still being discussed.

	Organ or method	Radiopharmaceutical	Effective dose equivalent mSv	Frequency %
	Schilling-Test	57 Co cyanocobalamin	0.032	
	Thyroid	99mTc pertechnetate	0.41	~ 30
	Kidneys	131 I Hippuran	0.57	
0.5 mSv				
1.5 mSv				
	Lungs	99mTc microspheres	2.0	
	Liver/Spleen	99mTc colloid	2.2	
	Bone	99mTc phosphonate	3.6	~ 60
	Kidneys	99mTc DTPA	3.7	
	Brain	99mTc DTPA	4.6	
	Brain	99mTc pertechnetate	4.6	
5 mSv				
	Myocardium	99mTc RBC	5.2	~ 10
		201 Tl chloride	7.0	

Table 2: Examinations most frequently performed in nuclear medicine, arranged in the order of increasing effective dose equivalent (compare table 1). The values of 0.5 and 5 mSv correspond to 1/100 or 1/10, respectively, of the annual dose limit recommended by the ICRP (2) for occupationally exposed persons; 1.5 mSv is the mean annual effective dose equivalent in the Federal Republic of Germany from natural sources (47).

8. LOCAL TISSUE DOSE

In a recent publication (49), the limitations of conventional mean tissue doses were again (50, 51) emphasized in relation to radiation induced biologic effects. When Tl-201 was injected into mouse testes, the low-energy Auger electrons from its electron-capture decay were found to be much more effective in causing loss of testicular weight and reduction of sperm heads than the energetic beta-particles from similarly distributed Tl-204. These results were contrary to expectations based on conventional dosimetry of tissue-incorporated radionuclides, and point to possible underestimation of risks by the mean tissue dose concept in the case of radionuclides decaying by electron capture and internal conversion.

Hofer (52) concluded from his investigations on the biological effects of Auger emitters, such as Tl-201, I-125, I-123, In-111, Tc-99m, Ga-67, Co-57, Cr-51, that the cytocidal effects to Auger emitters result exclusively from deposition of radiation energy in the cell nucleus, and the absorption of radiation energy in the cytoplasm or at the plasma membrane contributed little, if anything, to these effects. Therefore the rational use of Auger emitters in nuclear medicine would require information on the intracellular distribution of the radionuclides. From the radiopharmaceuticals discussed in (52) and used currently in diagnostic nuclear medicine, only Co-57 bleomycin appears to localize in the cell nucleus. However, more attention to the intracellular distribution of currently used or future radiopharmaceuticals would be justified in view of its biological consequences.

9. AGE DEPENDENCE OF DOSE (39, 53, 11, 54)
9.1. Administered activity
For imaging procedures the activity administered to children may be derived from the activity administered to adults according to a (body weight) $2/3$ relationship, yielding an approximately equal count rate density.

9.2. Effective dose equivalent
The effective dose equivalent approximately shows an inverse linear relationship to the total body mass, when assuming constant administered activity and biokinetic data. For activities according to the (body weight) $2/3$ rule, the mean ratios of effective dose equivalents in newborn or children and in adults are: 2.7 for the newborn, 1.7 for age 5, 1.6 for age 10 and 1.2 for age 15.

9.3. Age dependent biodistribution and retention
Only relatively few age dependent biokinetic data are available, e.g. for iodine in the newborn and in the adult, where thyroidal activity concentration and half time are age-dependent in a reverse sense. The activity concentration of Tc-99m MDP and thus the local radiation exposure of the

epiphyseal growth complexes appears to be higher for equal activities per kg body weight than in the epiphyses of adult patients.

10. PATHOPHYSIOLOGY AND DOSE

Organ masses greater than those for reference man result in lower organ doses at otherwise identical conditions. This may be particularly important for the dose to thyroid, spleen or liver. The dose dependence on residence time has been documented, e.g. for the kidney dose in cases of renal disease. A recent detailed biokinetic and dosimetric study of Tc-99m HIDA (55) demonstrates that a disease and its stage may determine the organ receiving the highest dose. While in healthy volunteers and in patients with normal serum bilirubin the gallbladder and the large intestine received the highest doses, the kidneys and the bladder were the organs of highest radiation exposure for bilirubin levels greater than 10 mg/%. The lower effective dose equivalent in icteric patients is compensated by the necessity of administering larger activities (370 instead of 74 MBq) at higher bilirubin levels.

11. BLOCKING AGENTS

Although, at first glance, the principle of preventing accumulation of activity in an organ by blocking agents appears promising, it is used in practice only in a few specific instances: e.g. blocking of the thyroid when administering iodine labelled radiopharmaceuticals, such as iodinated fibrinogen, or blocking of thyroid, parotis and plexus choreoideus when administering pertechnetate for brain studies. The degree of successfully blocking an organ depends on the amount of the blocking agent and time of administration. Respective theoretical considerations and results may be found in (56).

12. RADIOCONTAMINANTS

Radiocontaminants may contribute to the radiation exposure of the patient and at the same time deterioriate the image quality. Some time ago, this problem was investigated in relation to generator eluates (57); presently it may be of concern for longer-lived contaminants of iodine 123 such as I-124 and I-125 (58), or Tl-201, such as Tl-202 and Tl-200 (59). An upper limit of the dose contribution from these radiocontaminants may be estimated by considering an administration at the recommended time of expiration.

13. RADIATION RISK

From a risk coefficient of 1.65 x 10^{-5} mSv, as given in ICRP Publication 26 (2), a calculated radiation risk of 5th order may be derived from data in Table 1 and 2 for nuclear medical examinations. This probably represents a conservative estimate, considering the differences of age distribution and child expectancy in occupationally exposed persons and in patients in whom radiation induced genetic defects or malignomas are expected to be manifest at a lesser degree. In Table 3 the calculated radiation risk of 5 x 10^{-5} from a typical nuclear medical examination is related to similarly low daily risks.

Activity	Cause of death
50 — 100 cigarettes smoked	cancer, cardiopulmonary disease
5 000 kilometers car ride	accident
1 1/4 hours mountain climbing	accident
1 1/2 years of work in a typical factory	accident
1 month of work in a coal mine	accident
17 hours of being 60 years of age	overall mortality

Table 3: Comparison of the calculated $5 \cdot 10^{-5}$ risk of a typical nuclear medical examination with other risks implying the same probability of death for 5 per 100 000 cases as a consequence of the activities as shown (60).

14. CONCLUSIONS

The essential elements of internal dose estimation for radiopharmaceuticals are described and may be employed for documenting the safety of a radiopharmaceutical regarding radiation exposure, as specified for instance by the American Guidelines for the Clinical Evaluation of Radiopharmaceutical Drugs (61):

" Projected human radiation dosimetry calculations should be shown for the primary organ(s) of concern, the organ receiving the highest absorbed radiation dose, the critical organs (whole body, active bloodforming organs, lens of the eye, gonads), and any other organs with significant radiation exposure from the radiopharmaceutical drug (e.g., bladder).

These calculations should include equations based on the highest dose of the radionuclide to be administered

The actual equation(s) used for the dosimetry calculations should be given in full. The system set forth by the Medical Internal Radiation Dose (MIRD) Committee of the Society of Nuclear Medicine or the system set forth by the International Commission on Radiological Protection for the calculation of radiation absorbed dose are the recommended methods of calculation. All underlying assumptions concerning distribution and effective half-lives should be documented. In general, biologic distribution studies for the radiopharmaceutical should be sufficiently complete to account for as much of the administered dose as possible".

These conventional mean organ doses are considered as characteristic radiopharmaceutical properties which should be documented, such as results from toxicological tests, for an assessment of the safety of the radiopharmaceutical. In addition, these may be supplemented by data for the effective dose equivalent and for the intracellular distribution in case of Auger-emitters. The radiation exposure from a new radiopharmaceutical will be judged in relation to the exposure from currently used radiopharmaceuticals (effective dose equivalent: typically a few mSv for imaging procedures) and in relation to the diagnostic benefit, considering established procedures that may or may not involve a radiation exposure of the patient.

Acknowledgements

Thanks are due to Mrs. R. LeMar for assistance in translation and to Mrs. I. Zeitlberger for preparing the manuscript.

REFERENCES
1. Loevinger R, Bergman M. A revised schema for calculating the absorbed dose from biologically distributed radionuclides. MIRD pamphlet No. 1, revised. New York, Society of Nuclear Medicine, 1976.
2. ICRP publication 26. Recommendations of the International Commission on Radiological Protection. Oxford, Pergamon Press, 1977.
3. Persson BRR. Effective dose equivalent concept in radiopharmaceutical dosimetry, in: E. E. Watson et al., eds. Third International Radiopharmaceutical Dosimetry Symposium (HHS Publication FDA 81-8166) 1981:616-624.
4. Roedler HD. Strahlenexposition von Patienten bei diagnostischer Anwendung von Radionukliden, in: O. Messerschmidt et al., eds. Strahlenschutz in Forschung und Praxis, Vol. XXIII, Stuttgart, Thieme Verlag 1982:79-94.
5. Roedler HD, Kaul A. Strahlenrisiko für den Patienten durch nuklearmedizinische Diagnostik, in: B. Glöbel et al., eds. Das Strahlenrisiko im Vergleich zu chemischen und biologischen Risiken, Stuttgard, Georg Thieme Verlag 1981:84-92.
6. Roedler HD. Accuracy of internal dose calculations with special consideration of radiopharmaceutical biokinetics, in: E.E. Watson et al., eds. Third International Radiopharmaceutical Dosimetry Symposium (HHS Publication FDA 81-8166) 1981:1-20.
7. Roedler HD. Radiation dose to the patient in radionuclide studies, in: Medical Radionuclide Imaging, Vol. 1. Vienna, International Atomig Energy Agency 1981:527-542.
8. Roedler HD, Kaul A, Berner W, Koeppe P, Glaubitt D. Development of an extended formalism for internal dose calculation and practical application to several biologically distributed radioelements, in: Assessment of Radioactive Contamination in Man. Vienna, International Atomic Energy Agency, 1971:515-541.
9. Roedler HD, Strahlenbelastung durch Radiopharmaka -Entwicklung eines mathematischen Dosiskonzepts und Ergebnisse von Neuberechnungen der Energiedosis. (Thesis) Berlin, Freie Universität, 1974.
10. Roedler HD. Internal dosimetry of Technetium 99m labelled radiopharmaceuticals used in clinical nuclear medicine. J Belge Radiol 1977;60:463-472.
11. Roedler HD. Biokinetik und Dosisermittlung, in: Medizinische Physik `79. Heidelberg, Dr. Alfred Hüthig Verlag 1979:279-284.
12. Roedler HD, Kragh P. Measurement of radiopharmaceutical biodistribution in patients, in: W. Bleifeld et al., eds. Proceedings of the World Congress on Medical Physics and

Biomedical Engineering 1982 Hamburg, (MPBE 1982 eV, 21.10.)

13. Berman M. Compartmental analysis and kinetics, in: R.W. Stacy et al. eds. Computers in Biomedical Research, Vol. 2 New York, Academic Press, 1965:Chapt.7.

14. Kaul A, Oeff K, Roedler HD, Vogelsang T. Radiopharmaceuticals - Biokinetic data and results of recalculations of internal dose. Berlin, Informationsdienst für Nuklearmedizin, 1974: 600 pp.

15. Kubassi F. Tierexperimentelle Untersuchungen zur Kinetik von Tc-99m Pertechnetat und Berechnung der Strahlenexposition von Patienten (Thesis) Berlin, Freie Universität,1975.

16. Berner W. Tierexperimentelle Untersuchungen zum Problem der Dekorporierung von radioaktiven Metallionen (Thesis) Berlin, Freie Universität, 1973.

17. MIRD Dose Estimate Report No. 5. Summary of current radiation dose estimates to humans from I-123, I-124, I-125, I-126, I-130, I-131 and I-132 as sodium iodide. J Nucl Med 1975;16:857.

18. MIRD Dose Estimate Report No. 8. Summary of current radiation dose estimates to normal humans from Tc-99m as sodium pertechnetate. J Nucl Med 1976;17:74.

19. Lathrop KA, Johnston RE, Blau M, Rothschild EO. Radiation dose to humans from Se-75 L-selenomethionine. MIRD pamphlet 9, J Nucl Med 1972;13:Suppl.6.

20. MIRD Dose Estimate Report No. 2. Summary of current radiation dose estimates to humans from Ga-66, Ga-67, Ga-68 and Ga-72 citrate. J Nucl Med 1973;14:755.

21. ICRP Publication 30. Limits for intakes of radionuclides by workers. Oxford, Pergamon Press, 1979.

22. Tsui BMW, L athrop KA, Harper PV. Extrapolation from animals to the human for the retention of radiothallium in the blood, in: E.E. Watson et al., eds. Third International Radiopharmaceutical Dosimetry Symposium (HHS Publication FDA 81-8166) 1981:283-291.

23. Stara JF, Nelson NS, DellaRosa RJ, Bustad LK. Comparative metabolism of radionuclides in mammals: A review. Health Phys 1971;20:113-137.

24. Richmond CR, Furchner JE, Trafton GA, Langham WH. Comparative metabolism of radionuclides in mammals - I. Uptake and retention of orally administered Zn-65 by four mammalian species. Health Phys 1962;8:481-489.

25. Furchner JE, Richmond CR, Drake GA. Comparative metabolism of radionuclides in mammals - III. Retention of manganese-54 in the mouse, rat, monkey and dog. Health Phys 1966;12:1415-1423.

26. Furchner JE, Richmond CR, Drake GA. Comparative metabolism of radionuclides in mammals - IV. Retention of silver-110m in the mouse, rat, monkey and dog. Health Phys 1968;15:505-514.

27. Furchner JE, London JE, Wilson JS. Comparative metabolism of radionuclides in mammals - IX. Retention of Se-75 in the mouse, rat, monkey and dog. Health Phys 1975;29:641-648.

28. Furchner JE, Richmond CR, Drake GA. Comparative metabolism

of radionuclides in mammals - V. Retention of Ir-192 in the mouse, rat, monkey and dog. Health Phys 1971;20:375-382.

29. Furchner JE, Drake GA. Comparative metabolism of radionuclides in mammals - VI. Retention of Nb-95 in the mouse, rat, monkey and dog. Health Phys 1971;21:173-180.

30. Furchner JE, Richmond CR, Drake GA. Comparative metabolism of radionuclides in mammals - VII. Retention of Ru-106 in the mouse, rat, monkey and dog. Health Phys 1971;21:355-365.

31. Thomas JM, Eberhardt LL. Extrapolation of animal radionuclide retention data to man - Use of similarity ratios, in: Biological and environmental effects of low-level radiation. Vienna, International Atomic Energy Agency 1976;235-245.

32. McAfee JG, Subramanian G. Interpretation of interspecies differences in the biodistribution of radioactive agents, in: E.E. Watson et al., eds. Third International Radiopharmaceutical Dosimetry Symposium (HHS Publication FDA 81-8166), 1981:292-306.

33. Tsui BMW, Lathrop KA, Harper PV. Extrapolation from animals to the human for the retention of radiothallium in the blood, in: E.E. Watson et al., eds. Third International Radiopharmaceutical Dosimetry Symposium (HHS Publication FDA 81-8166), 1981:283-291.

34. Crawford DJ, Richmond CR. Epistemological considerations in the extrapolation of metabolic data from non humans to humans, in: E.E. Watson et al., eds. Third International Radiopharmaceutical Dosimetry Symposium (HHS Publication FDA 81-8166), 1981:181-197.

35. Lathrop KA. Collection and presentation of animal data relating to internally distributed radionuclides, in: E.E. Watson et al., eds. Third International Radiopharmaceutical Dosimetry Symposium (HHS Publication FDA 81-8166), 1981:198-203.

36. ICRP Publicaton 23. Report of the task group on reference man. Oxford, Pergamon Press, 1975.

37. Snyder WS, Ford MR, Warner GG, Watson SB. "S", absorbed dose per unit cumulated activity for selected radionuclides and organs. MIRD pamphlet No. 11. New York, Soc of Nucl Med, 1975.

38. Henrichs K, Kaul A. Dosimetrie inkorporierter radioaktiver Stoffe - Altersabhängige Werte der spezifischen absorbierten Bruchteile. StH-Bericht 1/1982 Berlin, Dietrich Reimer Verlag, 1982.

39. Henrichs K, Kaul A, Roedler HD. Estimation of age-dependent internal dose from radionuclides. Phys Med Biol 1982;27:775-784.

40. Roedler HD, Kaul A, Hine GJ. Internal radiation dose in diagnostic nuclear medicine. Berlin, Hildegard Hoffmann Verlag, 1978.

41. Kaul A, Henrichs K, Roedler HD. Radionuclide biokinetics and internal dosimetry in nuclear medicine. La Ricerca Clin Lab 1980;10:629-660.

42. Kaul A, Roedler HD. Dosimetrie, in: D. Emrich, ed. Nuklearmedizin - Funktionsdiagnostik, Stuttgart, Georg

Thieme Verlag 1980:107-120, 482-498.
43. Kaul A, Roedler HD, Hine GJ. Internal absorbed dose from administered radiopharmaceuticals, in: Medical Radionuclide Imaging, Vol. II. Vienna, International Atomic Energy Agency, 1977:423-453.
44. ICRP Publication 17. Protection of the patient in radionuclide investigations. Oxford, Pergamon Press, 1971.
45. Johansson L, Mattsson S, Nosslin B. Stråldoser fran radioaktiva ämnen i medicinskt bruk. Stockholm, Statens strålskyddsinstitut, 1981.
46. Smith T, Veall N, Altman DG. Dosimetry of renal radiopharmaceuticals: the importance of bladder radioactivity and a simple aid for its estimation. Brit J Radiol, 1981;54:961-965.
47. Jacobi W. Dosisgrenzwerte für berufliche Strahlenexposition - biologische Grundlagen, Festlegung, Interpretation - , in: G. Möhrle et al., eds. Kurslehrbuch für ermächtigte Ärzte, Berlin, Hildegard Hoffmann Verlag 1980:41-58.
48. Johansson L. S-values for bone surfaces with a source distributed homogeneously in bone volume or with a surface deposited source, in: E.E. Watson et al., eds. Third International Radiopharmaceutical Dosimetry Symposium (HHS Publication FDA 81-8166), 1981:554-562.
49. Rao DV, Govelitz GF, Sastry SR. Radiotoxicity of Thallium-201 in mouse testes: Inadequacy of conventional dosimetry. J Nucl Med 1983;24:145-153.
50. Reddy AR, Nagaratnam A, Kaul A, Haase V. Microdosimetry of internal emitters: A necessity? in:RJ. Cloutier et al., eds. Radiopharmaceutical Dosimetry Symposium (HEW Publication FDA 76-8044), 1976:174-185.
51. Hofer KG. Toxicity of radionuclides as a function of subcellular dose distribution, in: E.E. Watson et al., eds. Third International Radiopharmaceutical Dosimetry Symposium (HHS Publication FDA 81-8166), 1981:371-391.
52. Hofer KG. Microdosimetry of labelled cells. Paper presented at the Satellite Symposium "Labelled Cells" in Graz of the World Congress of Nuclear Medicine and Biology, 1982.
53. Henrichs K, Kaul A. Strahlenexposition von Kindern und Jugendlichen in der nuklearmedizinischen Diagnostik. Nucl Med 1980;19:228-231.
54. Roedler HD. Strahlenexposition des Patienten durch Radiopharmaka - Grenzen der Genauigkeit von Dosisberechnungen (Thesis) Berlin, Freie Universität, 1977.
55. Brown PH, Krishnamurthy GT, Bobba VVR, Kingston E. Radiation dose calculation for Tc-99m HIDA in health and disease. J Nucl Med 1981;22:177-183.
56. Wootton R, Hammond BJ. A computer simulation study of optimal thyroid radiation protection during investigation involving the administration of radioiodine-labelled radiopharmaceuticals. Brit J Radiol 1978;51:265-272.
57. Herzberg B, Kaul A, Meinhold H, Roedler HD. The additional radiation dose in patients due to radioactive impurities

178

in radionuclide generators, in: H.W. Pabst et al., eds. Nuklearmedizin-Ergebnisse in Technik, Klinik, Therapie Stuttgart, Schattauer Verlag 1974:639-642.

58. StH-Bericht 20/77. Ersatz von Jod-131 in der nuklearmedizinischen Diagnostik durch kurzlebige Radionuklide, insbesondere durch Jod-123. Berlin, Neuherberg, Institut für Strahlenhygiene des Bundesgesundheitsamtes, 1977.

59. Watson EE, Coffey JL. Radiation dosimetry of thallium-201 and its contaminants. Personal Communication, 1979.

60. Upton AC. Strahlenrisiko im Alltag. Spektrum der Wissenschaft, April 1982,28-37.

61. Larson SM, Siegel BA, Robinson RG. Guidelines for the clinical evaluation of radiopharmaceutical drugs. J Nucl Med 1978;19:1359-1362.

11. CLINICAL TRIALS OF RADIOPHARMACEUTICALS

PER JUUL

1. INTRODUCTION

A drug is any substance or product that is used or intended to be used to modify or explore physiological systems or pathological states for the benefit of the patient (1). Accordingly radiopharmaceuticals whether intended for scientific investigational purposes or for diagnostic or therapeutic purposes are covered by the definition and subject to the professional principles underlying the development of drugs in general - including the clinical trials. In this respect therapeutic radiopharmaceutical drugs do not differ from ordinary drugs, whereas particular problems are involved concerning diagnostic drugs, and mainly the latter ones shall be discussed.

Although clinical trials have been carried out for centuries the principles and practice employed today only dates back to 1960 (2). Numerous textbooks and monographs have been published on this topic (3, 4, 5, 6, 7). Despite the efforts in clinical pharmacology a large number of trials are still poorly performed and inadequately published (e.g. 8, 9, 10, 11, 12, 13).

Publications on diagnostic procedures focus on general problems in medical decision making (14, 15, 16, 17, 18), whereas no effort is spent on the principles of clinical trials of diagnostic drugs. The quality of published data and material accompanying new drug applications concerning diagnostic compounds are often too insufficient to allow an evaluation of clinical relevance, and the adaptation of some of the major principles behind the testing of ordinary drugs may prove valuable.

Apart from being used in diagnosis the use of diagnostic drugs form an integral part of the investigation of new methods of treatment, including new drugs (e.g. with regard to definition of patient material, patient selection, and evaluation of the effects of treatment), which makes a proper evaluation even more important.

2. DRUG REGULATION

In the majority of the Western countries the undertaking of clinical trials and the marketing of radiopharmaceuticals imply a notification or registration procedure based upon scientific evidence - as it is the case concerning other drugs. Apart from the national and international rules and regulations issued by official agencies and organizations and covering drugs in general, specific recommendations and requirements deal with the risks of ionizing radiation (e.g. 19) and specific guidelines for the clinical evaluation of radiopharmaceutical drugs have been issued (20).

As to be expected the restrictions caused by the official rules and regulations and the paperwork involved in notifications and applications to national regulatory agencies, ethical review committees, adverse reactions committees et cetera have been met with opposition by industry, experts, and clinicians due to the resulting constraint on the development and clinical use of new drugs (e.g. 21, 22). However, past experience with ordinary drugs as well as with radiopharmaceuticals demonstrates the necessity to investigate both efficacy and safety according to updated scientific standards. Furthermore clinical trials have become a matter of public concern, and finally political interest is involved in the evaluation of the ressources spent on health-care activities.

3. CLINICAL TRIALS
3.1. Definitions

A clinical trial is an investigation in man intended to provide new information or to confirm existing knowledge of the pharmacokinetics and/or -dynamics of a drug. In the present context pharmacodynamics comprise "diagnostic value" and toxicity. When the experiment is conducted as a comparative investigation it is described as a controlled clinical trial. A randomized clinical trial (RCT) is an investigation comparing two or more procedures to which the patients are randomly allocated, based upon a systematic collection of clinically relevant data, the nature and number of which enable a conclusive numerical analysis, and following an experimental design which -as far as possible -excludes the influence on the result by unrelated conditions.

3.2 Strategy

Traditionally the clinical investigations are divided into four phases: Phase 1 comprising the initial studies in a few healthy volunteers (immediate safety and kinetics), phase 2 comprising a limited number of patients (detailed kinetic analysis with regard to "diagnostic accuracy"), phase 3 forming more comprehensive, preferably controlled studies, and phase 4 dealing with postmarketing surveillance (clinical relevance under routine conditions and detection of adverse reactions; final cost/benefit analysis). A distinct separation does not exist between the various phases, but the phase-system contains the important elements to be considered when a new diagnostic procedure is being developed.

The investigations from the early animal experiments (the preclinical investigations) throughout the various clinical phases including postmarketing surveillance must follow a particular, coherent plan consisting of a logical sequence of steps ("the chain of prediction") based upon a superior, well-considered and careful schedule leading to a final, conclusive evaluation (Fig. 1).

The "flow-sheet" developed by the responsible principal investigator should allow a stepwise progression of the trials based upon preceding results. The common lack of adherence to the plan causes needless investigations (e.g. unnecessary repetitions), invalid conclusions and delayed marketing. Under normal conditions the development of a new drug takes several years and may require millions of dollars. Therefore the

stepwise progression should also allow the earliest possible
cessation of the development in case of unforeseen adverse
reactions or lack of efficacy.

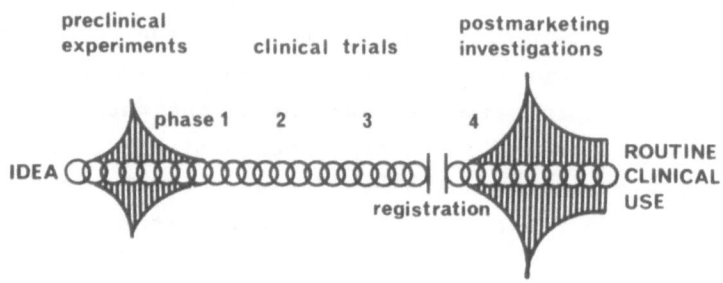

FIGURE 1. The strategies including the clinical phases
involved in the development of a new drug.

3.3. Protocol

The preparation of a meticulous protocol for each clinical
trial is the prerequisite for an acceptable result (23). The
question to be answered by the trial must be specified and
should preferably be simple. The design of the trial must be
tailored to the solution of the actual problem. A few points
of particular interest shall be commented upon.

3.3.1. Selection. Initially a well defined sample of
patients must be studied. Even this apparently simple approach
may create problems, since the criteria used for the
definition of the disease entity are often variable and the
object of discussion, perhaps even the purpose of the new
diagnostic procedure (e.g. the diagnosis of alcoholic
cirrhosis "verified" by anamnesis, clinical signs and
symptoms, a series of clinical chemical analyses, liver
function tests, liver biopsy et cetera (24). The selection
criteria are crucial, since the conclusion is only valid
concerning this subpopulation. Very strict inclusion criteria
often improve the possibility of a conclusive result -but with
a narrow application, whereas wide inclusion criteria may lead
to a "negative" result. It is most often difficult to
establish a suitable balance between these two extremes. As a
general rule the inclusion criteria should widen during phase

3 studies.

3.3.2. Design. Although retrospective investigations may give valid information and concerning certain diagnostic procedures may be the only way to obtain conclusive results, the advantages of prospective trials with consecutive patient recruitment shall be stressed. To ensure the important consecutive recruitment according to the inclusion criteria a close collaboration with a responsible clinician is necessary.

Part of the clinical trials must be carried out as controlled trials - though not necessarily as randomized clinical trials.

3.3.3. Safety. The requirements with regard to preclinical toxicity studies are modest concerning drugs intended for a single or a few administrations (e.g. 1, 3, 20). With ordinary drugs the inevitable risk during the early phase 1 studies is extremely small (25). With diagnostic radiopharmaceutical drugs the risk of adverse reactions caused by a few mg of "active" ingredient is even smaller. However, allergic reactions, febrile reactions due to pyrogens, certain vascular effects caused by macromolecules, and effects caused by excipients may be observed. It is therefore important that at least part of the animal toxicity studies as well as the clinical trials involve the radiopharmaceutical prepared in the final form intended for marketing (including the instrumentation involved). Taking into account an average, overall incidence of adverse reactions of 1-6 per 100,000 diagnostic examinations (26) it is obvious that such reactions are almost never encountered in the small-scale premarketing trials (27, 28). The potential risks of low level radiation exposure have been discussed in detail elsewhere (e.g. 19, 29).

3.3.4. End-point. In clinical trials of ordinary drugs it is often difficult to define and measure the end-point, i.g. the efficacy. However, the problems are much bigger when dealing with diagnostic drugs. Any clinical evaluation of diagnostic performance involves a comparison with the "truth", which is only rarely known. An unsophisticated view of "diagnostic value" would be the measure of diagnostic decision resulting in a treatment that would improve the condition and/or prognosis of the patient. However, the end-point of a trial of diagnostic drugs involve a whole series of concepts that will influence the final evaluation of cost/benefit: Nosographic and diagnostic sensitivity and specificity, diagnostic efficacy, management efficacy and outcome efficacy, within and between observer variation, kappa statistics, receiver operating characteristic analysis et cetera (14, 15, 16, 17, 18, 30, 31 ,32, 33, 34). To most clinicians the "diagnostic value" of a test is a vague synthesis of the above mentioned (often difficult) concepts. The use of an unexplained, sophisticated nomenclature in published reports may invalidate the possible clinical utilization of the results.

3.3.5. <u>Withdrawal of subjects</u>. A major problem in any drug trial is the number of patients available for investigation and follow-up (Fig. 2).

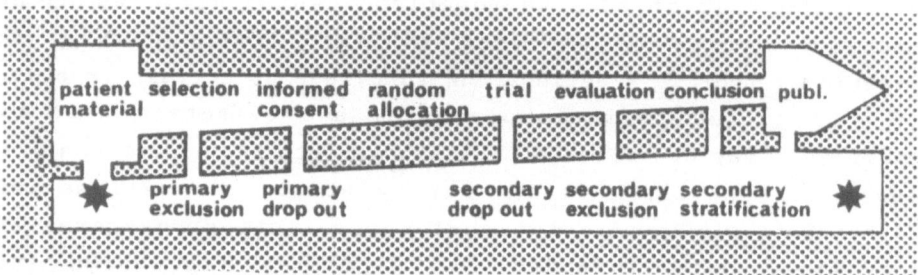

FIGURE 2. Withdrawal of patients during a clinical trial.

The assumed number of patients diminishes for various reasons at the initiation of the trial. If strict selection criteria are applied a number of patients will deliberately be excluded. Some patients refuse to participate in connection with the informed consent. During the trial a number of patients drop out, among other things due to the severity of the disease. During the evaluation phase some patients may be excluded because of lack of adherence to the original inclusion criteria, unforeseen errors during the trial et cetera. Secondary stratification of the material may increase the possibility of erroneous conclusions. Finally negative results are published more rarely than positive ones. Thus the

final information available to the reader of scientific
journals may represent a very distorted picture comprising a
group of patients not being representative for the patient
population originally described - and the paper may not even
disclose what has really happened from idea to publication.

These problems cannot be solved in general, but at least
any published paper on clinical trials should include a
careful account for the original and resulting patient
material including the reasons for exclusions and drop-out.

3.3.6 Ethics. Clinical trials of diagnostic drugs are
covered by the declaration of Helsinki II (35, 36), which
among other things implies the use of informed consent. This
point may give rise to particular problems due to public
animosity against ionizing radiation (37).

4. CONTROLLED CLINICAL TRIALS
4.1. Reference group

Every medical decision involves an element of comparison.
Part of the clinical trials of a new drug - including a
diagnostic drug - must be comparative. The most obvious
question is: What may be achieved by the use of a new
diagnostic method compared with existing ones? The existing
methods (the reference) may be radiopharmaceutical,
radiological, clinical, pathological, clinical chemical et
cetera or a combination of some of these.

The simplest form of reference group is the historical
control. Assuming that no diagnostic method exists to detect a
certain disease and that a new method is developed which
possesses high diagnostic sensitivity and specificity (e.g. a
cancer tag), then a historical control would be acceptable.

More likely is the situation that a new diagnostic method
is added to a battery of existing ones. The change of
diagnosis, patient management and clinical outcome as a result
of the addition of the new method may be measured as the
efficacy of the new method in comparison with a reference
group not being subject to the new diagnostic examination.

4.2. Number of patients

With an estimate of the diagnostic value of existing

methods, a selection of minimum clinically relevant difference and choice of 2 alfa and beta, the number of patients necessary for the trial may be estimated (38, 39).

5. RANDOMIZED CLINICAL TRIALS

The design of a randomized clinical trial is schematically shown in Fig. 3.

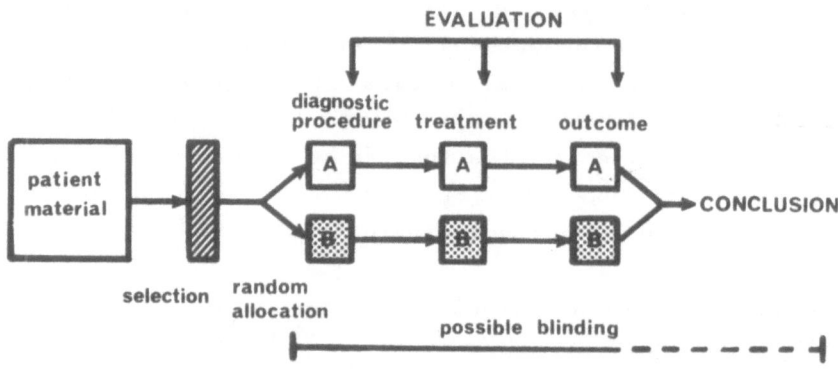

FIGURE 3. The design of a randomized clinical trial of a diagnostic drug.

The obvious advantage of the randomized clinical trial is the random allocation of the patients to two or more groups, which - if performed correctly - minimizes the risk of many types of bias otherwise involved in clinical trials. The trial may be "blinded" in various ways, but this is not prerequisite. The design may be modified, e.g. by using a cross-over technique. The results may be calculated at the end of the trial concerning groups of patients, or the design may use matched pairs and a sequential analysis.

To answer the question: Is the new method better than the existing ones? the randomized clinical trial is ideally the relevant tool (provided that a clinically relevant end-point can be defined and measured).

The risk of an erroneous positive conclusion (i.e. the finding of a difference that does not exist) is called a type I error. The size of this probability is always stated in the publications. The risk of an erroneous negative conclusion (i.e. the finding of no difference that in fact does exist) is called a type II error. The probability of a type II error in negative trials should be calculated. However, the risk of a type II error is often not published (11).

The randomized clinical trial is rightly the best tool for the evaluation of new therapeutic drugs. However, it is far from being the ideal or only tool, and in some ways it seems less suited to evaluate diagnostic drugs. One of the major problems is that the often complicated trial situation in itself changes the diagnostic and therapeutic performance in a way that makes an extrapolation to routine clinical conditions invalid. Blinding procedures may involve an external observer and create further unrealistic circumstances. In the present context it is furthermore unrealistic to compare a single new diagnostic method with an existing one, since normally the method will be only a single piece of the jig-saw puzzle.

However, considering the definite advantages of the randomized clinical trial, the performance of at least a few trials of this kind (part of which using a blinding technique) during the development of a new radiopharmaceutical is indispensable.

6. POSTMARKETING SURVEILLANCE

6.1 Purpose

Large-scale studies performed after the marketing of a new radiopharmaceutical have two main objectives: To perform a cost/benefit analysis of the method when employed under routine clinical conditions and to reveal possible adverse reactions. The value of the diagnostic method may rely on uncontrolled studies, which sometimes may even advantageously be retrospective.

Another important postmarketing activity is the collection of papers published on a particular diagnostic method in an attempt to assess the actual diagnostic value (e.g. 40, 41, 42). Striking features of these literature surveys are: The limited number of papers fulfilling the basic criteria for evaluation, the small sample sizes in most reported series, and the considerable inhomogeneity in results. Superficially the results may seem frustrating. However, often the actual value of the diagnostic method in the individual clinical situation cannot be evaluated on the basis of these literature surveys. The results furthermore should be an incitement to perform future studies according to well-defined and accepted criteria and to include the interpretative criteria in the final publication.

7. SUMMARY

The clinical pharmacological principles and practice involved in the development of ordinary drugs may profitably be adopted to the evaluation of radiopharmaceuticals for diagnostic use. The strategy comprising a coherent plan extending from the preclinical experiments to postmarketing surveillance is emphasized. The importance of a meticulous clinical trials protocol is stressed. It is necessary that at least part of the clinical documentation consists of controlled trials. The recruitment of the patients must be consecutive, and particular attention should be paid to selection criteria, definition of a clinically relevant end-point (diagnostic value), reference group, number of patients included and withdrawals. Final evaluation of cost/benefit can only be obtained by further postmarketing surveillance studies and critical reviews of published reports.

REFERENCES
1. Principles for preclinical testing of drug safety: report of WHO Scientific Group. WHO Technical Report Series, No. 341, Geneva 1966.
2. Hill AB.Controlled clinical trials. Blackwell 1960.
3. Guidelines for evaluation of drugs for use in man: report of a WHO Scientific Group. WHO Technical Report Series, No. 563, Geneva 1975.
4. Harris EL, Fitzgerald JD, eds. The principles and practice of clinical trials. Livingstone, Edingburgh and London 1970.
5. Good CS, ed. The principles and practice of clinical trials. Churchill Livingstone, Edingburgh, London and New York 1976.
6. Wardell WM, Velo G, eds. Drug development, regulatory assessment, and postmarketing surveillance. Plenum Press, New York and London 1980.

7. Cavalla JF, ed. Risk-benefit analysis in drug research. MTP Press Limited, Lancaster, Boston, The Hague 1981.
8. Lionel NDW, Herxheimer A. Assessing reports of therapeutic trials. Brit med J 1970;3:637-640.
9. Christensen E, Juhl E, Tygstrup N. Randomized clinical trials of a decade (1964 to 1974). Gastroenterol 1977;73:1170-1178.
10. Christensen E, Juhl E, Tygstrup N. Treatment of gastric ulcer. The randomized clinical trials from 1964 to 1974 and their impact. Amer J Gastroenterol 1978;69:272-282.
11. Freiman JA, Chalmers TC, Smith H. Kuebler RR. The importance of beta, the type II error and sample size in the design and interpretation of the randomized control trial. Survey of 71 "negative" trials. New Engl J Med 1978;299:690-694.
12. Tygstrup N, Christensen E, Juhl E. Randomisierte klinische Therapiestudien in der Hepatologie. Internist 1979;20:565-570.
13. DerSimonian R, Charette L, McPeek B, Mosteller F. Reporting on methods in clinical trials. New Engl J Med 1982;306:1332-1337.
14. Lusted MB. Introduction to medical decision making. CC Thomas, Springfield 1968.
15. Lindley DV. Making decisions. Wiley & Sons, New York 1971.
16. Koran LM. The reliability of clinical methods, data and judgements. New Engl J Med 1975;293:642-646.
17. Koran LM. The reliability of clinical methods, data and judgements. New Engl J Med 1975;293:695-701.
18. Wulff HR. Rational diagnosis and treatment. Blackwell Scientific Publications, London 1976.
19. Use of ionizing radiation and radionuclides on human beings for medical research, training, and nonmedical purposes: report of a WHO Expert Committee. WHO Technical Report Series, No. 611. Geneva 1977.
20. Guidelines for the clinical evaluation of radiopharmaceutical drugs. Food and Drug Administration 1981.
21. Gross F. Constraints of drug regulation on the development of drugs. Arch Toxicol 1979;43:9-17.
22. Gottschalk A. Radiopharmaceuticals: Admiration, enthusiasm, and despair. Year Book of Nuclear Medicine 1982:183-186. Year Book Med Publ Inc, Chicago and London 1982.
23. Maxwell C. Clinical trials protocol. Stuart Phillips Publ., Surrey 1969.
24. Shreiner DP, Barlai-Kovach M. Diagnosis of alcoholic cirrhosis with right-to left hepatic lobe ratio: Concise communication. J Nucl Med 1981;22:116-120
25. Zarafonetis CJD. Rilej PA, Willis PW, Power LH, Werbelow J, Farhat L, Beckwith W, Marks BH. Clinically significant adverse effects in phase I testing program. Clin Pharmacol Ther 1978;24:127-132.
26. Rhodes BA, Cordova MM. Adverse reactions to radiopharmaceuticals: Incidence in 1978 and associated symptoms. J Nucl Med 1980;21:1107.

27. Mitchell AA, Slone D, Shapiro S, Goldman P. Adverse drug effects and drug surveillance. In: Yaffe SJ, ed. Pediatric pharmacology. Grune & Stratton Inc. 1980.
28. Newbould BB. The effect of industry. In: Cavalla JF, ed. Risk-benefit analysis in drug research. MTP Press Limited, Lancaster, Boston, The Hague 1981:17-26.
29. Bond V. Radiation cancer risk; What is "safe" exposure? Proc Conf Known Effects of Low Level Radiation Exposure. NIH Publ No. 80-2087. 1980: 123-137.
30. Yerushalmy J. Statistical problems in assessing methods of medical diagnosis with special reference to X-ray technics, In: Neyman J, ed. Outline of statistical treatment of the problem of diagnosis. Pub Health Rep 1947;62:1431.
31. Conn HO, Spencer CP. Observer error in liver scans. Gastroenterol 1972;62:1085-1090.
32. Metz CE. Basic principles of ROC analysis. Sem Nucl Med 1978;VIII:283-298.
33. Lusted LB. General problems in medical decision making with comments on ROC analysis. Sem Nucl Med 1978;VIII:299-306.
34. Bell RS. Efficacy. Whats that?? Sem Nucl Med 1978;VIII:316-323.
35. Declaration of Helsinki. Recommendations guiding medical doctors in biomedical research involving human subjects. Tokyo 1975.
36. Research involving human subjects. WHO Drug Information. October-December 1980:2-14.
37. McNeil BJ, Pauker SG, Sox HC, Tversky A. On the elicitation of preferences for alternative therapies. New Engl J Med 1982;21:1259-1262.
38. Halperin M, Rogot E. Gurian J. Ederer F. Sample sizes for medical trials with special reference to long-term therapy. J chron Dis 1968;21:13-24.
39. Feinstein AR, Clinical biostatistics XXXIV. The other side of "statistical significance": alpha, beta, delta, and the calculation of sample size. Clin Pharmacol Ther 1975;18:491-505.
40. Teates CT, Bray ST, Williamson BRJ. Tumor detection with 67-Ga-citrate: A literature survey (1970-1978). Clin Nucl med 1978;3:456-459.
41. Fritz SL, Preston DF, Gallagher JH. ROC analysis of diagnostic performance in liver scintigraphy. J Nucl Med 1981;22:121-128.
42. Christensen M, Rødbro P. The diagnostic value of liver scintigraphy to disclose metastases in patients with suspected or proven gastrointestinal cancer. A critical review of the literature. Dan Med Bull 1982;29:206-208.

12.   EVALUATION OF CLINICAL INFORMATION

HARRIET DICE-PETERSEN

1. INTRODUCTION

Evaluating the clinical utility of diagnostic radiopharmaceuticals is a complicated process, considering - among other things - adverse reactions, radiation dose, stability in vitro and in vivo, drug interaction, pharmacokinetics, costs, acceptability and clinical efficacy. The latter point is the main subject of this paper, which aims at defining a logic structure for clinical evaluation.

However, conclusions based on even well structured clinical information may be hampered by fundamental problems of medical practice, first of all related to the fact that an objective diagnostic truth and/or specific therapy are often non-existent. Disease classifications are man-made, and the final health outcome may not be a simple result of the therapy chosen. This means that logic reasoning during the evaluation procedure may not be founded on solid ground. Accordingly, terms like specificity and sensitivity refer to no more than to-days medical practice, and are no more meaningful than the end-point available.

Other problems arise when the making of rational decisions must be superseded by ethical necessities or financial costs. Nuclear medicine has been born into these impediments, considering radiation dose problems, increasing financial costs, and series of medical rituals -including diagnostic tests - of which the benefit has never been measured, but which form the yardstick of to-day.

2. CLINICAL DECISION MAKING

Evaluation of clinical information obtained from trials of

"new" diagnostic radiopharmaceuticals should be viewed as part
of the complete process of clinical decision making. As an
example of such strategy fig. 1 goes through the hypothetico-
deductive method, which is probably the most wide spread in
clinical practice (1,2). From the figure it appears that new
tests may be compared to other diagnostic tests, either used
at the same level of the diagnostic procedure or at a "higher"
level (1.-n.). The hypothetico-deductive system implies that
the "diagnosis" be revised by the successive steps in the
procedure (fig. 1, dotted lines), i.e. primary and secondary
tests, effect of treatment, final health outcome etc. The
reference "diagnosis" used during a trial may thus be 1) a
single test result or preliminary hypothesis, or 2) may be
based on certain test outcomes, or 3) may include the
treatment outcome. Finally 4) the health outcome, ranging from
cure to death, may be the final reference.
Accordingly, diagnostic information obtained from trials
include a variable proportion of the complete clinical
decision making procedure. Both when planning the trial and
when evaluating the information obtained the degree of
complexity, necessary for any specific problem should be
considered - and reconsidered.

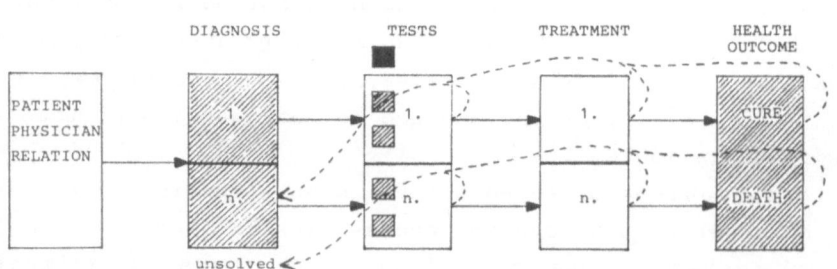

FIGURE 1. HYPOTHETICO DEDUCTIVE METHOD
The trial test ■ must not be part of the clinical diagnosis
used as clinical end-point. The test may be compared to other
tests, to the diagnosis, or to health outcome.▨

3. TYPES OF CLINICAL INFORMATION

The design of clinical trials determines not only the amount and the quality of information supplied, but also the type of information to be obtained.

Table 1 relates the different types of trials to the type of information given. The subdivision is far from complete or ideal, and comprises only phases 2 - 4.

Table 1. RELATION BETWEEN TRIAL DESIGN AND TYPE OF INFORMATION OBTAINED

TRIAL	REFERENCE TEST	CLINICAL END-POINT	TYPE OF INFORMATION CONSEQUENCE
"PILOT"	NONE	DIAGNOSIS BY OTHER MEANS	PRELIMINARY INFORMATION ON TEST QUALITY (DESCRIPTIVE) DISCARDED/FURTHER TRIALS
COMPARATIVE	NUCLEAR MED. OTHER	REFERENCE TEST	TEST PRECISION TEST "ACCURACY" ACCEPTED/DISCARDED
COMPARATIVE	NUCLEAR MED. OTHER	DIAGNOSIS BY OTHER MEANS	TEST PRECISION TEST ACCURACY ACCEPTED/DISCARDED DIAGNOSTIC STRATEGY
SCIENTIFIC	?	HEALTH OUT-COME	SCIENTIFIC PATHOBIOCHEMISTRY-PHYSIOLOGY POTENTIALS: CHOOSE/ADJUST THERAPY REVISE DIAGNOSTIC SYSTEM DEVELOP NEW THERAPY ETC.

3.1. "Pilot" studies, as defined here, are not controlled trials, but consist of "pattern recognition evaluation" in single patients. Most often minor variants of well-known radiopharmaceuticals are subjected to this type of testing. The result of any one test is referred to the diagnosis or clinical problem of the patient, and no statistical evaluation can be performed. Usually the individual study is classified as "excellent, fair, bad ....." regarding diagnostic information and test quality. This type of documentation is poor, and should not be accepted as the final trial when essentially new drugs are concerned - and in fact should never be accepted as the only type of trial prior to registration.

3.2. Comparative studies (including all sorts of randomized trials) should be planned in such a way that sufficient statistical information as to test reliability is available. One or more of these types of trials are to be chosen whenever essentially new diagnostic agents are marketed. The reference method may be other nuclear medicine studies, radiology, ultrasound, computerized tomography, biochemistry etc. In the simplest form such studies may show, if a new test gives similar information as a reference test, e.g. does liver scintigraphy classify patients into the same groups as ultrasound. In this case the liver diagnosis has been defined as the ultrasound diagnosis, which is, accordingly, the clinical end-point. However, usually an independent clinical end-point is settled by means of one or more other techniques, biopsy, surgery or autopsy, i.e. independently of both test and reference test. Large groups of patients with a diagnosis thus "verified" may, however, be hard to obtain. Nevertheless, for planning of future diagnostic strategy this latter type of information is clearly necessary.

3.3. The last type of information to be mentioned may be called scientific. It results from trials of essentially new radiopharmaceuticals, synthesized according to hitherto unknown principles, which may be based on biochemical science rather than conventional diagnostic experience. Promising examples are radioactive tracers measuring brain blood flow, oxygen metabolism or deoxyglucose metabolism. The role of such tracers may be mapping of brain function as a guide for surgical or radiation therapy, or they may be used for monitoring treatment effect. Another example is monoclonal tumourspecific antibodies. Last but not least, scientific information thus obtained may be the starting point of new pathobiochemical understanding and a subsequent development of pharmacotherapy. The evaluation of this type of clinical information is a long and demanding process, for which definite rules cannot be given.

4. EVALUATION OF TRIAL QUALITY
4.1. Patients and controls

The number of and the selection of patients and controls as to age, sex, associated disease and other factors is - of course- highly important for the quality of any trial. It is worth while to keep in mind that the group of controls may heavily influence the statistical results. They may be strictly normal or they may be selected among patients who present relevant differential diagnostic problems. Bone scintigraphy in children suspected of osteomyelitis and purulent arthritis has in some papers a close to one hundred per cent nosographic specificity (3). In our hands (to be published) the figure was 50%, without doubt because the controls were chosen among children presenting similar clinical symptoms, the final diagnoses including e.g. other types of arthritis. Thus, false positive ratios may be misleading without a thorough definition of control diagnoses. In studies known to be non-specific but highly sensitive -such as bone scintigraphy - a false positive result must be defined according to the clinical situation.

4.2. Test procedure

The complete study protocol including test procedure, detailed description of technical equipment and performance, counting statistics etc. should be given. An inappropriate technical performance may invalidate the results of otherwise well planned trials.

4.3. Description and classification of results

The method of classifying results, binary, graded or a continuum, must be part of the trial plan, and never a post-trial agreement, which would make bias much too likely.

"Blinding" of observers is a classical way to avoid bias, which may arise due to knowledge of patient diagnosis, symptoms, other tests etc. As a worst case may be mentioned "circular" diagnostic reasoning where the results of the test in question is used as part of the clinical end-point. Looking once again at the situation with bone scintigraphy in osteomyelitis in children: "Blinded" evaluation implies that the observer does not know which part of the body is suspected, he may not know anything about difficulties during the examination such as movements or positioning. Thus, blinding techniques may certainly test the procedure even harder than every-day life.

Observer variation should be handled as a special part of the study. In addition it must be decided whether statistical values describing the test accuracy should be based on single-observer results or on a "conference" result in order to simulate the routine of nuclear medicine departments. Obviously, there is no simple answer to these questions, but it seems important to point out that the evaluation procedure as such must be carefully described.

5. DECISION MAKING

The rather simple basic problem is to find methods - and to describe the reliability of these methods - which can detect disease in diseased persons and exclude disease in those without, considering also financial and health benefit/cost relations and the amount of diagnostic information provided. In the following a brief introduction to some methods is given; for a more extensive review, see references.

5.1. The decision matrix

The matrix shown in Table 2 can be used for binary data which are often related to a binary clinical end-point as well (yes/no). From such data we may calculate the ratios indicated in the table (4,5,6).

Table 2

TEST	DISEASE		
RESULT	Yes	No	Total
Abnormal	a	c	a + c
Normal	b	d	b + d
Total	a + b	c + d	

TP = true positive ratio: $\dfrac{a}{a + b}$ (sensitivity)

FP = false positive ratio: $\dfrac{c}{c + d}$

TN = true negative ratio: $\dfrac{d}{c + d}$ (specificity)

FN = false negative ratio: $\dfrac{b}{a + b}$

Predictive Value of positive test = $\dfrac{a}{a + c}$ (PV pos)

Predictive Value of negative test = $\dfrac{d}{b + d}$ (PV neg)

The true positive ratio is the (nosographic) sensitivity of the examination and the true negative ratio is the (nosographic) specificity. Obviously, tests with a high sensitivity and specificity are wanted in clinical practice.

However, practically no test is perfect. So the terms given are not a sufficient description of the test quality in the bedside situation. We should ask for the following probabilities: What is the probability that a patient has the disease, if the test is positive (predictive value of positive test). If the result is negative, what is the probability of no disease (predictive value of negative test). These probabilities efficiently characterize the test in the clinical situation. The predictive values are, however, dependent on the prevalence of disease in the study group, that is the prior probability of disease. Theoretical examples are given below, symbols as in Table 2.

$$\text{Ex. 1: } a = 50, \ b = 50, \ c = 10, \ d = 90$$

$$\frac{a + b}{a + b + c + d}$$

Prevalence 50%

TP = 0.50,　　　TN = 0.90

PV pos = 0.83

PV neg = 0.64

Example 1 shows that a test with a sensitivity of (only) 50% may be acceptable in a selected study group, i.e. relatively high prior probability of disease. The post-test probability of disease is 83% for a positive result. A supplementary test is, however, needed with a negative result, because it gives only 64% probability of no disease.

$$\text{Ex. 2: } a = 10, \ b = 10, \quad c = 20, \ d = 160$$

Prevalence 10%

TP = 0.50,　　TN = 0.89

PV pos = 0.33

PV neg = 0.94

Example 2 illustrates the change in predictive values due only to a change in prevalence.

5.2. ROC analysis

Few results are adequately expressed as dichotomous values, but rather as a continuum. The Receiver Operating Characteristic curve (ROC analysis) (4,5,7,8) describes the relation between the false-positive ratio (FP) and the true-positive ratio (TP) for a range of data (fig. 2). The proportion of patients classified as "diseased" or "not-diseased" depends upon where the cut-off point is placed on the result scale. The selection of a proper cut-off point depends on the prior possibility of disease prevalence and on the benefit/cost relationship of the disease. If e.g. a serious but curable disease is looked for, one would probably choose a high true positive ratio (sensitivity) whereas some false positives may be accepted. Accordingly a cut-off point close to a true positive ratio of 1.0 is selected.

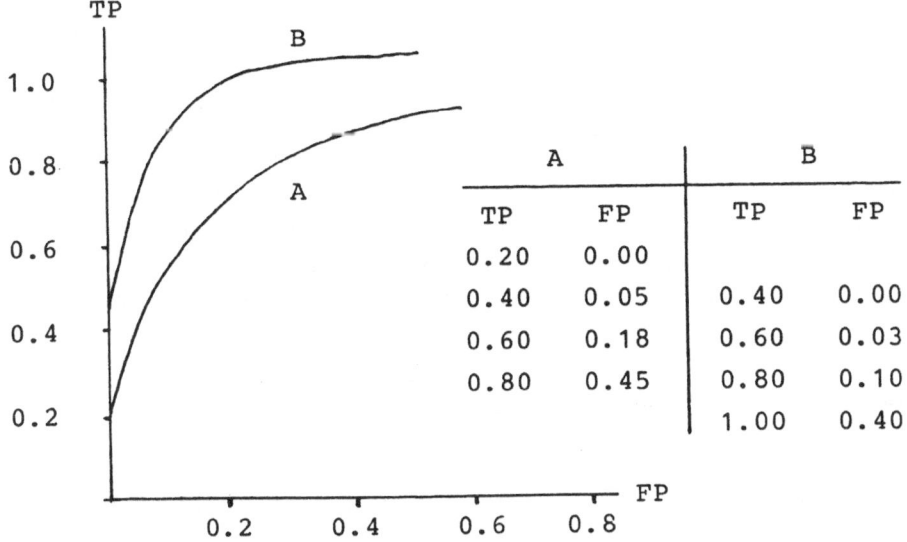

FIGURE 2. HYPOTHETICAL ROC CURVES
TP = true positive ratio, FP = false positive ratio
At the left extreme both tests have poor sensitivity and high
or relatively high specificity. At the upper extreme the tests
show the opposite characteristics. The improvement from test A
to B is illustrated.

5.3. Bayes´ Theorem

Bayes´ theorem is a technique that allows us to calculate
post-test probabilities of disease, i.e. predictive values of
the test, once a diagnostic test has been characterized as to
(nosographic) sensitivity and specificity, and when the prior
probability of disease is known (4,5,7,8). Thus, for
consecutive tests, the predictive value of the first test is
defined as prior probability and the result as posterior
probability and so forth. If trial design is ideal, we can
obtain a quantitative estimate of the diagnostic improvement
obtained by supplementary tests. It is necessary to know the
true positive (TP) and false positive (FP) ratios and the
false negative (FN) and true negative (TN) ratios as well as
the prior probability of disease (PD+) or not disease (PD-).
The formula is as follows:

$$\text{Posterior probability of disease (positive test)} = \frac{TP \times PD+}{TP \times PD+ + FP \times PD-}$$

$$\text{Posterior probability of no disease (negative test)} = \frac{FN \times PD+}{FN \times PD+ + TN \times PD-}$$

In order to illustrate these formulas we may use the hypothetical ROC curve B (fig. 2). Assuming that we study a group of patients in whom the prior probability of disease is 30% and that we use a cut-off point corresponding to a true positive ratio of 0.90, the posterior probability of disease is as follows:

$$\text{Posterior probability (positive test)} = \frac{0.90 \times 0.30}{0.90 \times 0.30 + 0.15 \times 0.70} = 0.72$$

$$\text{Posterior probability (negative test)} = \frac{0.10 \times 0.30}{0.10 \times 0.30 + 0.85 \times 0.70} = 0.048$$

An abnormal test changed the probability of disease from 30% to 72%, whereas a negative test reduced the probability of no disease from 30% to 4.8%. This test design would be well suited for excluding disease in this group of patients.

Obviously, this type of evaluation is highly important when planning diagnostic strategy.

5.4. Intra- and interobservervariation

The reliability of methods is described not only in terms of accuracy (sensitivity, specificity and predictive values) but also by precision. Some intra- and interobservervariation can hardly be avoided when the results - such as evaluation of scintigrams - is a matter of judgment. There are several statistical ways of defining observervariation, e.g. (7).

5.5. Benefit/cost relations

Knowledge of, not only the reliability of available tests, but also the benefit/cost relation for a given hypothetical diagnosis, allows the physician to make a rational choice between "treatment" or "no treatment" at any step in the diagnostic procedure (10,11). If the benefit of treatment is high as compared to the risk of untreated disease (high health cost) the "threshold probability" of disease may be very low (e.g. 10% or lower) for choosing immediate therapy. If, on the contrary, benefit is low in relation to cost, the diagnosis should be very safe (high threshold probability) prior to treatment.

To-day the use of benefit/cost "analysis" is often more intuitive than detailed and rational. Nevertheless, useful theory on this part of clinical decision making has been developed, although only introductory remarks can be given in this paper.

6. CONCLUSION

Evaluation of clinical information obtained in trials may be more or less complex, as it may include only one - or in extreme cases - all steps of the clinical decision making process relevant to the problem.

The type of information obtained in trials must be defined, e.g. it may be merely descriptive, it may define test reliability as compared to the results of other studies on several levels, or it may be scientific.

The statistical treatment of data must describe both the precision and the accuracy of the test, and if possible lead to decisions on diagnostic strategy, regarding also benefit/cost relations.

The final conclusion as to clinical efficacy should be an intelligent synthesis of all relevant clinical information, related to to-day's medical practise and/or the potentials of tomorrow.

REFERENCES
1. Campbell EJM. Basic science, science, and medical education. Lancet 1976; i: 134-136.
2. Editorial. The value of diagnostic tests. Lancet 1979; i: 809-810.
3. Duszynsky DO, Kuhn JP, Afshani E, Riddlesberger MM jr. Early radionuclide diagnosis of acute osteomyelitis. Radiology 1975; 117: 337-340.
4. McNeil BJ, Keeler E, Adelstein SJ. Primer on certain elements of medical decision making. N Engl J Med 1975; 293: 211-215.
5. McNeil BJ, Adelstein SJ. Determining the value of diagnostic screening tests. J Nucl Med 1976; 17: 439-448.

6. Vecchio TJ. Predictive value of a single diagnostic test in unselected populations. N Engl J Med 1966; 274: 1171-1173.
7. Metz CE. Basic principles of ROC analysis. Sem Nucl Med 1978; 8: 283-298.
8. Lusted LB. General problems in medical decision making with comments on ROC analysis. Sem Nucl Med 1978; 8: 299-3o6.
9. Koran LM. The reliability of clinical methods, data and judgement (First of two parts). N Engl J Med 1975; 293: 642-646.
10. Schwartz WB, Gorry GA, Kassirer JP et al. Decision analysis and clinical judgement. Am J Med 1973; 55: 459-472.
11. Pauker SG, Kassirer JP. Therapeutic decision making: A costbenefit analysis. N Engl J Med 1975; 293: 229-234.

13. COMPARATIVE EVALUATION OF DRUGS

ROLF DE JONG AND WIM B. HUISING

1. INTRODUCTION

In most countries radiopharmaceutical drugs have now become recognized as substances which require reviewing and acceptance by a governmental agency before the medical profession is allowed their unrestricted use. However many uncertainties still exist about the basis for reviewing. Usually radiopharmaceuticals do not fit the concepts which apply to pharmaceuticals in general. Therefore it is often extremely unsatisfactory to apply the rules, developed for the evaluation of drugs to the process of evaluating a radioactive drug. In this presentation we will try to explore to what extent evaluation procedures accepted in the evaluation of pharmaceuticals may or may not be used in evaluating radio-pharmaceuticals.

2. GOVERNMENTAL REQUIREMENTS

Almost invariably governmental agencies require proof of safety and efficacy of a drug before it is being released to the public. As far as radiopharmaceuticals are concerned the Food and Drug Administration in USA have probably been the first to formulate a set of proposed rules, later followed by a set of guidelines for the clinical evaluation of radio-pharmaceutical drugs(1,2). These guidelines state that scientific evidence is to be provided to substantiate the safety and efficacy of the radioactive drug under investigation for its proposed diagnostic or therapeutic indications. If not in exactly the same wording the majority of other countries have adopted similar rules. The opinions of how the formal requirements for proof of safety and efficacy must be met, tend to differ considerably from country to country, and notably with time. Both the concept of radio-pharmaceuticals as such, and the experience with their registration is under steady development. Obviously every opinion, every approach is mainly based on the experience obtained with and the procedures involved for pharmaceuticals used for therapeutic purposes. At this time radiopharma-ceutical drugs which are supposed to exert a therapeutic action are very rare, so rare that it is not worthwhile to consider them in the scope of this presentation.Radiopharma-ceutical drugs are essentially intended for diagnostic purposes and this fact has great influence on the approach to proving safety and efficacy.

The IFPMA publication "Requirements for Drug Registration" (3) presents a survey to what extent other criteria than quality, safety and efficacy are applied in various countries to refuse registration of a drug. The aspect of interest here is the criterion of comparative therapeutic and safety advantages. Because this publication is mainly written for the manufacturers of therapeutics it is not in all aspects fair to translate therapeutic advantages into diagnostic advantages and to assume that the safety aspect may be neglected for radiopharmaceuticals. But we believe that - in a general sense - the rules in various countries will apply for radiopharma-ceuticals in the same way as for therapeutic drugs. From this publication we selected the policy with respect to comparative evaluation in 21 countries: 15 Western European countries, USA, Canada, Australia, New Zealand, Japan and Israel. In 11 of these countries comparative advantages are not taken into consideration in the registration of a new drug. However, for the UK it has been indicated that refusal may be possible in case of safety disadvantages, but explicitly not on the basis of comparative efficacy advantages. The US FDA policy is expressed most explicitly: "a new drug registration cannot be refused on the basis of relative effectiveness, provided the drug is proven to be safe and effective".Of the 10 countries where registration may be refused on the basis of comparative evaluation Norway has taken the most extreme point of view: a drug is not accepted unless it shows safety and efficacy superior to similar (probably already accepted) products. Israel consider comparative safety advantages. That the attitude in a country to require and/or consider comparative evaluation in general to radiopharmaceuticals as well may be illustrated by our recent experience in the registration of antimony sulfide colloid in Australia, where a comparative efficacy study with sulfur colloid was asked for. Australia is one of the countries where registration of a drug may be refused on the basis of comparative evaluation. We think that it is interesting to note that the countries with -in our opinion- the largest experience with drug registration, the USA and the UK, indicate that comparative efficacy advantages are no factor in refusing registration.

3. COMPARATIVE EVALUATION.

The architecture of a clinical evaluation involves three elements (4), which occur in the logical sequence:

initial state - maneuver - subsequent state.

In the evaluation of radiopharmaceuticals the maneuver is the administration of the radiopharmaceutical drug, and the process determining its behaviour temporarily as well as spatially in the body. In the following paragraphs it will be shown how this principle is applied to comparative evaluation.

3.1. Safety evaluation

In single evaluations little or nothing will be learned about the safety of a maneuver. During the preclinical evaluation of the radiopharmaceutical, margins of safety have been assessed while- as explained elsewhere - the design of what is usually called a phase I study has been aimed at proving the negligibility or absence of pharmacological effects. This leaves us with the adverse reactions which may occur with a certain, but usually very low,frequency. When following the sequence "initial state - maneuver - subsequent state" the objective of research will define whether a comparative maneuver needs to be considered. When the objective is of purely descriptive purpose a comparative maneuver would not be necessary. Such an objective would be the assessment of the occurrence or the incidence of adverse reactions in a patient population receiving a certain radio-pharmaceutical.A comparative maneuver will be required for a completely different - not solely descriptive -objective. Since we are dealing with a maneuver of a diagnostic nature the objective might be whether the degree of unsafety involved is justified by the importance of the information obtained. It will be clear that it is nearly impossible, if not impossible at all to define a set of scientific parameters which could provide an acceptable answer to such an objective.A more limited objective which does require a comparative evaluation of safety is the assessment of the frequency of adverse reactions in the clinical application of different radio-pharmaceuticals in the maneuver leading to the same subsequent state.In itself this objective is very relevant to the safety aspect of a new radiopharmaceutical drug.The design of a scientifically acceptable protocol to satisfy this objective is not impossible. However, it is not a very practicable undertaking as the frequency of adverse reactions is very low. The comparative maneuver would comprise a choice between the administration of "A" or "B" in a population with a comparable initial state and subsequent state. Because of the very low expected frequency of adverse reactions the size of the study will be almost unmanageable.

We therefore firmly believe that comparative evaluation of safety must not form part of the clinical evaluation of a radiopharmaceutical drug in the pre-marketing phase. The evaluation of benefits versus risks can be undertaken only by the scientific community and can never be the subject of a comparative evaluation within the scope of providing information for registration.

3.2. Efficacy evaluation

The second aspect for which a manufacturer of a radio-pharmaceutical drug must provide scientific proof of: the efficacy of the drug. It is necessary to etablish first what might be meant by the term efficacy. Bell (5) presents three different approaches, the most important, but at the same time the most elusive one is the "outcome efficacy" of a procedure. This is a systematic comprehensive evaluation of risks and benefits, which in practice is beyond the capacity of nearly every organisation. This is already illustrated by the fact that this evaluation, in which both diagnosis and therapy are tightly knitted together might well require 10 and more years of patient follow-up to arrive at conclusions.

Less unworkable would be to limit the concept of efficacy to "diagnostic efficacy" or to "management efficacy". Diagnostic efficacy tries to determine the influence of a diagnostic test on the probability of the various possible differential diagnoses in a quantitative way. Management efficacy is probably the least difficult concept. It tries to measure whether and to what extent a diagnostic procedure changes patient management. The most attractive aspect of this concept is the relative simplicity of the study as the number of variables is limited.

It seems that for none of these concepts of efficacy a comparative evaluation is essential. Feinstein (3) has stated that in dealing with the question of efficacy of an experimental maneuver the appropriate comparison should be either no maneuver at all or the application of placebo. Only when in reality not efficacy but efficiency is asked for, the evaluation process should comprise a deliberately comparable maneuver.

3.3. Comparative evaluation in practice

We want to present and discuss here the three most usual approaches to comparative evaluation:

a. comparison of a radiopharmaceutical to an accepted radiopharmaceutical, aimed at the same diagnosis;

b. comparison of a radiopharmaceutical to a non-radioactive diagnostic method which yields the same or similar information;

c. comparison of a radiopharmaceutical to relevant, but completely different diagnostic methods.

Comparative evaluation of radiopharmaceuticals has been done and is being done on a rather extensive scale. One of the most favoured subject seems to be substances for bone scintigraphy.We have taken for the literature 26 studies, published between 1973 and 1982, in which every known bone scanning agent has been compared with one or more other bone scanning agents in humans in almost every conceivable combination. We have tried to extract some information from these publications. Of the 26 studies 8 originate from USA,18 from Europe. In 11 studies the agents have been compared in the same patients.Of these 11 studies 7 originate from USA and 4 from Europe.The various agents were considered to be of equal efficacy by 14 investigator groups, although "cosmetic" superiority for one agent or another was often indicated. Of these studies 7 originated from the USA and 7 from Europe, but 6 of the US studies were done in the same patient whereas only 3 of the 7 studies done in Europe compared the same patient.In the other 12 studies preference as to one agent or another was expressed, often very assuredly; 1 study came from the USA and 11 studies were of European origin. The one US study and one European study were done in the same patients and both were aimed at myocardial infarct detection. These were the only two studies aimed at that aspect in the total of 26 studies.

We feel that from these results we learn that comparative evaluation of various agents can very easily turn into an exercise of doubtful value. Obviously it is efficiency and not efficacy these studies try to demonstrate.In demonstrating differences in efficiency the method of comparison chosen should be scientifically sound. The bone agent comparison studies, we found, often suffered from the problem that observer subjectivity could play a role.Where more objective methods were chosen the results were either inconsistent or even contradictory. We must seriously consider the possibility that our methods are not sufficiently refined to determine the relative efficiency of diagnostic agents with comparable action and a proven efficacy.

It is not necessary to discuss here the growing reluctance against the administration of radiation to a patient when this radiation is not compensated by obtaining information of potential importance to that patient. Obviously comparisons in the same patient are undesirable. We believe that for registration purposes the comparison of different radiopharmaceuticals of the same class should not be requested - neither in the same nor in different patients. In countries where registration authorities do request comparative evaluation for non-radioactive drugs, this policy must not automatically be extended to radiopharmaceuticals.

As illustration for the comparison of a radiopharmaceutical to a non-radioactive, equivalent method we present a clinical trial organised to evaluate a method for measuring fat absorption. The radioisotope test method makes use of two components: iodinated triolein (I-125) and a triether, labelled with Se-75. The ratio between I-125 and Se-75 in the test meal is compared with the ratio in samples of stool passed in the days following the ingestion. From the two ratios the percentage of absorbed triolein may be calculated. In the trial these amounts were compared to the amounts of fat absorbed as determined by the classical chemical method. Gastro-enterological departments from several European countries participated in the trial. Where errors of a technical nature in performing the isotope study could be detected from the reports, all patients from that particular participating institution were eliminated. In the final evaluation the results of 204 patients were included. When the results of the chemical fat absorption determination are taken as the standard the results of the isotope study may be expressed in the following way:

chemical test	isotope test		
	+ (> 1%)	- (< 1%)	
+ (> 7 g/d)	87	12	99
	true pos.	false neg.	total
- (< 7 g/d)	51	54	1o5
	false pos.	true neg.	total

These results may be used to demonstrate the results of this trial in terms of sensitivity and specificity

$$\text{sensitivity} = \frac{\text{true positives}}{\text{true positives + false negatives}} = \frac{87}{87+12} = 87,8\%$$

$$\text{specificity} = \frac{\text{true negatives}}{\text{true negatives + false positives}} = \frac{54}{54+51} = 51,4\%$$

A clinical value of the isotope test may not be concluded from the high value for sensitivity. Neither may a low clinical value be concluded from the low value for specificity. Assessment of efficacy from the values for both sensitivity and specificity requires that the patient population is known with regard to the prevalence of the disorder to be diagnosed. The clinical value of this test is illustrated by considering that the near-50% specificity means that only 50% of all patients without fat malabsorption are identified, and that further diagnostic procedures are necessary to identify the other 50%, which showed a false positive test results. This test was supposed to replace another test, the chemical method.When in an actual patient population the incidence of fat malabsorption is not high further diagnostic tests would be required in a very high number of patients. This would probably have to be the chemical method.On the basis of the unsatisfactory correlation betwen the isotope test and the chemical test the development of this test was not continued. If the radiopharmaceutical, or the way it is used, or its administration or measurement would be redesigned, comparative evaluation would require a repetition of the clinical trial using the same"initial state". This means that the same patient selection criteria must be applied, and the same chemical test method is to be used for comparison. The major problem of such an evaluation is the necessity to be able to duplicate the "initial state". Unless the second study is managed by the same group or the same institution, the probability of arriving at acceptable results stands or falls with the completeness of the knowledge of the design of the first study. Many of the diagnostic procedures avaible in the practice of nuclear medicine are not directly comparable to diagnostic tests,aimed at the same mechanism in the same pathological condition.Assessment of

myocardial quality by scintigraphy with thallium-201 has no
equivalent test to be compared with. The evaluation of these
procedures and the radiopharmaceuticals involved will require
an approach which allows the use of results from other
incomparable test as standard. This approach starts from the
assumption that a medical diagnosis has a degree of
probability - any diagnosis is almost 100% sure at autopsy
only. If, for a given population of patients the probability
of a diagnosis can be changed by the execution of a
radioisotope test, one can ascribe a level of efficacy to that
test. This diagnostic efficacy may be measured if it is
possible to obtain estimates of the probability of the
different diagnoses before and after the radioisotope test was
performed.

Bayes´ theorem as applied to medical diagnosis states that
the probability that the patient with a given set of symptoms,
signs and test results has a particular disease is directly
proportional to the probability of occurrence of that given
set in that particular disease, multiplied by the a priori
prevalence of the disease and inversely proportional to the
probability of that given set to occur in the general
population (6,7).The fact that this approach is only accepted
in limited circles as a model for the process of arriving at a
diagnosis is not important to our problem. The a priori
prevalence of disease is a constant factor, which, however,
may differ from institute to institute.Moreover the
probabilities of a given set of signs, symptoms and test
results in the general population and in the population of
persons suffering from a particular disease is also constant
and should be available from literature and experience.

Consequently Bayes´ theorem may be a tool for the
evaluation of the efficacy of a diagnostic test by measuring
pre- and post-test probability. Obviously this model is only
applicable if a method is available to establish post-test
probability. But the fact that within one given institution
the factors of a priori prevalence and the probabilities are
constant factors means that both efficacy and comparative
evaluation of the efficacy of different tests may be

212

estimated.

From a managerial point of view the major problem is that
very strict adherence to the study protocol must be assured.
Pre-and post-test probability must be recorded in proper
sequence and independent from knowledge of the final
diagnosis. The study is probably not excessively time-
consuming but requires a considerable patient throughput and
therefore a large institution.

4. Conclusion.

Summarising we may state that

1. Comparative evaluation turns an efficacy estimation into
   a determination of efficiencies.
2. Comparative evaluation is not an efficient tool for
   proof of safety.
3. For proof of efficacy
   - comparison of agents is undesirable
   - comparison to similar diagnostic information is
     suitable
   - comparison on the basis of shift in probabilities of a
     diagnosis is a useful tool.

REFERENCES
1. General considerations for the clinical evaluation of
   drugs.1977 HEW(FDA) 77-3040.
2. Guidelines for the clinical evaluation of radiopharmaceutical drugs. 1981 HEW(FDA) 81-3120.
3. Legal and practical requirements for the registration of
   drugs. 1980, Zurich, I.F.P.M.A..
4. Feinstein AR. The architecture of clinical research. Clin
   Pharm Ther 1970;11 : 432-41
5. Bell RS. Efficacy. What 's that. Sem Nucl Med 1978; 8 :
   316-23
6. Wagner HN. Bayes ' Theorem: an idea whose time has come?
   Am J Cardiol 1982; 49 : 875-77
7. Hamilton GN, Trobaugh GB, Ritchie JL et al. Myocardial
   imaging with Thallium-201: an analysis of clinical
   usefulness based on Bayes' Theorem. Sem Nucl Med 1978; 8 :
   358-64
8. Nosslin B. Quality control and data evaluation in nuclear
   medicine. Proc. 13th Int. Annual Meeting of the Soc. of
   Nucl.Med. Sept. 1975, Copenhagen. 307-15.

14. THE PAPER WORK WITH APPLICATIONS FOR REGISTRATION OF RADIOPHARMACEUTICALS IN DENMARK

THOMAS MÜLLER

1. INTRODUCTION

The term paper work here is attributed to the work connected with preparation and handling of an application for registration of a radiopharmaceutical product. The material to be presented derives from applications for registrations submitted in Denmark since 1976 with the exception of applications later withdrawn. It is considered of general interest since the registration material in most cases seems to be identical to that submitted to registration authorities in other countries. At the start of the Danish registration system for radiopharmaceuticals (January 1 1976) a grand-father clause was granted for products, which were well known and well established and had been in regular use for several years. For these products registration could take place without full documentation with respect to the pharmacological, toxicological and clinical developing work. With respect to these points such products of course too are excluded from the present study of quality of the applications. The questions raised by the registration authority according to the first review are considered to represent the most open defects and errors and thus form the basis of most of the presented material.

2. HANDLING OF THE APPLICATION

According to the Ministry of the Interior Order of November 28, 1975, and later of July 7, 1978, it is the National Board of Health, which handles the application for registration. This board takes the final decisions on the basis of recommendations of The Board of Registration. The different stages of handling are as follows:

1. Preliminary handling by the Radiopharmaceutical Secretariat
2. Supplementary information provided by the applicant according to the questions raised on the basis of the first review by the Secretariat
3. Final handling by the Radiopharmaceutical Secretariat
4. Handling by the Board of Registration
5. Final handling by the National Board of Health

Applications for registration of radiopharmaceutical products or labelling kits are to be submitted to The Isotope-Pharmacy, where the preliminary handling by the Radiopharmaceutical Secretary takes place. Immediate decisions are taken with regard to obvious deficiencies or errors in the application, and the questions raised are submitted to the applicant. Often severe problems are demonstrated with regard to the size of the material. At this early stage the applicant is informed on these and similar facts in order to promote the handling. Then the secretary's handling continues at the Radiopharmaceutical Secretariat at the Isotope-Pharmacy as well as by an associated secretary in the field of nuclear medicine. Both the National Institute of Radiation Hygiene, the National Laboratory of the National Board of Health, and the pharmaceutical and medical Secretary of the Board of Registration may be consulted with regard to radiation-hygienic questions and common pharmaceutical and clinical problems. Responsa on the overall value and efficacy of the product may be obtained from "ad hoc" nuclear medical and radiobiological experts. On the basis of all the collected material the Radiopharmaceutical Secretariat prepares a report for discussion by the Board of Registration which then give a recommendation to the National Board of Health. After this the application is processed to its end at the Isotope-Pharmacy.

As can be seen clearly the greatest importance is attached to the Secretariat level with expert advice and responsa. The Board of Registration performes the final weighing e.g. by means of a general evaluation to make sure, that the decisions to be taken will be in harmony with other decisions taken in

the rest of the drug field. The basis of registration of
radiopharmaceuticals etc. is efficacy, safety and quality. To
convince the authority of registration that the product is
safe and effective in use many points have to be considered
which will be handled in the following. These points have been
grouped arbitrarily in an attempt to give an impression of
where the main problems are in preparing an application for
registration and to what extension they occur.

3. OVERALL CONDITIONS

A synopsis shall be given of the submitted material and
conclusions drawn with regard to safety and efficacy.
Information must be given about applied, granted, withdrawn or
refused registrations in other countries. All material
submitted must be indexed and must together with reprints and
other submitted literature be in Danish, Norwegian, Swedish,
English, French or German. The extent of the submitted
documentation shall be reasonable. This means, that from the
summary and the prepared material it should be feasable to
evaluate the characteristics of the product. The summary must
be aggregated, not spread round in the heap of papers as we
sometimes see. Of course the summary must be objective and of
reasonable size, i.e. 15-20 pages. The references from the
synopsis to the file itself are best done by means of volume
number, enclosure number and page number. We believe that
these three things are reasonable to claim in order to make
proper orientation in the file possible. It would too be of
real advantage to have the synopsis prepared by a person
familiar with the subject.

Another problem is, that all investigations, reports,
conclusions and summaries etc. have to be dated. The
evaluation of an investigation is not too seldom dependent on,
whether it was performed before or after certain other
investigations presented in the file. Laboratory reports must
explicitly show the identity of the investigated product and
the batch number. Overall conditions also comprise
handwritten, undated and unsigned amendments and supplements
on laboratory precepts as well as missing signature on release

protocols and similar things. This often gives an interesting insight as to what extent GMP-rules are adopted or complied with. References to publications and investigation reports not enclosed and contradictory information and limit values in different parts of the file round off this kind of problems. It may seem obvious, that the greater and more voluminous an application is, the more important is it, that it appears in a physical easy accessible form. It should be possible to open the material and it should be possible to close it again after reading. Sometimes the quite grotesque files cannot be opened, sometimes it is impossible to close them again. If a wish is accepted here, we would ask for the material being paper-bound, a wish which has been promoted earlier in the field of registration of ordinary drugs too (1).

As of legibility the attention is drawn to simple problems which nevertheless often occur: The left margin being too small. One must guess the content of the first left part of the lines. It is obvious, too, that photocopies of articles with scintigrams etc. only should be used in the cases, where original material is not available. Handwritten values on laboratory reports and release protocols often are illegible on the photocopies. The quality should be controlled before they are inserted in the file. It should be evident from the previous, that collections of loose pages in closed folders is an abomination for those who have to work with the application and one can only hope, that it is understood, that the "technical" problem is a quite considerable one. In fact every third file shows up one or more of these technical deficiencies, which is felt meaningless and absurd if one realizes, that the material has been collected with the purpose for use and not for being buried in an archive.

An application for approval of a new valuable radiopharma-ceutical will never be rejected alone pleading technical and formalistic deficiencies. But deficiencies often result in prolonged treatment which is unsatisfactory for all those involved. Applicants capable of solving the "technical" problems may expect a reward in the form of an easier and more flexible progress of their application. "Technical" excellent applications do exist, but there is a needless number of inadequate and poorly prepared applications.

4. PHARMACEUTICAL/CHEMICAL PART

4.1 Manufacture

Information must be given in details about production, control and handling of the product in all companies involved in production and control. Attention is drawn to the guidelines in Good Practices in the Manufacture and Quality Control of Drugs (2). Reference is also made to A Proposal from a Nordic Group on Practices in The Manufacture of Radio-pharmaceuticals (3). A manufacturer with no prior registered products in Denmark must submit information on production facilities and the organisation of work. Information must be given about the persons having overall responsibilities for production and quality control. A statement from the National control authority might be enclosed.

Experiences from the daily work with the applications show that every 4th application has been encumbered with deficiencies concerning production. A total loss of information on the applied mode of production or defective descriptions with scarce details referring only to a method described in literature is often found. A detailed description step by step of the production process is indispensable. This leads to another point: Too often information on applied GMP-guidelines is missing, maybe because GMP-thinking has become a natural thing during the past 10 years. On the other hand we often can see from the attached documents, that this might not be so at all levels.

4.2 Raw material

According to the guidelines attached to the application form of December 1975 for registration of radiopharmaceuticals in Denmark (4) monographs must be given for all components including physical and chemical constants, purity tests, identity tests as well as methods for quantitative determination. The reason for the different purity tests must be stated. Reference to a pharmacopoeia monograph may be sufficient.

More than half of the submitted applications show deficiencies on this point. Several of them have even more than one question raised on this subject. Some applicants have deficiencies in each application, others in every third application. The most frequent deficiencies are defective information on identity, purity, quantitative analysis and methods. Unfortunately in many cases the question of raw materials has not been touched at all though explicitly mentioned in the attached guidelines of the application form. Often specifications etc. are missing for the radioactive solution used in the manufacturing process, probably because this raw material erroneously is not considered to be a raw material. The same considerations apply to the containers, stoppers, labels and the packing material. In the case of labels and packing material it is considered sufficient to present samples. Also attention is drawn to dyes, buffers, bacteriostatica etc. and so-called indifferent gases as i.e. nitrogen. With compounds pretended indifferent the problem might be to prove, that they really are indifferent in this connexion e.g. that the quality applied does not change the bioavailability of the radiopharmaceutical.

4.3 Stability

Methods for and results from stability studies performed on a number of batches shall be given, if possible also including identification of degradation products. It is difficult to have general rules for the extent of the necessary investigations as well as for the number of batches to be studied. In any case more than one batch should be studied. It is desirable that degradation products are identified or characterized and evaluated with respect to their possible degree of toxicity. As for preparation kits stability documentation for the labelled product as well as for the inactive product is required.

Apparently this point too has created difficulties for the applicants. In more than every second application there have been raised questions on this subject. Most frequently there has been observed a totally missing stability documentation for the product or for the labelled product prepared with kits. Documentation for one batch only or no investigations performed on matters apparently having influence on stability is considered insufficient. This concerns f.ex. aggregation of particles, absorption, pH-change with time, bacteriological stability etc. If the applicant may be convinced of or has any previous experience that certain factors have no influence on stability the subject should at least be discussed. It is the task of the applicant to convince the registration authority that the product really is stable and of sufficient quality. And not to say it is useless to submit stability studies not capable to hold specification limits set by the applicant himself.

With regard to accelerated stability studies, the following practice has been adopted. If the claimed stability is one or two years it may be difficult to present normal results for such a long period together with the application. In these cases accelerated stability studies may be accepted provided that studies based on storage under the actual circumstances also will be carried out. After reformulation of a product the National Board of Health only will accept short shelf lives for the new product and only permit prolongation along with submission of further stability results obtained under actual circumstances. A certain degree of extrapolation from accelerated studies might be accepted, provided the system is homogeneous.

4.4 Final vial

The questions raised within this group concern deficient information and documentation of the ready-to-use product. The pharmaceutical form of the final product including the range of the radioactive concentration and specific activity shall be described e.g. by reference to a pharmacopoeia monograph. The material accompanying an application for registration shall contain detailed information on production control, i.e. unambiguous identification and quantitative determination of the principal contents. Results from the analytical quality control of the final product must be presented in order to make evaluations possible of the proposed limits. Special demands as to sterility etc. must be accompanied with control methods. Claims for the pharmaceutical/technical properties of the product must be documented by description of or reference to control methods. Considering preparation kits information must be given for control methods for the labelled preparation in order to be able to perform a full control of all parameters. Control methods considered necessary as a control for the labelling process must be given in the application as well as in the pack-leaflet.

Only with every sixth application questions have been raised on this subject. Dominating is lack of methods for quality control of the final product. Other typical examples are no practicable method for quantitative determination of the active ingredient in the freeze-dried preparation kits, or no methods for determination of radiochemical purity in radio-pharmaceuticals. Sometimes the method is so incomplete, that it is impossible to verify it in the laboratory. Other applications have incomplete specifications e.g. no information on pH, degree of iodination, total number of particles or missing discussion with regard to the possibility and/or limits for certain radionuclidic impurities to be expected in the product.

4.5 Other problems

Finally in the pharmaceutical/chemical chapter there is a group of problems, which could not become incorporated in the previous groups but which occured frequently enough to justify them to be mentioned. It has been demonstrated (5) that the quality of the pertechnetate (Tc-99m) injection used for labelling sometimes may have influence on the quality of the labelled product (compatibility). Therefore the applicant must discuss this problem both in the documentation submitted and in the pack-leaflet. Here there may be given specifications for the pertechnetate (Tc-99m) eluate to be used by referring to a pharmacopoeia monograph or it may be indicated, that eluates from one or several specified generators can be used.

These matters should be documented and discussed in the application for a preparation kit. Another problem is full declaration of all components with respect to nature and quantity on both label and package and indicating at least the main constituent on the label of the vial of the final labelled product with kits. The above mentioned problems and problems of similar nature have been observed in every fourth application.

4.6 Conclusion. Pharmaceutical/chemical deficiencies.

Table 1 demonstrates the number of the above mentioned groups of problems relative to the total number of applications. As can be seen the most frequent deficiencies lie in the field of raw material and stability documentation.

Table 1. Number of applications with questions raised on deficiencies concerning the PHARMACEUTICAL/CHEMICAL part including "overall conditions". (Total of 66 applications)

RAW MATERIAL	38
STABILITY DOCUMENTATION	38
(OVERALL CONDITIONS	25)
MANUFACTURE	17
OTHER PROBLEMS	17
FINAL VIAL	11

But of course there exist differences between the different applicating companies. A total of 66 applications by a total of 9 applicants form the basis of this investigation and only the first questions raised to the applicant by the registration authority are considered. Fig. 1 demonstrates the profile of the companies with the predominant types of deficiencies characteristic for the single company. For obvious reasons it has not been possible to put company names on that scheme. The figure only shows six companies because the other companies would have been represented by too few applications to become representative.

In total it can be derived from the investigation, that the number of pharmaceutical/chemical deficiencies ranges from less than one to about four per application.

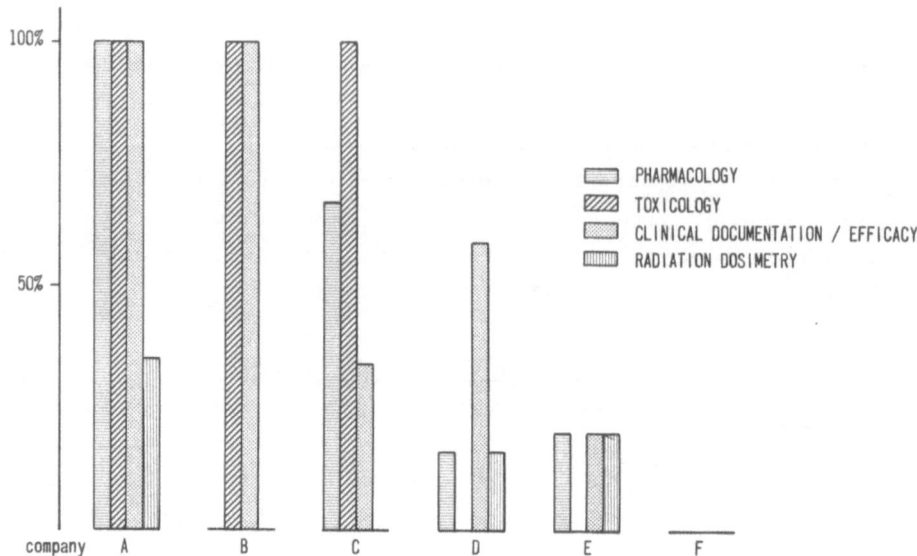

Figure 1. Frequency of applications with different deficiencies.

5. CLINICAL/PHARMACOLOGICAL PART

5.1 Introduction

The basis of this review consists of 27 applications and six companies, not all of them identical with those involved in the first chapter. The reason for the decreased number of applications considered is the grand-father clause of 1976 when the Danish registration system was introduced. It must be underlined, that all questions have been raised by the clinical experts in this field. With respect to a detailed discussion of the nature and extent of the requirements there shall be made reference to the treatment of these problems in chapter 11 and 12.

5.2 Clinical documentation/efficacy

Questions raised on this subject belong to the most frequent, namely in more than half of all applications. Generally a documentation is required, which is capable of giving an objective basis to evaluate the real value of the radiopharmaceutical. The answer is very closely connected with the documentation for the claimed indications, under which the product is to be marketed and with the documentation of efficacy. It is obvious that the nature and the extent of that documentation material may vary very much, however the results must be presented in a prepared form, i.e. with evaluations and conclusions. Case reports, laboratory journals, undocumented evaluations and similar untreated material alone is considered to be inexpedient. The most often raised questions during the past 5-years period is on insufficient documentation for the claimed indication and in some cases even a total absence of documentation. Occasionally only references to other products of a similar type are made. If they are of different composition then this reference is considered to be insufficient documentation. Special attention shall be drawn to questions concerning documentation of efficacy because one would expect a documented evidence of the intentional effect to be very essential. Nevertheless in every fourth application questions had been raised by the clinical experts on efficacy. This problem seems to be specific for some companies, as three applicants had no problems at all, one had problems with every sixth application, but two of the applicants had problems in each application.

5.3 Toxicology

Questions raised on toxicology belong as well as questions on clinical documentation to the most frequent ones in two out of five applications. However, it has to be pointed out, that only three of the applicants had problems in each application while all other applicants had presented a full satisfactory documentation. Besides information on toxicity the requirements of the registration authority includes undesired side-effects. The extent of the information will depend greatly on the use of the radiopharmaceutical. When the preparation earlier has been in use as a non-radioactive drug or it is a labelled form of a natural compound occurring in the organism, chronical toxicological studies normally are not required. The same applies for compounds without a real pharmacodynamic effect and to be used for diagnostic purposes. The material on this subject shows most often an insufficient handling of problems concerning human-toxicological conditions. Information on registered or known adverse reactions may be missing or there are no discussions of the frequency of side-effects to be expected. With blood-protein products there often is insufficient or even missing evaluation of the risk of sensibilisation. It shall be mentioned, that subacute toxicity studies comprising only four animals and of only one species have been rejected as being unacceptable.

5.4 Pharmacology

In this section studies are required to demonstrate the pharmacokinetics and pharmacodynamics of the product. The questions raised in this section concern for a great deal the metabolism and the excretion from the organism. Both total missing information and inadequate documentation as well as missing systematic studies have been seen. These deficiencies have been criticised in one third of all applications, though there are applicants whose applications have been without any problems as well as applicants who had no application without this type of problem.

5.5 Radiation dosimetry

Calculations of radiation dose to the sick as well as the healthy organism must be presented, preferably according to the MIRD-system. This of course includes impurities and possible degradation products with significant contributions to the radiation dose. In the case of doubt this question must be discussed. If relevant, different age groups must be considered. Dosimetry data were totally absent in relatively few applications, less than in every sixth. This almost must be ascribed to an oversight, though one could wonder how this could happen in an application for a radioactive drug.

5.6 Conclusion. Clinical/pharmacological deficiencies

Concluding reference is made to table 2 demonstrating the above mentioned problems according to the number of applications.

Table 2. Number of applications with questions raised on
deficiencies concerning the CLINICAL/PHARMACOLOGICAL
part (Total of 27 applications)

CLINICAL DOCUMENTATION/EFFICACY	18
TOXICITY	11
PHARMACOLOGY	9
RADIATION DOSIMETRY	4

More than one third of all applications showed problems
with every type of the clinical/pharmacological problems
mentioned here. However the problems concentrate most on half
of the companies (fig.2), as the other three companies had
submitted fairly good applications. It is obvious, too, that
every applicant again seems to have some sort of fingerprint,
which in some cases is highly significant.

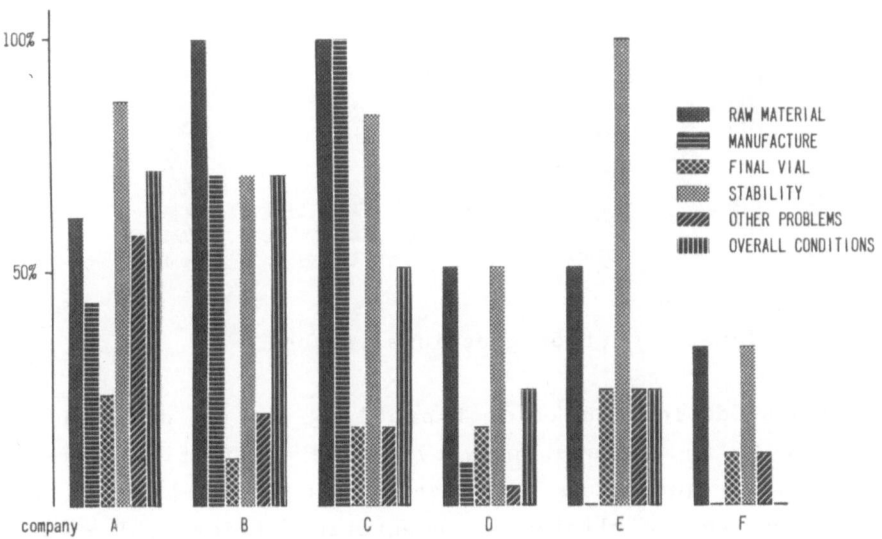

Figure 2. Frequency of applications with different deficiencies.

6. SUMMARY AND CONCLUSIONS

Fig. 3 shows the total number of questions raised on both
parts of the application. Nearly all companies have problems

with both the pharmaceutical/chemical part and the
clinical/pharmacological part. Thus the secretary in the
initial handling of the applications in the past as a mean at
least has dealt with two pharmaceutical/chemical and with
between one and two clinical/pharmacological main deficiencies
in each application.

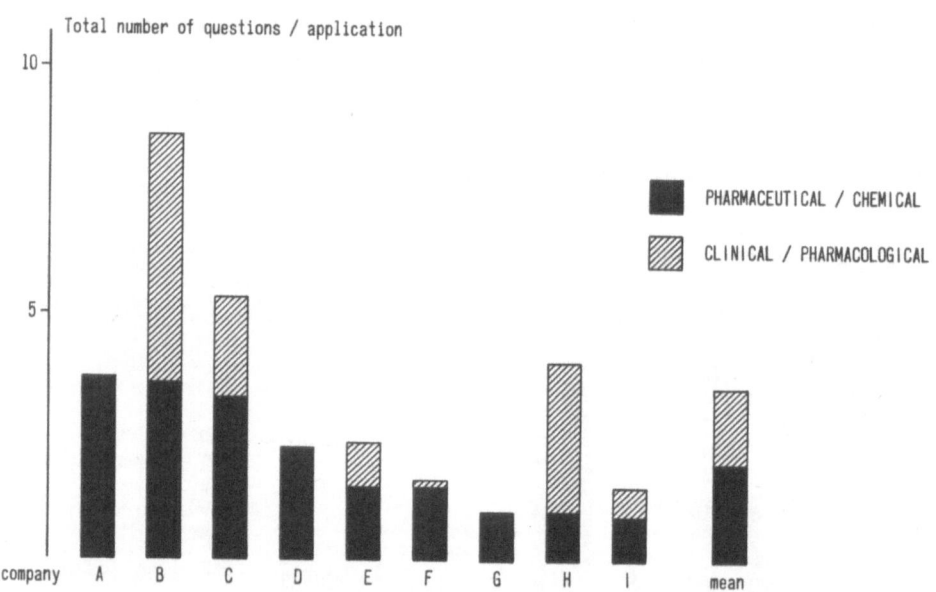

Figure 3. Total number of questions raised.

The most dominating kind of problems can be derived from
table 3. As an average in every second application there had
been raised questions both on raw material, stability,
toxicology and on clinical documentation/efficacy. The value,
quality and safety of a radiopharmaceutical last not least is
considered to be close dependent on a good and sufficient
documentation of these points. This makes the result of this
investigation quite surprising.

Table 3	Questions raised on deficiencies concerning	
In every	Pharmaceutical / chemical problems	Clinical / pharmacological problems
2nd application	RAW MATERIAL STABILITY	TOXICOLOGY CLINICAL DOCUMENTATION / EFFICACY
3rd application	(OVERALL CONDITIONS)	PHARMACOLOGY
4th application	MANUFACTURE OTHER PROBLEMS	
6th application	FINAL VIAL	RADIATION DOSIMETRY

From the subsequent handling of the applications it seems obvious that many of the companies have been in the possession of the required information at the time of the submission of the registration material. Much money and a lot of time has been spent and a good deal of work has been undertaken, before a product can reach the stage of registration. One can wonder why it is so difficult to do this last effort properly. After all nobody is interested in marketing poor products, and the problem often seems to be, that the additional required information might be buried somewhere else in other files at the company.

The present quality of the applications for registration of radiopharmaceuticals demonstrate a spectrum one would expect could become better with time. Comparing with the situation in the field of ordinary drugs in 1981, there had been initial refusals in one third of all submitted applications because of insufficient documentation in the pharmaceutical/chemical part (6), which means there had been questions raised to be answered before further treatment of the application could take place. In this comparison radiopharmaceutical applications seem to be more defective by a factor of at least three with regard to the pharmaceutical/chemical documentation. Comparing with another investigation in the field of ordinary drugs from 1977 (7) there had been raised three times less questions on stability and twice less questions on toxicology and pharmacology (table 4).

Table 4. APPLICATIONS FOR REGISTRATION IN DENMARK

REFUSALS IN THE FIELD OF ORDINARY DRUGS IN 1977		INITIAL QUESTIONS (=REFUSALS) RAISED ON RADIOPHARMACEUTICALS 1976 - 1981
RAW MATERIAL	41 %	58 %
FINAL VIAL	13 %	17 %
STABILITY	18 %	58 %
CLIN. DOC.	45 %	67 %
TOXICOLOGY	22 %	41 %
PHARMACOLOGY	16 %	33 %
TOTAL NUMBER OF APPLICATIONS	109	66 (pharmaceutical/chemical part) 27 (clinical/pharmacological part)

Preparation of a good application for registration of course requires years of experience, which some of the companies concerned not yet have had the opportunity to attain. However, even experienced companies sometimes demonstrate incomprehensible poor documentation material too. Maybe a change might require a different organisation in the company.

Paper work comprises both preparing of an application for registration and the subsequent handling by the registration authority. The load of work of the applicant can never become less by submitting poor applications if they shall result in a finally granted registration, because the stepwise supplementation demands disproportional efforts by both the applicant and the registration authority and violates the principle that the application must be accompanied by a complete synopsis. Good prepared applications are worth-while for the applicant in the form of shorter handling time etc., so the advantages should be obvious. Therefore let this presentation be an attempt to get better applications by having motivated the applicants critical to examine their applications according to the given rules and proposals.

REFERENCES
1. Engelund A. In: Registrering af lægemidler (Registration of drugs). Proceedings Symposium Lyngby (Copenhagen) 1972: 36. (in Danish).
2. Good Practices in the Manufacture and Quality Control of Drugs. In: WHO Expert Committee on Specifications for Pharmaceutical Preparations. 25. Report. WHO Technical Report Series 567, Geneva 1975: 16.
3. Good Practices in the Manufacture of Radiopharmaceuticals. A Proposal Put Forward by a Group of Pharmacists from the Nordic Countries. Arch Pharm Chemie 1971;78:1002-1009.
4. Application form for radiopharmaceuticals. Obtainable from The Isotope-Pharmacy, 378 Frederikssundsvej, DK-2700 Brønshøj, Denmark.
5. A Comparative Test of Tc-99m Liver Scanning Agents. The Isotope-Pharmacy Report IA-1, January 1975.
6. Kyllingsbæk H. In: Lægemidler Registrering og Klinisk Afprøvning (Registration and Clinical Evaluation of Drugs). Proceedings Symposium Copenhagen 1981:45. (in Danish).
7. Andersen H O. In: Registrering af Lægemidler (Registration of Drugs), Proceedings Symposium Lyngby (Copenhagen) 1977:19-21. (in Danish).

15. DRUG-RADIOPHARMACEUTICAL INTERACTIONS AND OTHER POSSIBLE
MODIFICATIONS IN RADIOPHARMACEUTICAL BIODISTRIBUTION

MARTIN G. WOLDRING

1. INTRODUCTION

Alterations in the biodistribution of radiopharmaceuticals used in nuclear medicine can have various causes. In the first place, the modified distribution may be the result of an intended pharmacological or physiological intervention. Such studies are an extension of nuclear medicine procedures for obtaining the desired diagnostic data and narrowing the differential diagnosis. On the other hand, as a result of patient medication, there is an increasing awareness of unexpected alterations in radiopharmaceutical biodistribution (1). These unexpected changes in the biodistribution of the tracer may reduce the diagnostic value of nuclear medicine imaging or, worse, give rise to misleading results or to the necessity of revising dosimetric calculations.

Not all treatment modalities involve the administration of different drugs but the net results of interaction with the radiopharmaceutical may be the same: i.e. the radiopharmaceutical reflects a new process secondary to the therapy (e.g. radiation therapy), which possibly provides misleading information about the primary disease of the patient. Other causes of totally "abnormal" results can be: unexpected pathophysiology, treatment modalities such as surgery, interference from radiodiagnosis, faulty injection techniques, interaction between radiopharmaceuticals and radiopharmaceuticals of inferior quality.

2. RADIOPHARMACEUTICALS OF INFERIOR QUALITY

The results of administration of inferior radiopharmaceuticals are usually predictable. Example are: -bone imaging with the presence of free pertechnetate in thyroid and stomach,

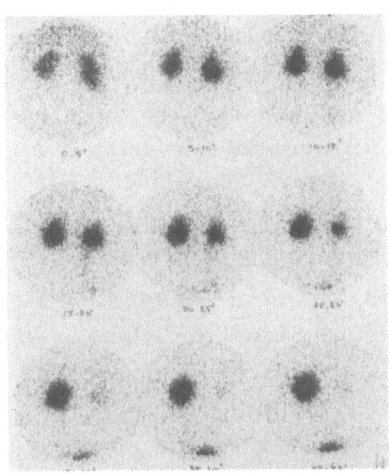

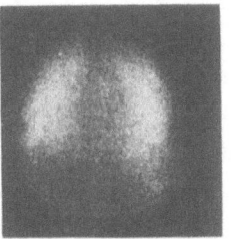

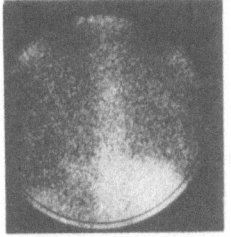

Fig. 1. A hippuran study in a patient with obstruction of the left ureter. Furosemide i. v. after 25[1] shows that at the right side there is no obstruction.

Fig. 2. In a patient with sarcoidosis, diffuse uptake of radiogallium in the lungs is seen before treatment; after treatment with corticosteoids a normal distribution pattern is seen (posterior view).

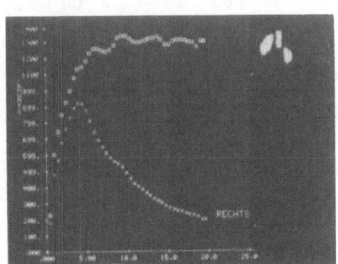

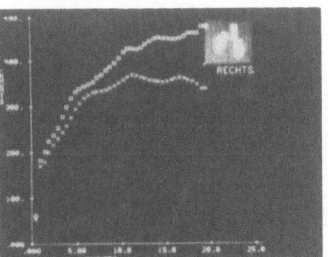

Fig. 3. In a patient with testicular carcinoma, the left ureter is obstructed due to metastases (left). After therapy with cis-platinum both kidneys demonstrate a disturbed hippuran accumulation (right).

- bone imaging with the presence of colloids in the reticulo-endothelial system,

- lung imaging showing perfusion defects caused by administration of too few radioactive particles, - lung imaging with asymmetric uptake and multiple foci of increased radioactivity caused by clumping of particles, - liver imaging with the presence of excessively large particles retained in the lungs, - liver imaging with the presence of under-sized particles in the bonemarrow.

3. EFFECT OF INTENDED PHARMACOLOGICAL INTERVENTION

Many examples of this can be found in endocrinology, especially in the diagnosis of thyroid disease. Other examples are in the field of cardiology, where cardioactive drugs are used. In nephrology, the introduction of the diuresis-renogram enables differentiation of mechanical and functional obstructive uropathy, thus assisting in the decision to manage the patient or not (Fig. 1).

Another possibility is that the nuclear medicine study is used to monitor the progress of a course of drug therapy. An example of the effect of such a therapy is shown in fig. 2.

Chemotherapeutic agents may have nonspecific effects, but compromise bone marrow reserves in the same way as radiation therapy. A modern chemotherapeutic agent is Cis-platinum, an inorganic platinum-containing compound, particularly effective against metastatic testicular carcinoma and carcinomata of prostate and bladder. The compound is found mainly in the liver after injection, but is also known to be nephrotoxic. (Fig.3).

4. INTERACTION BETWEEN RADIOPHARMACEUTICALS

An interaction between radiopharmaceuticals is the well-known case of pertechnetate administration - e.g. for brain scanning - after a previous bone scan. The result is that the stannous ions from the bone imaging kit - remaining within the red blood cells - reduce the sodium pertechnetate, thus labelling the cells in vivo. The labelled cells are apparently not able to penetrate possible blood-brain barrier defects. The advice still basically applicable is that the use of radiopharmaceuticals containing stannous ions should be

performed after all other nuclear medicine studies requiring
sodium pertechnetate.

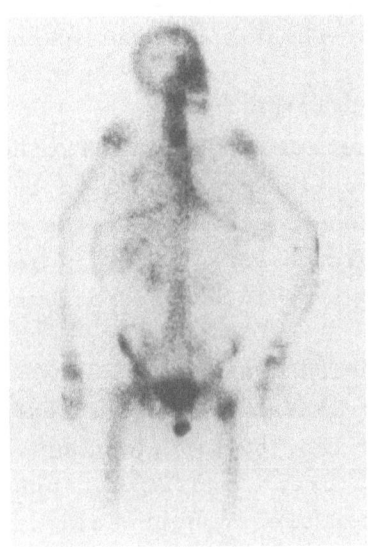

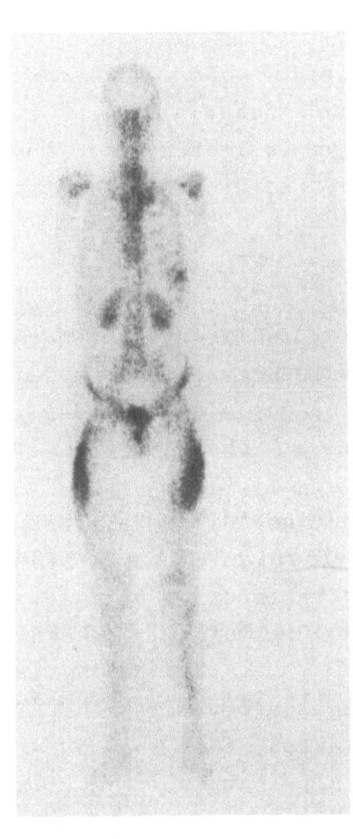

Fig. 5. Bone-scintigraphy in a
patient with breast carcinoma
after irradiation bilaterally.
Increased uptake of the
radiopharmaceutical in the soft
tissue is seen.
Fig. 4. (Left) Interference of
i.m. iron-dextran in bone-
imaging

5. RADIOPHARMACEUTICAL - DRUG INTERACTION

A typical drug interaction is illustrated by the
administration of intramuscular iron-dextran. The excess body
iron saturates the plasmatransferrin and has considerable
potential to modify the biodistribution of the
radiopharmaceutical. It prevents e.g. binding of indium
chloride and thus invalidates plasma space measurements or

bloodpool imaging. It also results in local accumulation of bone-imaging radiopharmaceuticals in the soft tissue at the site of the intramuscular iron-injection (Fig. 4). The mechanism is not quite clear, but may involve hyperaemia or formation of a dextran-Tc-phosphate complex.

6. RADIATION THERAPY

Therapeutic irradiation of patients has different implications for the behaviour of radiopharmaceuticals. It is reported, that the uptake of radiogallium is increased in the irradiated soft tissue. A local effect of radiotherapy is also often seen in bone-scintigraphy (Fig. 5).

7. RADIOGRAPHY

Radiographic contrast agents containing iodine are known to alter the thyroid gland uptake of radioactive sodiumiodide. Scintigraphic examinations after radiography also may result in cold areas on the scintigram because of the presence of barium sulphate (Fig. 6).

In the past, colloidal solutions of thoriumdioxide have been used as X-ray contrast medium. Its elimination is very slow and incomplete and because of its long radioactive half-life the accumulation is dangerous. The phenomenon of this effect of thorotrast is named thorotrastosis; scintigraphy with Tc-99m colloid shows longterm sequelae including cirrhosis of the liver (Fig. 7). Nowadays it is considered, that the use of thorotrast is never justified.

8. SURGERY

In surgery, gallium citrate localizes markedly in operative sites as do bone-seeking radiopharmaceuticals to a lesser degree. We have noted on occasion the uptake of technetium-methylene-diphosphonate (MDP) in patients with a scar due to gastrectomy(2). Similar findings can be anticipated, f.i. after pneumectomy, but also in trivial "surgical" lesions such as i.m. injections of antibiotics as well as pressure lesions on skin or other physiotherapeutic effects (Fig 8). After urologic surgery like urinary deviation operation abnormal accumulation of the tracer can be found (Fig. 9)

9. INACCURATE ADMINISTRATION

Inaccurate administration of radiocolloid may cause a troublesome clumping of the collodial particles with subsequent entrapment in the vasculature of the lungs.

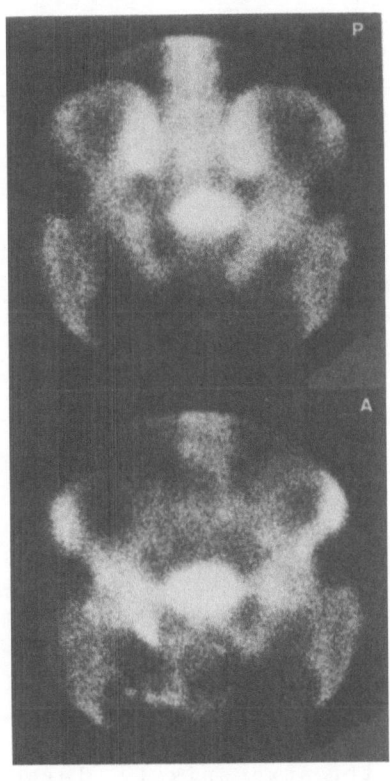

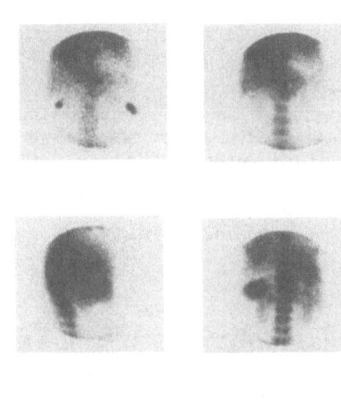

Fig. 6. Bone scan in a patient after a gastrointestinal X ray contrast study. Anterior view with cold area near L5 due to the presence of barium sulphate in the colon is seen.

Fig. 7. In a patient with thorotrastosis diminished irregular uptake to radiocolloid in the liver and high uptake in bone and lungs is seen (top anterior, left bottom right lateral, right bottom posterior view).

236

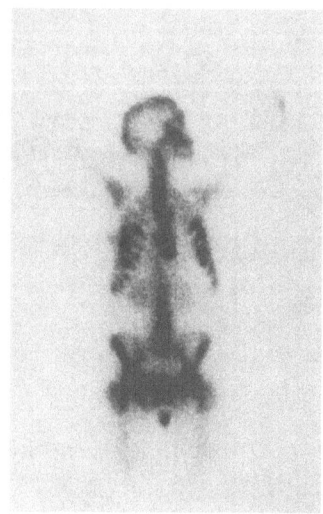

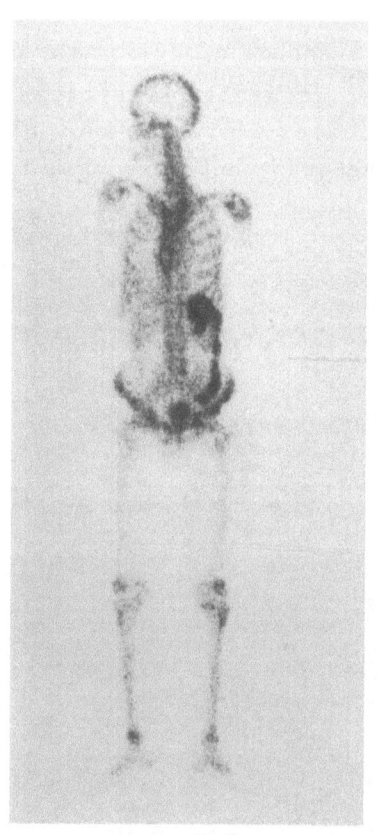

Fig. 8. Bone scintigraphy in a
patient with osteoporosis.
Traumatic lesions (broken
ribs) are seen after
physiotherapy.
Fig. 9. (Right) A bone scan in a
patient with bladder cancer.
After surgery a left kidney
drainage via colon is seen.

Mixing the colloid f.i. with some blood during intravenous
injection causes such clumping; the excessively large
particles are retained by the lungs (Fig. 10).

   The possibility of an inadvertent extravenous injection
also causes modifications in the distribution pattern of the
radiopharmaceutical (Fig. 11). The nature of the altered
distribution depends upon the physiology of the localization
of the specific radiopharmaceutical. It is one of the many
artifacts that must be born in mind to explain the occasional
perplexing image.

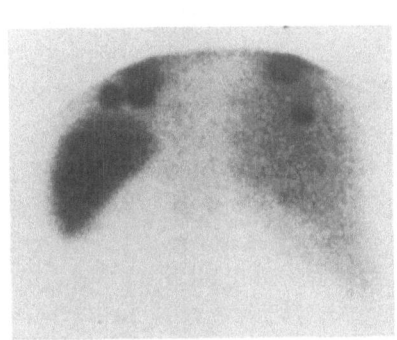

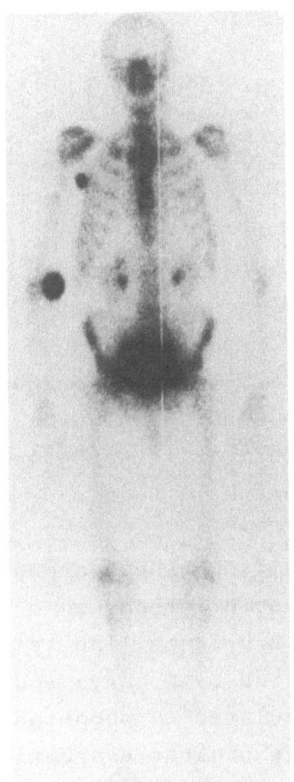

Fig. 10. Inaccurate administration
of radiocolloid; clumping of
colloidal particles causes
embolisms.

Fig. 11. (Right) Bone scan.
Radiopharmaceutical
injected extravenously;
uptake in axillary lymph
node is seen.

10. OTHER CAUSES

Finally causes of totally abnormal biodistribution can be:
unexpected pathology or pathophysiology of the patients. There
are numerous examples of this unexpected biodistribution in
for instance oncology, hepatology or urology. Examples are
shown in fig. 12 and fig. 13.

11. CONCLUSION

The introduction of new drugs such as cis-platinum and the
use of existing drugs in greater dosages imply that the future
may lead to more unexpected observations due to variations in

238

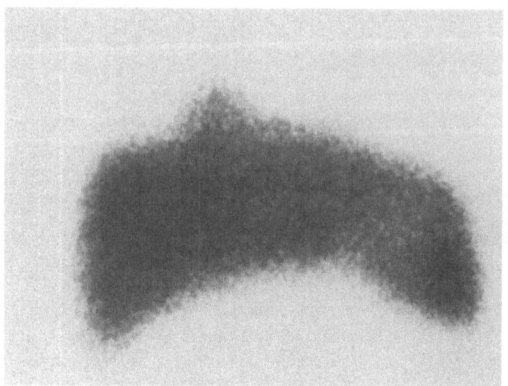

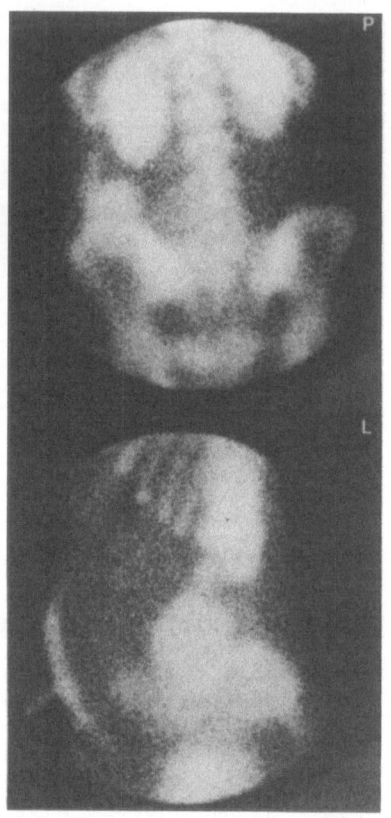

Fig. 12. Unexpected image.
Liver scan: Herniation of a
part of the liver through the
diaphragm is seen.

Fig. 13. Unexpected pathology.
Bone scintigraphy in a patient
with a urinoma. The tracer is
excreted by kidneys and is
accumulated in abdominal tissues
due to urether dysruption.

the biology of the lesions. It may happen that alterations in biodistribution modify the anticipated behaviour of the radiopharmaceutical to the point at which it is misleading in diagnosis, or even of no value.

The effect of drugs or treatment, or of drug toxicity on radiopharmaceutical distribution seem to be very important in the field of nuclear medicine imaging. In conventional pharmaceutical practice, there is a growing realization of the importance of drug interaction or drug incompatibilities. The same applies for the application of radiopharmaceuticals on the understanding, that its biodistribution can be influenced by concomitent drug administration and other treatment modalities. The identification and recording of intervening interactions seems to be potential function of the nuclear pharmacist.

REFERENCES
1. Hladik WB, Nigg KK, Rhodes BA. Drug-induced changes in the biological distribution of radiopharmaceuticals. Sem Nuclear Med 1982; 12: 184-210.
2. Woldring MG. Pitfalls in nuclear medicine and radiopharmacy practice. Proceedings of the third world federation of nuclear medicine and biology. Paris: Pergamon, 1982: 1671-74.

16. ADVERSE REACTIONS TO RADIOPHARMACEUTICALS

DAVID H. KEELING

In any report or survey of adverse reactions to radiopharmaceuticals, difficulties arise in the interpretation of what constitutes an adverse reaction. For medicines in general, adverse drug reactions have been conventionally classified into over-dosage, intolerance, side-effects, secondary effects, idiosyncrasy and hypersensitivity. They can also be divided into those that arise from the normal pharmacological action of a drug and those that represent a totally abnormal and novel response (1).

The U.S. Code of Federal Regulations (2) quotes as a definition, "any adverse experience associated with the use of a drug, whether or not considered to be drug related and includes any side effects, injury, toxicity or sensitivity reaction or significant failure of expected pharmacological action". Because of the radically different pattern of use of radiopharmaceuticals from normal therapeutic drugs, not to mention the difference in total quantities, it is inevitable that problems arise in adapting systems and definitions designed for normal therapeutic drugs to radiopharmaceuticals. There has been no shortage of definitions of adverse reaction -whether to radiopharmaceuticals or drugs in general, but, whilst there is general agreement, there are many minor points of difference such as whether or not to include mal-distribution or radiation problems. In addition it must be realised that the chance of getting reports back to any system are closely related to the severity of the reaction; minor transient manifestations are almost certainly grossly under-reported whereas fatalities are probably rarely missed.

Cordova et al (3) at a recent U.S. meeting have used a

definition for radiopharmaceuticals that includes all unexpected or unusual and undesirable clinical manifestations due to a radiopharmaceutical which excludes `failure of expected action` noted in the U.S. Code. They also exclude, as do most writing on the subject, reactions due to radiation rather than the pharmaceutical as a chemical entity. The logic behind this is not entirely clear though the practical reason is: they also exclude reactions due to an overdose or to faulty administration technique. The present author, whilst excluding the (statistical) risks associated in the long-term with normal doses of radiation, has nevertheless included short-term radiation dose problems produced either by altered biological handling - such as with some intrathecal preparations held back by a spinal block or subcutaneous colloids clearing excessively slowly due to lymphatic blockage. These highlight the problems associated with some longer lived radionuclides in which the biological clearance is vital in keeping the radiation dose either locally or generally, within acceptable limits (4).

In the past, reported series from both the U.S. Atkins et al (5); Ford et al (6); Rhodes & Cordova (7) and Cordova et al (8) and the U.K. by Williams (9); Keeling (4); Sampson & Keeling (10) have highlighted certain types of radiopharmaceutical implicated in significant numbers of adverse reactions. Colloids have usually headed the list though the incidence is certainly small because of their widespread use. Particulates principally designed as micro-emboli and used mainly for lung perfusion imaging have also featured: the iron hydroxide particles, with their serotonin-type reactions (4), have now been discontinued and it was the successful introduction of the Limulus pyrogen test which finally solved the problem of aseptic meningitis from intrathecal radiopharmaceuticals. (11, 12). A full review of the early literature on the subject is given by Shani et al (13).

In the U.K., the British Institute of Radiology together with the British Nuclear Medicine Society, the Hospital Physicists` Association and the Radiopharmacists Group of the

Pharmaceutical Society of Great Britain have been operating a centralised reporting system for the last ten years. Experience in the last five years has shown a notable change in the pattern of reports though colloids continue to feature but in place of the serotonintype reactions with iron particulates and the pyrogen reactions from intrathecal preparations, we now find a group of skin reactions to methylene diphosphonate emerging with a smaller series of reactions to albumin particulates.

There are now forty-eight cases of adverse reactions reported in the five year period 1978-82 inclusive.

TABLE 1

| | U.K. SERIES 1978-82 | | U.S. SERIES 1967-81+** | |
	CASES	PERCENT	CASES	PERCENT
COLLOIDS	15 (13)*	31%	72 (65)**	26%
MAA/HAM	6 (5)	13%	72 (71)	26%
MDP/EHDP/PyP	13 (13)	27%	40 (35)	14.5%
OTHER RP	14 (10)	29%	93 (87)	33.5%
TOTAL	48 (41)	100%	277 (258)	100%

* Present author's assessment to exclude `unlikely` reports.
+ Cordova et al (8)
** Cordova et al (3) excluding `unlikely` reports.

Once again it can be seen that the largest single group (15 cases; 31% of total) is associated with the use of intravenous colloids for reticuloendothelial (`liver`) scans. The recent U.S. series (8) showed 26% of their total of 277 cases related to colloids. The five year period of the recent U.K. series corresponds to the introduction of MDP for bone scanning and very considerable numbers of patients have now been scanned with this agent: it has featured in 13 adverse reaction reports (27% of the total) in the U.K. whereas in the American series it accounts for only 14.5% of the total. Some at least of the difference is probably due to the fact that the American series starts two years before the widespread use of

MDP and stops one year earlier than the U.K. survey.

A difference is also seen in the third other major group -that due to albumin particulates. This accounts for only six reports (13% of the total) in the present U.K. series whereas it is proportionately twice as numerous in the U.S. series. This group includes both macro-aggregated albumin as well as microspheres of human albumin and millimicrospheres. It is likely that the marketing and pattern of use show significant differences either side of the Atlantic. Microspheres account for the great majority of the American series and for three of the six in the United Kingdom. It would seem from the report of Rhodes and Cordova (7) that there is over a tenfold difference in risk between these preparations.

Cordova et al (3) have analysed the most recent U.S. data with a modified algorithm to get a more objective assessment of the responsibility of the radiopharmaceutical for the reported reaction. The totals, excluding those reckoned `unlikely` to be causally related, are shown separately for the U.S. series in Table 1. The factors taken into account include general experience with the radiopharmaceutical, alternative aetiological candidates, the timing of events and a modified version of dechallenge. Rechallenge is rarely encountered in the series.

TABLE 2. U.K. SERIES 1978-82:Adverse Reaction Reports and
        Colloids all Tc-99m labelled

TOTAL	15/48	31%
Less `unlikely` reports	13/41	31%
Antimony sulphide colloid		7
Sulphur colloid		6
Other		2
Wheeze, dyspnoea, bronchospasm		4
Flush, pallor, pulse changes,		4
hypotension		6
Sweats, fever		1
Aches, paints		6
Rash		2
(distribution to lungs)		3

Using similar criteria but without the same rigorous scoring techniques and being admittedly purely subjective, I have personally reviewed the U.K. series and, in the separate column noted, excluded those I thought to be `unlikely` due to the radiopharmaceuticals.

Amongst the symptomatology mentioned for colloid reactions, it can be seen that vasomotor changes account for a significant group.

Non-specific aches and pains - head ache and back ache were specifically mentioned - are also common and slightly less common was the problem of wheeziness, dyspnoea or bronchospasm. With this latter allergic type of reaction it was felt that there was a significantly raised number of patients with asthma or other atopic problems.

The reports of reactions for albumin particulates are all this time associated with lung perfusion scanning. (Table 3).

TABLE 3. U.K. SERIES 1978-82: Adverse Reaction Reports and Albumin Particulates all Tc-99m labelled

TOTAL	6/48	13%
Less `unlikely` reports	5/41	12%
MAA		3
HAM		1
mHAM		2
Chest pain		3
`Collapse`, syncope		1
Flush, pallor		1
Dyspnoea		1
Sweating, cold		2
Nausea, malaise		2
Trembling, shivering		2

TABLE 4. U.K. SERIES 1978-82: Adverse Reaction Reports and MDP (and HEDP and PyP) all Tc-99m labelled

TOTAL	14/48	27%
Less `unlikely` reports	13/41	31.5%
Rash - erythematous		
(often delayed)	7)	9
- urticarial, `hives`	2)	
Itching		5
Faintness, pallor, hypotension, bradycardia		3
Nausea, malaise		4

None of the serotonintype reactions noted with iron

preparations are seen with albumin but chest pain or discomfort, nausea, malaise and shivering attacks all feature. With the methylene diphosphonate reports (Table 4) there is high proportion showing a rash, most frequently a delayed erythematous rash appearing within two to twenty-four hours after injection and itching is also a prominent feature. Less frequently an urticarial type of reaction (`hives`) was noted and a small number showed a vasomotor reaction plus a small number of patients complained of nausea or malaise.

The miscellaneous group which make up the remainder (Table 5) are seen to be extremely diverse and feature most of the less commonly used radiopharmaceuticals though with such small numbers, no pattern can be seen and the question of cause and effect becomes tenuous. The serotonin-type reaction noted with the In-111 Tropolone labelled platelets is not entirely surprising as they are known to contain this chemical at high concentration. It is likely that this reaction will be seen more frequently if Indium platelet studies get into more general use.

TABLE 5. U.K. SERIES 1978-82. Adverse Reaction Reports and Other Radiopharmaceuticals.

TOTAL		14/48	29%
Less `unlikely` reports*		10/41	24.5%
Cases			
1	Tc-99m pertechnetate		(1* patient died of) haemorrhage
1	Tc-99m DTPA		
1	Tc-99m Glucoheptonate		
1	I-131 HSA		
1	I-131 Hippuran		
1	I-123 Hippuran		(1* patient on Frusemide and beta blocker
1	I-125 HSA		
	Cr-51 Chromate/red cells		
2	Ga-67 Citrate		
1	In-111 DTPA		(1* symtoms from the) cisternal puncture
1	In-111 Tropolone/platelets		
1	Se-75 Methyl norcholesterol		
1	Fe-59 Desferrioxamine		(1* poor injection) technique

Amongst this group, four of the fourteen patients were thought `unlikely` due to the radiopharmaceutical. In one, a patient who died 20 minutes after the injection of sodium pertechnetate for a brain scan was felt to have died of her subarachnoid haemorrhage and to be totally unrelated to the pharmaceutical. The only intrathecal problem reported was with Indium-111 DTPA and the symptoms were those not infrequently encountered after simple cisternal puncture with changes in CSF pressure; there was no evidence of meningism. The desferrioxamine was inadvertently given by relatively fast intravenous injection and produced a not unexpected result. The fourth case involved hippuran renography in which the patient was undergoing a diuretic stress. She was already taking a beta blocking drug and on being given intravenous Frusemide became hypotensive with associated symptoms. It seems very likely that the effect was entirely due to the alteration in fluid volumes and blood pressure and not related to the hippuran. Another fatality followed 20 minutes after the intravenous injection of sulphur colloid with a reaction in an already seriously ill patient. One lung perfusion scan done with Tc-99m macroaggregated albumin resulted in apparent immediate cardiac arrest but successful resuscitation was carried out promptly. A third fatality in the present U.K. series occurred three days after the injection of human serum albumin millimicrospheres for a liver scan. It was noted that a high proportion of the dose was retained in the lung fields though no complaint was made by the patient at that time. The patient was not thought to be seriously ill but died three days later of "cardiovascular disease".

It is noteworthy that with the awareness of the problems of pyrogens at very low concentrations in intrathecal preparations, there have been, with the introduction of the limulus test, no reactions in the present series due to pyrogens and there have been none due to sterility problems for many years. Very few radiopharmaceuticals are found to provide good growth conditions for bacteria or fungi and the time between production and use is at most a few hours so that microbial multiplication does not occur (14, 15).

True incidence figures are very difficult to obtain. In the U.S. the incidence of radiopharmaceutical reactions has been

quoted as 1 to 6 per 100,000. In Japan a slightly higher
figure of 6 to 20 per 100,000 was quoted though here it was
noted that I-131 labelled cholesterol reactions were reported
at a higher incidence of approximately 3 to 5 per 1,000.
Centralised statistics are not available for Nuclear Medicine
investigations in the U.K. and I have therefore attempted to
get some estimate by looking in detail at my own two
Departments covering the west of Devon and Cornwall. Here two
Departments under my own supervision report, I hope, the great
majority of all adverse reactions including the relatively
trivial ones. In this five year period 8 of the present series
of U.K. reports emanate from these Departments and we serve a
population of very close to threequarters of a million.
Multiplied up to the population of the United Kingdom we would
expect therefore on this basis a total of approximately 550
adverse reaction reports: we received less than one tenth of
this total. An alternative approach using the total number of
radiopharmaceutical doses given in my two Health Districts
would suggest a figure of approximately one adverse reaction
per 4,000 administrations, covering a wide variety of
radiopharmaceuticals. I think these figures become too
inaccurate for finer analysis but if our own experience was
indeed a true reflection of the larger scale, it would suggest
that antimony sulphide colloids show some reaction - mostly
very minor - at approximately one case per thousand
injections. These figures are very much higher than those
usually quoted in other reports e.g. 1 to 6 per 100,000 (8); 3
per 100,000 (16); but I suspect are considerable more
accurate.

The design of the pro-formas to be used for the reporting
of adverse reactions is seen to vary considerably from system
to system. Not infrequently they seem to reflect the
professional interests of their authors: those that have
involved pharmacists usually and quite understandably
introduce questions of drug defects and packaging and
formulation problems. I must declare a bias, having designed
the U.K. pro-forma (9). This is relatively short and
clinically orientated as might be expected from a doctor. The

shortness is also intentional and designed simply to elicit a
response in the first place. It is known that the incidence of
these adverse reactions to radiopharmaceuticals is small - in
the U.K. we scarcely get one a month - and it is no problem to
go back to people making reports for further details (17). It
was felt that some would be put off making reports if there
were many more questions to be filled in and recent experience
with the European Joint Committee on Radiopharmaceuticals
report for 1980/82 (18) might not be irrelevant. Table 6 is
taken from this report and it can be seen that the only
sizeable numbers in relation to population would seem to come
from the German Democratic Republic, Denmark and the United
Kingdom. These are the three countries involved who have
existing national systems for the collection of
radiopharmaceutical reactions.

TABLE 6. Nationality of Adverse Reaction Reports

	CH	DDR	DK	I	NL	UK	Total
1980	0	12	1	0	2	10	25
1981	1	4	3	0	1	7	16
1982 (first half)	0	1	2	1	1	5	10
Total	1	17	6	1	4	22	51

The collection and publication of this type of data can
have several useful effects. By pooling our experience, first
at national level and then internationally, we can expect to
identify a radiopharmaceutical with either unduly frequent or
serious side effects. This has already happened, but perhaps
just as useful is the recognition of patterns of adverse
reactions to particular agents. With this foreknowledge
doctors are much more likely to recognise an adverse reaction
when one occurs and appropriate treatment instituted without
delay. Particular types of patient at risk may be given, for
example, steroid cover if a sensitivity reaction is
anticipated.

At present it is taking us several years to recognise these patterns of adverse reactions; about the same time scale we see with the change to yet newer radiopharmaceuticals. Awareness of the value of reporting reactions must be spread more widely - this way will come much quicker recognition of problems to the benefit of all.

REFERENCES
1. Rawlins M D, Thompson J W. Pathogenesis of Adverse Drug Reactions in Davies, D.M. ed. Textbook of Adverse Drug Reactions: 2nd Ed Oxford Med Publ 1981.
2. CFR 21, Code of (U.S.) Federal Regulations 1979;21:310.301.
3. Cordova M A, Hladik W B, Rhodes B A. Validation and characterization of adverse reactions to radiopharmaceuticals. Presented at Annual Western Regional Meeting, Society of Nuclear Medicine. San Diego, California, 1982.
4. Keeling D H. Side-effects associated with the use of Radiopharmaceuticals in J.W. Gorrod ed. Drug Toxicity: London Taylor & Francis Ltd., 1979.
5. Atkins H L, Hauser W, Richards P, Klopper J. Adverse reactions to radiopharmaceuticals. J Nucl Med 1972;13:232-3.
6. Ford I, Shroff A, Benson W, Atkins H L, Rhodes B A. SNM Drug Problem Reporting System. J Nucl Med 1978;19:116-17.
7. Rhodes B A, Cordova M A. Adverse Reactions to Radiopharmaceuticals: Incidence in 1978 and associated symptoms. J Nucl Med 1980;21:1107-9.
8. Cordova M A, Rhodes B A, Atkins H L, Glenn H J, Hoogland D R, Solomon A C. Adverse Reactions to Radiopharmaceuticals. J Nucl Med 1982;23:550-51.
9. Williams E S. Adverse Reactions to Radiopharmaceuticals: a preliminary survey in the United Kingdom. Brit J Radiol 1974;47:54-9.
10. Sampson C B, Keeling D H. Adverse Reactions to Radiopharmaceuticals; a follow up survey in the U.K. presented at Annual Scientific Meeting, British Nuclear Medicine Society, London. 1982.
11. Cooper J F, Harbert J C. Abstract in J Nucl Med 1973;14:387.
12. Cooper J F, Harberg J C. Endotoxin as a cause of aseptic meningitis after radionuclide cisternography. J Nucl Med 1975;16:809-13.
13. Shani J, Atkins H L, Wolf W. Adverse Reactions to Radiopharmaceuticals. Sem Nucl Med 1976;6:305-28.
14. Sørensen K, Kristensen K, Frandsen P. Microbial contamination of radionuclide generators. Eur J Nucl Med 1977;2:105-7.
15. Abra R M, Bell N D S, Horton P W. The growth of micro-organisms in some parenteral radiopharmaceuticals. Int J Pharmaceutics 1980;5:187-93.
16. Abra R M, Bell N D S, Horton P W, McCarthy T M. A survey

250

of radiopharmaceutical manufacture in United Kidngdom
hospitals. J Clin Hosp Pharm 1980;5:11-20.

17. Keeling D H. `Radiopharmaceuticals` in: W.H.W. Inman ed.
Monitoring for Drug Safety: Lancaster U.K. M.T.P. Press
Ltd. 1980.
18. Kristensen K. First Report on the system for `Reporting of
Adverse Reactions and Drug Defects 1980-82` from the Joint
Committee on Radiopharmaceuticals of the European Nuclear
Medicine Society and the Society of Nuclear Medicine,
Europe. Nuklearmedizin 1982;21:274-77.

17. DRUG DEFECTS

BENTE PEDERSEN

1. INTRODUCTION

Radiopharmaceuticals are characterized by a number of parameters such as chemical composition and purity, apyrogenicity, sterility, pH, radiochemical purity, radionuclidic purity, radioactive concentration, specific activity, optical purity, particle size and numbers. When one or more of these parameters fall outside specified limits, we have a drug defect. Under the term drug defects we also include errors in labels and package inserts, external contaminations of vials etc.

The effect of drug defects may vary from small problems to severe problems such as pyrogenreactions during cisternography and erroneous biodistribution. Information about the quality of radiopharmaceuticals can be accomplished in two ways. Either by collecting information about drug problems from the users of these drugs or by systematic testing of the drugs against specifications. Reports from hospitals about drug defects are important to regulatory agencies as well as manufacturers. Regulatory agencies needs the knowledge when setting standards and for drug surveillance. Manufacturers needs the information for product improvements and manufacturing adjustments. Centralized registration of drug defects is also valuable for the clinician when he needs information about similar problems at other hospitals. It is often difficult to distinguish between adverse reactions and drug defects and so far little is published about the nature and frequency of drug defects. Present information can be separated in drug defect reporting and compliance testing.

2. DRUG DEFECT REPORTING

From Japan Radioisotope Division we have unpublished survey data from 1975-1979. (1). Table 1 gives the number of defects. The frequency varies between 0 and 0.14% of administered doses. The nature of these defects is not mentioned.

Table 1. Defects to Radiopharma-ceuticals in Japan 1975-79

PRODUCT	NUMBER OF DEFECTS
^{57}Co- BLEOMYCINS	-
^{67}Ga- CITRATE	7
^{75}Se- SELENOMETHIONINE	2
^{111}In- CHLORIDE	2
^{111}In- DTPA	-
^{131}J - BSP	-
^{131}J - MAA	-
^{131}J - SODIUM IODIDE	-
^{131}J - HSA	-
^{131}J - JODOHIPPURATE	-
^{131}J - JODOALDOSTEROL	-
^{131}J - ROSE BENGAL	-
^{131}Cs- CHLORIDE	5
^{169}Yb- DTPA	-
^{197}Hg- CHLORMERODRIN	2
^{198}Au- GOLD COLLOID	8
^{99m}Tc- GENERATOR	12
^{99m}Tc- PERTECHNETATE	1
^{99m}Tc- EHDP	8
^{99m}Tc- GLUCONATE	3
^{99m}Tc- DTPA	1
^{99m}Tc- HIDA (DIETHYL) *	1
^{99m}Tc- DMSA	17
^{99m}Tc- SULPHUR COLLOID	4
^{99m}Tc- TIN COLLOID	18
^{99m}Tc- RBC *	1
^{99m}Tc- MAA	19
^{99m}Tc- HSA	7
^{99m}Tc- PYRIDOXYLIDENE ISOLEUCINE *	1
^{99m}Tc- PYROPHOSPHATE	4
^{99m}Tc- PHYTATE	33
^{99m}Tc- HIDA (P-BUTYL) *	3
^{99m}Tc- MDP	55

* NO APPROVAL

Table 2. Drug defect in USA 1976-78

COMPLAINT	NUMBER OF DEFECTS
pH	-
RADIOCHEMICAL PURITY	37
RADIONUCLIDIC PURITY	6
RADIO ASSAY	7
PACKAGE LABEL	15
PARTICLE SIZE	7
PYROGENS	1
BIODISTRIBUTION	33
STERILITY	3
PARTICULATE MATTER	5
CONTAMINATIONS	12
CONTAINER DAMAGE	6
OTHERS UNKNOWN	29

The Society of Nuclear Medicine (SNM), U.S.A. established in 1976 a Drug Problem Reporting System as a cooperative arrangement between SNM, USP and FDA. The number of defect products in 1976 have been published (2). 37 defective radiopharmaceuticals were reported. Poor Tc-99m labelling was the major defect reported for liver, lung and bone agents. Other problems were incorrect radioassay, wrong particle size, inadequate radiochemical purity and external contamination of vials. FDA established a computerized data base with information from this system (3). This data base can give a list of drug product defects arranged by manufacturer and radiopharmaceutical. Table 2 lists the number and types of major complaints during the first 2 1/2 years. SNM and FDA reported in 1979 a major concern about continuous decline in adverse reaction and drug defect reporting (4). In July and August 1979 only four reports about drug defects were received. This probably indicates improvements in the quality of radiopharmaceuticals as well as declining interest in the programme. Assuming 1 million administrations per month the sampling of defects was estimated to 0.1%.

A new approach has been tried in U.S.A. since 1978 (5). Drug problem reporting materials are mailed by USP to hospital pharmacies, clinics, community pharmacies and to members of SNM several times a year. Members of SNM also receives a report of previous findings. Reporting can be done either by mailing a form or by telephone. A special telephone number has been established. The information collected is the identity of the products, lot number, manufacturer and a brief description of the problem. Approx. 45% of all reports came by telephone.

Table 3. Reports on defective radiopharmaceuticals from Danish hospitals 1980

PRODUCT	COMPLAINT	CONFIRMED BY QUALITY CONTROL STUDIES
^{99m}Tc- ELUATE	COLLOIDAL	No
^{99m}Tc- ELUATE	RADIOCHEMICAL PURITY	No
^{99m}Tc- ELUATE	LABELLING PROBLEMS	Yes
^{99m}Tc- SULPHUR COLLOID	LUNG UPTAKE	Yes
^{99m}Tc- TIN COLLOID	LUNG UPTAKE	Yes
^{99m}Tc- TIN COLLOID	LABELLING PROBLEMS (EMPTY VIAL)	Yes
^{99m}Tc- MAA	HOT SPOTS-RADIOCHEMICAL PURITY	Yes
^{99m}Tc- MAA	LARGE PARTICLE AGGREGATES	Yes
^{99m}Tc- PYROPHOSPHATE	VIAL NOT CLOSED	-
^{99m}Tc- PYROPHOSPHATE	NO BONE UPTAKE	No
^{99m}Tc- MDP	THYROID VISUALIZATION	No
^{99m}Tc- MDP	LIVER UPTAKE	Yes
^{99m}Tc- GENERATOR	COULD NOT BE ELUTED	-
^{99m}Tc- GENERATOR	LOW ELUTION YIELD	-
^{57}Co/^{58}Co- CAPSULES	CLINICAL RESULTS	No
^{125}J - SODIUM IODIDE	RADIONUCLIDIC PURITY	No
^{131}J - SODIUM IODIDE	CONTAMINATION	Yes
^{131}J - SODIUM IODIDE	NOT A CLEAR SOLUTION	-
^{131}J - HIPPURANE	ANAPHYLACTIC REACTION	NOT STUDIED
^{131}J - ALBUMIN	CLINICAL RESULTS	No
^{133}Xe- INJECTION	LEAKING AMPOULE	Yes

Table 4. Reports on defective radiopharmaceuticals from Danish hospitals 1981

Product	Complaint	Confirmed by quality control studies
^{99m}Tc- Eluate	^{99}Mo in first eluate	No
^{99m}Tc- Eluate	^{99}Mo in second eluate	No
^{99m}Tc- MDP	1 patient abnormal,1 patient normal	No
^{99m}Tc- MDP	High tissue background	No
^{99m}Tc- MDP	Free pertechnetate	No
^{99m}Tc- Tin colloid	Lung uptake	Not studied
^{99m}Tc- Tin colloid	Bone uptake, lung uptake	Not studied
^{99m}Tc- Tin colloid	Rubber particles,High kidney uptake	- , No
^{99m}Tc- DTPA	Empty vial	-
^{99m}Tc- DMSA	Yellow colour (leaking vial)	Yes
^{99m}Tc- Albumin	Solubility problems	-
^{99m}Tc- MAA	Large particle aggregates	Yes
^{99m}Tc- Gluconate	Lung uptake (solubility)	Yes
^{99m}Tc- Generator	Low elution yield (2 reports)	No , Yes
^{99m}Tc- Generator	Label	-
^{99m}Tc- Generator	Lot number	-
^{99m}Tc- Generator	Could not be eluted (2 reports)	Yes
^{51}Cr- Sodium chromate	Radioactive concentration	No
^{57}Co/^{58}Co- Capsules	No activity	No
^{123}J - Hippurane	High tissue background	No
^{125}J - Fibrinogen	Low countrate	No
^{125}J - Hippurane	Anaphylactic reaction	No
^{131}J - Hippurane	Brown colour	No
^{131}J - Hippurane	Radioactive concentration	No
^{131}J - Sodium iodide	Label	-
^{133}Xe- Gas	No activity	Not studied
^{133}Xe- Gas	Vial to big for dispenser	-

Table 5. Reports on defective radiopharmaceuticals from Danish hospitals 1982

Type of product	Complaint	Confirmed by quality control studies
^{99m}Tc- DPD	Rubber particles	-
^{99m}Tc- DPD	Large unsoluble particle	-
^{99m}Tc- DPD	High tissue background	No
^{99m}Tc- MDP	Rubber particles	-
^{99m}Tc- Pyrophosphate	Low RBC labelling	No
^{99m}Tc- Tin colloid	Rubber particles	-
^{99m}Tc- Albumin	Rubber particles	-
^{99m}Tc- Microspheres	Free pertechnetate (slow labelling)	Yes
^{99m}Tc- Generator	Frozen during transport	-
^{47}Ca- Chloride	Leaking vial	-
^{90}Y - Silicate	Large particle	-
^{123}J - Fatty acids	Lung uptake (2 reports)	Yes
^{125}J - Albumin	Radioactive concentration	Yes
^{131}J - Sodium iodide	Frozen during transport	-
^{133}Xe- Gas	Vial to big for dispenser	-

Approximately 1-2 recalls pr year are one of the results of this programme. The reports are entered into as computerized data base. The data are readily accessible and thus of great importance to FDA and other interested parties.

Danish hospitals have been encouraged to report drug defects to the Isotope-Pharmacy. Depending upon the nature of these reports we try to test if the problem is related to the drug. We believe the frequency of reporting is very high and for more serious defects it is approx. 100%. Results from 1979 have been published (6). Tables 3-5 lists major complaints for product types 1980-1982 and column three of the tables indicates if it has been possible to confirm the complaint by analysis. The frequencies of defects in % of total shipments reported to the Isotope-Pharmacy were 1.0% in 1979, 1.1% in 1980, 1.4% in 1981 and 0.6% in 1982. These percentages indicates an increase in quality of radiopharmaceuticals in 1982. Comparison between results from different reports is difficult. The method of collection varies and the nature and frequency of complaints are not present in all the reports.

3. COMPLIANCE TESTING BY REGULATORY AGENCIES

Reports are available from three countries U.S.A., Canada and Denmark.

3.1. U.S.A.

From Bureau of Drugs, FDA we have a Radioactive Drug Survey from 1977-1979 (7).

Table 6. Compliance testing Bureau of Drugs, FDA, USA, 1977-79

	NUMBER OF FIRMS	NUMBER OF SAMPLES	NUMBER OF SAMPLES FAILED
	2	7	0
1977	1	22	6
	3	27	5
	1	14	6
	1	22	5
1978	1	13	4
	1	9	6
	7	27	5
	8	32	0
1979	1	19	4
	1	12	2
	3	?	3

Table 6 gives the number of firms covered, samples tested and number of failures. The frequency of defects varies from company to company between 0 and 67%. Table 7 lists reasons for failure for different products. The National Institute of Health, U.S.A. have published (8) results from ten years (1962-1971) quality control of radioactive products for patient administration. Methods and reasons for defects are thoroughly described. Results are given as the deviation of assays from specified values. If assay values outside ± 20% are considered errors then approx. 6% of all shipments were defective. If assay values of ± 10% are considered errors then approx. 16% were defective. This paper though twelve years old gives a good description of a thorough quality control system.

Table 7. Compliance testing, Bureau of Drugs, FDA, USA, 1977-79

Product	Reasons for failure
^{99m}Tc- MAA	Particle size - biodistribution - radiochemical purity - specific activity - pH
^{99m}Tc- Sulphur colloid	Biodistribution - radiochemical purity - specific activity
^{99m}Tc- EHDP	Biodistribution - radiochemical purity -
^{99m}Tc- DMSA	Biodistribution
^{99m}Tc- Pyrophosphate	pH
^{99m}Tc- Generator	Radionuclidic purity
^{32}P - Chromic phosphate	pH
^{51}Cr- Sodium chromate	Specific activity - chromate content - labelling
^{57}Co- Cyanocobalamin	Specific activity - radiochemical purity
^{67}Ga- Citrate	pH
^{75}Se- Selenomethionine	Radiochemical purity
^{111}In- DTPA	Specific activity
^{123}J - Sodium iodide caps.	Radiochemical purity - labelling
^{125}J - Sodium iodide caps.	Specific activity
^{131}J - Sodium iodide caps.	Radiochemical purity
^{131}J - Sodium iodide sol.	Specific activity - radiochemical purity - pH - labelling
^{131}J - HSA	Radiochemical purity
^{131}J - MAA	Radiochemical purity - specific activity

3.2. Canada

Environmental Health Directorate, Health Protection Branch,

Canada has published two reports (9, 10) on compliance testing
of drugs (table 8). The frequency of defects varies in these
two reports, mainly due to change of specifications.

Table 8. Compliance testing, Environmental Health Directorate,
Canada

PRODUCT	NUMBER OF FIRMS	NUMBER OF BATCHES	NUMBER OF FAILURES
1976 - 1977			
^{99M}Tc- MAA	6	24	1 (BIODISTRIBUTION)
^{99M}Tc- MICROSPHERES	1	4	4 (BIODISTRIBUTION)
^{99M}Tc- HSA	3	14	6 (BIODISTRIBUTION AND FREE $\overline{TcO_4}$)
1978 - 1979			
^{99M}Tc- MAA	5	35	0
^{99M}Tc- MICROSPHERES	1	9	0
^{99M}Tc- HSA	3	16	3 (BIODISTRIBUTION)
^{99M}Tc- MDP	3	1o	NO SPECIFICATION
^{99M}Tc- EHDP	2	7	NO SPECIFICATION
^{99M}Tc- PYROPHOSPHATE	1	4	NO SPECIFICATION
^{99M}Tc- PYRO-TRIMETA-PHOSPHATE	1	2	NO SPECIFICATION

3.3. Denmark

Compliance testing at the Isotope-Pharmacy, Denmark is
mentioned in five reports (6, 11-14). The Isotope Pharmacy is
a national governmental institution supplying about 60% of all
radiopharmaceuticals used in Denmark in percent of number of
samples. The postmarketing surveillance of these commercially
available drugs is based on three systems: supply control,
compliance testing and drug defect reports from danish
hospitals.

3.3.1. Supply control. All products received at the
Isotope-Pharmacy are inspected, papers and labels are compared
with specifications, radionuclidic identity is measured with a
simple test in the form of measurements in a brass shielding
and a plastic shielding and comparing these with an unshielded
measurement in an ionization chamber. External contamination
is checked by smear-testing of all products. The number of
defect radiopharmaceuticals received at the Isotope-Pharmacy
1979-1982 have been published (12-14). The frequencies of
defects in % of total number of shipments are summarized in

table 9.

Table 9. Percentage of defects found among Radiopharmaceuticals received at the Isotope-Pharmacy

	1979 TOTAL	ACTION TAKEN	1980 TOTAL	ACTION TAKEN	1981 TOTAL	ACTION TAKEN	1982 TOTAL	ACTION TAKEN
FORMAL ERRORS (LABELS AND THE PAPER-WORK)	2.6	1.5	3.7	2.0	4.2	2.8	3.3	2.0
EXTERNAL CONTAMINATION	3.1	0.6	4.6	1.0	3.6	0.5	2.4	0.3
OTHER DEFECTS INCLUDING INVALIDATING ERRORS	2.4	1.4	3.0	2.4	2.0	1.3	2.4	1.6
ALL ERRORS	8.1	3.5	11.3	5.4	9.8	4.5	8.1	3.9
TOTAL NUMBER OF SHIPMENTS	1912		1855		2155		2591	

Minor and more formal errors will only cause action if they
are repeated over a period of time. However many small errors
can indicate a lack of efficiency in the manufacturers quality
assurance programme. During the period 1976-1980 a continuous
increase in these minor errors were seen. The Isotope-Pharmacy
therefore urged manufacturers to look at their quality
assurance programme. During the last period of 1981 and in
1982 a decrease in numbers have been recorded. Our supply
control represents a unique chance to follow a large part of
the production in this area. We still find changes in labels
and package inserts which for registered radiopharmaceuticals
should be approved beforehand. Half of the defects caused
direct action in form of a telephonecall or a letter to the
manufacturer. Only few cases were considered to be of a more
serious character. These defects include radioactive
concentration, volume, particle contamination, calibration and
expiry dates. Table 10 gives a list of product invalidating
errors found by the supply control. Half-closed vials causing
sterility problems and external contaminations, and errors in
labelling have been the dominating errors.

Table 10.   Supply control-product invalidating errors 1979-82

DELIVERY OF WRONG PRODUCT

BROKEN VIALS AND AMPOULES

DEFECT RUBBER CLOSURE

DEFECT METAL CLOSURE

EMPTY VIALS

LEAKING VIALS

LEAKING SYRINGES

HIGH PRESSURE IN SYRINGES

MISSING SYRINGES

SOLVENT FOR DILUTION MISSING

MISSING LABEL

NO DECLARATION OF CONTENT

WRONG LABEL

ERRORS IN LOT NUMBER

WRONG CALIBRATION DATE

PARTICLES

STERILITY

UNIFORMITY OF DOSAGE FOR CAPSULES

RADIONUCLIDIC PURITY

3.3.2. Compliance testing. All radioactive products apart from Tc-99m generators and preparation kits are sampled on a random basis for a complete analysis of all parameters in the product specification. Results of compliance testing of these radiopharmaceuticals from 1977-1982 are summarized in table 11.

Table 11. Results of compliance testing at the Isotope-Pharmacy 1977-82 (Tc-99m generators and preparation kits not included)

| | NUMBER OF PRODUCTS TESTED | NUMBER OF DEFECT PRODUCTS | FREQUENCY % | NUMBER OF DEFECTS | TYPES OF DEFECTS | | | |
					RAD.CONC.TOTAL RADIOACTIVITY	RAD.CHEMICAL IMPURITY	RAD.NUCLIDIC IMPURITY	OTHER DEFECTS
1977	46	6	13	6	2	-	-	4
1978	64	1o	15,6	1o	4	-	-	6
1979	35	1o	28,6	1o	6	2	-	2
1980	45	9	2o	9	2	2	1	7
1981	79	14	17,7	21	6	4	1	1o
1982	77	13	16,4	15	3	-	1	11

"Other defects" include pH, sterility, uniformity of dosage in capsules, osmotic pressure etc.. The frequency of

these defects in percent of number of samples varies from
13-29% with the highest frequency in 1979. In 1981 Tc-99m
generators (one from each manufacturer on the danish market)
were tested. No defects were found. Tc-99m labelled
radiopharmaceuticals based on Tc-99m generators and
preparation kits have been subjected to a systematic
compliance testing. Labelling was carried out with eluate from
a 100 mCi generator. For each product three batches were
analysed. For each batch labelling was carried out on three
different days. From January 1982 this was reduced to
labelling on two days. If these labellings are not identical a
third preparation is included. Appearance, pH and isotonicity
were recorded for each preparation. Analytical methods
includes methods from manufacturers and pharmacopoeias as well
as methods of our own choice. Methods were chosen to show free
pertechnetate, reduced-hydrolized Tc-99m and if possible
labelling efficiency directly. All results were double
determinations. Particle size and number were included where
relevant (12-14).

Table 12. Summary of the results of quality control of Tc-99m
labelled radiopharmaceuticals 1976-82.

	Products	Batches	Prep.	Batches Defect	Single prep. Defect	Single analytical parameter deviating	Single analytical result deviating
1976 - 1978	66	171	513	16	6	95	38
1979	34	47	141	4	4	1o	14
1980	3o	32	94	4	1	6	7
1981	29	42	112	1	4	9	19
1982	42	5o	96	o	o	9	9

Table 12 summarizes the numbers of defect batches and single
preparations and deviating analytical results from 1976 -
1982. Errors have not been concentrated on certain products or
firms. No clear relation between the age of the generator and
the quality of the products were seen. The frequency of
defects decreased during the period. In 1982 no defects were
found. Our results show two things; first we have eliminated
most of the analytical errors and second there has been an
increase in the quality of radiopharmaceuticals in use. This
have been accomplished in two ways. The hospitals have changed
to better preparation kits within the same type of kits and

better types of kits have been developed.

    3.3.3. Errors found in one of the three systems are always reported to the manufacturer. Consequences for the users of these radiopharmaceuticals are considered and the necessary action is taken in form of a letter or telephonecall. It would be nice to have an exact way to measure the effect of our quality control. This is of course not possible but we can give some examples. Frequent contaminations of certain products have been eliminated, Tc-99m-MAA preparation kits have been recalled due to large particles, errors in labels have been cleared up before the products are used, Tc-99m colloid kits have been recalled due to lung uptake, J-123 fatty acid was recalled due to particle impurities causing lung uptake etc. We think that all the three parts of our quality control programme are of importance and we will continue this type of system.

4. CONCLUSION

    Comparison of results from the different reports shows that the nature of defects are very much the same. The frequency of drug defects judged from collected hospital reports is very much dependent upon the frequency of reporting. We realize that it is difficult to keep a continuous interest in a reporting programme but it looks as the new system in U.S.A. and the danish system are rather good. Compliance testing in U.S.A. shows that errors are concentrated on certain firms while danish results apart from supply control shows no concentration. Errors found by supply control however are very much connected to certain manufacturers and they are periodical in appearance indicating leakage in quality assurance programs. Results from U.S.A. and Denmark may demonstrate an effect of compliance testing in the form of a decreasing number of defects. Judged from results shown in this paper the quality of radiopharmaceuticals in general is not inferior to the quality of other drugs but the number of small and formal errors could be decreased considerably.

REFERENCES
1. Kasida Y. Personal communication. Japan Radioisotope Association.1981.
2. Ford L, Shroff A, Benson W, Atkins H, Rhodes BA. SNM Drug Problem Reporting System. J Nucl Med 1978; 19:116-117.
3. Ford L. Drug product defects by manufacturer and radiopharmaceutical. FDA, unpublished. 1978.
4. Rhodes BA. Adverse Reaction and Product Problem Reports Decline. SNM Newsline, 1979:5.
5. Valentino J G, Kerwin C M. Product Problem Reporting System for Drugs and Radiopharmaceuticals. Unpublished. 1982.
6. Kristensen K. Quality Control of Radiopharmaceuticals. Medical Radionuclide Imaging 1980, IAEA, Vienna. 1981:59-78.
7. Halperin J A. Radioactive Drug Survey. FDA, Personal communication. 1980.
8. Vacca P C, Farcas R J, Semler M O. Quality Control of Radioactive Products for Patient Administration at the National Institutes of Health. J Label Compounds Radiopharm 1973; 9:755-768.
9. Health Protection Branch. Results of Quality Control Studies of Tc-99m labelled Radiopharmaceuticals Prepared from Kits. Report 78-EHD-24, Canada. 1978.
10. Health Protection Branch. Results of Quality Control Studies of Tc-99m labelled Radiopharmaceuticals Prepared from Kits. (1978-79). Report 82-EDH-75, Canada. 1982.
11. Kristensen K. Quality Control at the Hospital. Radiopharmaceuticals (Proc. 2nd Int. Symp. Radiopharmaceuticals 1979) 2. SNM. New York. 1979.
12. Isotope-Pharmacy. Reports on Activities 1978-79. 1980 Copenhagen (in danish).
13. Isotope-Pharmacy. Reports on Activities 1980-81. 1982 Copenhagen (in danish).
14. Isotope-Pharmacy. Reports on Activities 1982-83. Unpublished.

18. ETHICS-RESPONSIBILITY IN DEVELOPMENT, CLINICAL TRIALS AND
    MARKETING

OLE WEIS-FOGH

1. INTRODUCTION

The main responsibilities of the pharmaceutical industry
are to develop new and better drugs, to search for the proper
use of existing drugs and to be an intermediary between
researchers, doctors and patients. When people buy a cake or a
coat they are able to judge for themselves what they are
buying. When a drug is prescribed for them they have to trust
other people's judgement. This makes a great difference
between the responsibilities of the baker or tailor and those
of the drug manufacturer. We are not just selling a commodity,
we are delivering a system. In this system the software is
just as important as the hardware: and it is the software we
are developing in the preclinical tests and the clinical
trials. We are confronted with a lot of ethical conflicts
during the development period, partly because ethics are not
the same to all people at all times, and partly because the
ultimate goal of drug research - the proof for safety and
efficacy involves a lot of necessary tests which bring us in
conflict with other aspects of "doing right in all relations
of life".

People involved in drug research are well trained in
natural science, but this is not enough today. Ethics also
form an important part of our instrumentarium, and ethics are
not concerned mainly with bare facts, but with values, with
estimates and other imponderables. So, our problem is to
combine positive science with normative science.

Ethical aspects are involved in choosing research
programmes, in the toxicity programmes, in the methods
selected for clinical trials, in the information we give to

physicians and patients, and in the way this information is given.We will be held responsible for product liability in the broader sense and in details, such as proper packaging systems, etc., and we are responsible for following all possible regulations. Is it possible to meet this big complex of responsibilities and ethical demands and, at the same time, to meet our main responsibility: the development of new drugs, the opening up of new therapeutic possibilities? There is no easy answer to this question, but it seems obvious that the greatest ethical conflict lies in the interplay between the need for new and better preparations and the steadily increasing demands to even greater safety.

2.PRECLINICAL TESTS

It is beyond all questions that drugs must be safe in use. But nowadays safe in use tends to be understood as absolute safety. What tools do we then use to predict safety? A range of more or less unspecific, orthodox toxicity tests in which we use an incredible number of animals. And still we have to realize that the results of the tests give a very weak basis for prediction in man. It is the requirement for absolute safety which causes most of the troubles in drug research and development. We are closing our eyes every time we trust the results of these orthodox testing programmes. And we are closing our eyes every time we even tend to believe that any drug will be absolutely safe. What we really are looking for in the preclinical tests is the risk/benefit factor.

This lead to the conclusion that more sophisticated tests should replace the orthodox testing programme and much more emphasis should be put on the pharmacological test programmes. It also leads to the conclusion that we stress the facts of life to the public: The use of drugs is a balance between effects and side-effects and a balance between new drugs and the ability to cure many diseases.

Safety, or rather people's feeling of safety, is not an absolute term. Everybody takes risks every day. People do not mind walking in the streets or driving a car, they even drink alcohol and smoke though they are well aware of the risks.If something goes wrong they won't blame the car dealer or the tobacconist. On the other hand, if they suffer from sideeffects of drugs they will blame everybody: the drug manufacturers, the authorities, society in general. Why so? Because nobody forces people to drive or to smoke, it's their own free choise. But, if you suffer from any disease or illness your doctor will tell you to take something you don't know a thing about, apart from one thing: now you will get well again. And look, your temperature goes down or your pain disappears -and then you suddenly have a skin rash. And you get furious and blame everybody, if you have not been told that this was a risk to be taken if you wanted to get the benefits of the cure.

There is little doubt that most of the people in this audience know much more about toxicology and pharmacology than I do. But I have the feeling that pharmacodynamics and pharmacokinetics should form a greater part of the animal safety studies than they do today, and that a great number of the orthodox toxicity studies could be abandoned. I know that it is extremely dangerous to suggest an extension of one section of studies at the expense of another section, the danger being that the other section is not reduced at all. We have seen what happened with the in vitro toxicity tests, they were just added to the prevailing conservative regimen. But what I am aiming at is well-founded specific toxicity tests to replace the non-specific tests which nearly kill modern drug research both from a financial and a temporal point of view without giving real value for the money. If we look at radiopharmaceuticals, especially radiopharmaceuticals for diagnostic use, the conservative toxicity studies are not regarded as the most important studies. Much more important are pharmacodynamic and, especially, pharmacokinetic studies. So would it be too optimistic to expect that scientists dealing with radiopharmarceuticals will blaze new trails in toxicity reserach?

3. CLINICAL TRIALS

Bearing in mind that we only have a feeling and not real

knowledge about safety and efficacy of a candidate new drug after the animal studies, it seems obvious that proper planning of the clinical trials is of the utmost importance. Proper planning includes precise specification of diagnostic criteria, patient allocation, parameters to be monitored, methods and time points for observations and analysis, the extent and length of the trial, all based on the statistical methods which form the background for the choice of test methods and analysis of the test results.

In short, to be able to obtain true and objective results without putting the patients at risk. Clinical trials which are not scrupulously planned cannot be considered as ethical. We must bear in mind that controlled clinical trials are only of potential value for half of the patients who take part in these trials. The purpose of a clinical trial is not directly to treat the patients involved better, but to find, hopefully, a better treatment for future patients. All concerned: the manufacturer, the authorities and the future patients are interested in achieving that goal. The dilemma, or the ethical conflict, is that the manufacturer and the investigator have the knowledge about the drug, but it is the patients and the patients only who lend their bodies to the clinical trial.

Attempts to solve this conflict have been made with the agreement of the Helsinki declaration (1) and a lot has been achieved, for one thing the rules about patient consent. My reason for mentioning the patients' consent especially is that this is the most important step towards a better understanding between the medical profession and patients. And, the closer we get to an understanding between these two groups, the closer we will get to a solution of the ethical conflicts in drug research and development. I called the Helsinki declaration only an attempt to solve the conflict, because obviously it is not enough to set rules for how a given clinical trial should be planned and performed. It is just as important to judge whether a trial should be performed at all or how often it should be repeated.There is, or should be, no doubt that the patients are well protected during a clinical trial.On the other hand, from a certain point it will become clear whether the new drug or treatment is better than the old drug or the old therapy. In other words whether the new drug or treatment will be of benefit to new patients. When this stage is reached, is it then ethical to continue with the trials well knowing that half of the patients would have been better treated if the blind trial had been discontinued and replaced by open trials, or the drug had been approved for general use?Normally a reasonable clinical trials programme is accepted within each country. But internationally we are still faced with requirements of performing local studies which means duplicating trials already performed elsewhere and where we often know what the results will be beforehand. Such duplication is justified where ethnic differences speak for it. But duplication is not always based on rational thinking, emotions are also involved in the writing of regulations and nationalistic undertones are not unknown.What can we do about it? Well, before we start blaming other people we should look into our own business. Are all clinical trials well planned? The answer is no. Do we always concentrate on the right mix of trials? Once again the answer is no. So the first thing we could do is to "clean our own house", and work out proper protocols for each clinical trial as well as a proper overall clinical plan. Naturally there is no unambiguous answer to what such a plan should contain. But, as with the preclinical test programmes I have a feeling that more emphasis should be placed on pharmacodynamic and pharmacokinetic studies. Just as with the preclinical tests, it is a limited knowledge we are to obtain within a reasonable clinical programme. We can't expose human beings to unlimited experiments and the more we know about the fate of a given drug before we continue to phase two or even phase three studies, the better the patients are protected and the better will our background be for predicting possible side-effects. Especially for the pharmacokinetic studies there should be more overlapping between phase one and phase two studies.

4. SIDE-EFFECTS

The most difficult thing in any drug development is to

elucidate the side-effects. We can't drag out the clinical trials infinitely, a system such as monitored release entails a lot of difficulties, and still it is our responsibility that the patients are not exposed to unknown or unpredicted side-effects if by any means we can avoid it. The official side-effect reporting systems, whether national or international, like the WHO system, often work very well, but now and then they simply collapse. So, valuable as they are, we can't rely on these systems alone.The fundamental shortcoming in the way we collect experience on side-effects and adverse reactions is that it is done passively. It should be possible to formulate the preclinical and clinical test programmes in a way which enables us to make better predictions on possible side-effects and adverse reactions. Any predictions or suspicions of possible side-effects should be explained in detail in the clinical protocol, thus enabling the investigators to look for signs or reactions which could predict possible side-effects.If we don't clean our own house, it will never come to a real dialogue between manufacturers and health authorities. If we do, it might be possible to influence the regulations and which is even more important, to come to an understanding with the general public. The latter process starts with our information - information on individual drugs and information on the basis for drug research and development.

5.INFORMATION

I think it is true that all manufacturers want to be in charge of information about their own products, not to leave it to a national or supranational body. Many attempts have been made to organize State information systems. None of them has been really successful and I don't think any further attempts will be. Three conditions are restraints to success, first: Product liability is closely connected to the information given and nobody wants to share product liability with the manufacturer. Secondly: the overwhelming amount of reports and documentation needed for proper information make it extremely difficult to handle thousands of products and finally, you can`t be your own watch-dog, and this is true also of official bodies.

And here we are again. If we claim our right we must meet our responsibility: proper information. The information on drugs and the soft-ware of the system we are selling, is just as important as the drug itself and if we look at it from an image point of view even more important. Information allows no escape route at all: it is a must that the information is true, it is a must that the information is complete, and it is a must that the information is given promptly, especially in case of bad news.I dare say that the most serious conflicts between drug manufacturers and the public have been rooted in improper or incomplete information, rather than in inferior drugs. The key word for ethical marketing of drugs is proper positioning of the drug, and proper positioning is a process which last for the entire life of the drug.

6.CONCLUSION

If we want to keep our freedom to meet our main responsibility - the development of new and better drugs and therapies - we have to be seen as honest and reliable people. The key word here is information, but not only on specific drugs. It is also vital that we devote part of our time to inform the public about the basic problems involved in the development of new drugs. The alternative is that the "absolute safety" -mill will accelerate until the possibilities for new development are completely pulverized. So, if we continue with the acceleration demands to absolute safety, we are indeed creating an unethical medical policy.

REFERENCE
1. Declaration of Helsinki. Recommendations guiding medical doctors in biomedical research involving human subjects 1964/1975. WHO Chronicle 1976; 3o:360-2.

19. UNITED KINGDOM REGULATIONS RELATING TO THE CONTROL OF SAFETY AND EFFICACY OF RADIOPHARMACEUTICALS

ROSEMARY J. SMITH

1. INTRODUCTION

The regulations applicable to radiopharmaceuticals fall into three main groups. Firstly, there are those which apply to all radioactive substances and cover the procedures and controls necessary to safeguard against radiation hazard. Secondly there are those which control safety, quality and efficacy of all medicinal products under the Medicines Act 1968. Finally there are regulations which apply specifically to radioactive medicinal products. These require authorisation to be obtained prior to the administration of named products for specified purposes and are also made under the Medicines Act 1968. Consideration will be given to each group separately followed by a summary showing how the combined application of these methods together provide the necessary control of the safety and efficacy of a radiopharmaceutical.

In a brief discussion of this nature it is only possible to give an overview of the regulations and guidelines applicable; full details may be obtained from the references listed in the bibliography.

2. LICENSING OF MEDICINAL PRODUCTS

Licensing of medicinal products for both human and animal use was introduced into the United Kingdom in 1971 following implementation of the Medicines Act 1968. In the following discussion only human medicines will be considered. The Medicines Act defines a Medicinal Product as a substance or article (not being an instrument, apparatus or appliance) which is used for administration to a human being for the purpose of treating or preventing disease, of diagnosis, of inducing anaesthesia, of contraception or of preventing or interfering with the normal operation of a physiological function.

Ingredients used for the preparation of medicines for dispensing in hospitals or pharmacies are also medicinal products although some qualify for exemption from detailed licensing control. Both generators and kits used in the production of radiopharmaceuticals are subject to the full licensing provisions of the Medicines Act.

Licences fall into the following categories:

1. Product Licences
2. Clinical Trial Certificates
3. Manufacturers Licences
4. Wholesale Dealers Licences

The licensing system is operated by the Health Ministers of the United Kingdom who act as the "Licensing Authority". However these functions are discharged on their behalf by the Medicines Division of the Department of Health and Social Security (DHSS).

A Product Licence is required before a medicinal product may be imported or manufactured and marketed. When licensing was introduced products already on the market were entitled to Product Licences of Right. These were issued without scrutiny of quality, safety or efficacy but are subject to review and may be suspended in certain circumstances, for instance, should new evidence come to light which proves the product is not safe.

For products introduced to the market since the commencement of licensing, the issue of a Product Licence depends upon provision of satisfactory evidence to support safety, quality and efficacy. The DHSS publishes notes for the guidance of applicants which detail the data required to support an application but it must be noted that each product is judged on its own merits in relation to the indications claimed. There are no separate notes for guidance relating to radiopharmaceuticals, generators or kits since it is felt that the existing notes form an adequate basis for an application for one of these products and such additional data as necessary, relating particularly to the radioactive component, can be added.

Evidence is required from animal pharmacological and toxicological studies, from clinical use in humans and from quality testing. Obviously products for diagnostic use on one occasion only would not require tests related to long-term use. Tests would need to demonstrate the suitability of the product for its intended function including studies of biological distribution and of factors which could affect tissue or organ uptake and in consequence the radiation dose received. The development work is therefore of critical importance. Purity and stability must also be demonstrated and physico-chemical factors which influence optimum biological distribution must be investigated and controlled. The evidence supplied for generators and kits must relate not only to the product as supplied but also to the finished product when prepared according to the instructions provided.

In judging the evidence provided, the Licensing Authority may be advised by committees of independent experts; it does not undertake any routine testing itself. For radiopharmaceuticals advice would be given by The Committee on Safety of Medicines and also by The Committee on Radiation from Radioactive Medicinal Products.

The Committee on Safety of Medicines (CSM) provides advice on questions of quality, safety and efficacy of new medicines for human use. It is also responsible for collecting and investigating reports on adverse reactions. The Committee is helped in its work by a number of Sub-Committees.

The Committee on Radiation from Radioactive Medicinal Products (CRRMP) provides advice with respect to quality, safety and efficacy in relation to radiation, of any substance or article for human use to which any provision of the Medicines Act is applicable. This Committee was formed in 1978 to cover the radiation aspects in relation to product licensing since sufficient expertise was not felt to exist within the CSM.

The two committees function independently but can draw to the attention of the other any aspects that are felt to warrant special attention. Representatives from the permanent secretariat of physicians and pharmacists within the DHSS who undertake initial assessment of applications also attend both committees.

Finally, before leaving the subject of product licensing, brief mention must be made of the review of licences of established products; certain licences, mainly but not exclusively Product Licences of Right, are subject to review in accordance with the European Community Directives. Although radiopharmaceuticals are specifically excluded from these provisions no formal exclusion has been issued in relation the the UK review but categories which are subject to EEC provisions would naturally be expected to take priority. The Committee on Review of Medicines advises the Licensing Authority on products being reviewed.

From this brief discussion it can be seen that radiopharmaceuticals are subject to normal product licensing requirements and that special provisions have been made to cover radiation aspects when safety, quality and efficacy are assessed. At the present time in the UK there are 63 Licences of Right and 47 Product Licences relating to radiopharmaceuticals, generators and kits; this represents only a small proportion of the current licences for medicinal products which now number just over sixteen thousand. The labelling and advertising of these products is also controlled under the Medicines Act. There are certain exemptions from the need for a Product Licence to be held. One that is sometimes met in connection with the use of radiopharmaceutical in hospital, is that granted to a physician who imports or has manufactured to his order an unlicensed product for administration to a "named patient". The doctor will carry complete responsibility for the administration of the product in these circumstances and will use his own clinical judgement to assess the risks involved against the benefits to be obtained.

Clinical Trial Certificates are necessary to authorize the supply of a medicinal product for the purpose of a Clinical Trial unless an appropriate exemption is granted. Certificates are issued on provision of satisfactory evidence relating to safety and quality plus information to support the trial rationale; the advisory committees will be consulted if necessary.

Manufacturers Licences authorize the holder to manufacture or assemble medicinal products, and are issued if the Licensing Authority is satisfied that production and control facilities are adequate for the operations to be carried out and that appropriate "Qualified Persons" are responsible for specified aspects. The Medicines Inspectorate visit the premises and advise the Licensing Authority on the facilities available, which would be expected to comply with the principles of Good Manufacturing Practice (GMP). The DHSS has published guidance on this aspect in the "Guide to Good Pharmaceutical Manufacturing Practice". The current edition does not refer specifically to radiopharmaceutical production but in future editions it is planned to refer to the need for modification of the guidance to take account of radiation aspects, particularly for sterile product production.

Inspections continue to be carried out at intervals after the licence is granted to ensure that standards are maintained. Inspection also takes place outside the UK; this is required by the provisions included in Product Licences for imported products. However, where mutual recognition of inspections is in operation between the UK and another country, inspection reports may be provided by the regulatory authority of the country concerned.

Hospital Manufacturing in the National Health Service (NHS) is not subject to the full licensing provisions of the Medicines Act. However, in 1975 Health Authorities were asked to introduce arrangements corresponding to the licensing procedures of the Medicines Act as applied to commercial undertakings. Dispensing by pharmacists is generally excluded from the activities which are controlled but an exception has been made for radiopharmaceuticals and all preparation of such products in hospitals is subject to the manufacturing control arrangements. Radiopharmacy departments are therefore subject to Inspection by the Medicines Inspectorate to ensure compliance with GMP. Special hospital guidance has been drawn up on "Premises and Environment for the Preparation of Radiopharmaceuticals". This guidance, published at the end of last year after a lengthy period of consultation, indicates where modification may be required to the standards applied to normal pharmaceutical manufacturing operations, in particular to the production of sterile products. Such modification takes into consideration the special characteristics of radiopharmaceuticals and the circumstances of their use in hospitals. Before official guidance was issued a number of different views on the subject had been stated or published and these did not agree in all aspects. The task confronting the DHSS was to maintain standards adequate to prevent production of unsafe or inefficacious products while preventing an over-strict approach which would result in unnecessary expenditure of resources. In the guidelines the standards normally required for aseptic manufacture are relaxed slightly in the case of a short-lived radiopharmaceutical prepared from a "kit" provided that this involves the addition of sterile ingredients via a "closed" system to a pre-sterilised closed container and the product is used within one working day.

3. POST-MARKETING SURVEILLANCE OF MEDICINAL PRODUCTS

Post-marketing surveillance is an important part of the control on safety, quality and efficacy of medicinal products. This takes the form of monitoring for both medical and pharmaceutical hazards.

Monitoring for Pharmaceutical Hazard is achieved by a programme of random sampling and by the maintenance of a Product Defect Reporting Centre to which reports may be sent at any hour of the day or night. Medical and Pharmaceutical staff are on call to advise on the action required in any particular case. There have only been a few defects relating to radiopharmaceuticals, perhaps the most serious being due to design defects. One such case related to a technetium-99m generator which was eluted the wrong way round. A subsequent design modification was introduced by the manufacturer and also a "Hazard Warning" was issued by the Department of Health to alert users to the need for care in assembly and for checking molybdenum breakthrough. In another case generator leakage problems necessitated a design modification. A few reports have related to incorrect tissue or organ uptake but, interestingly, on investigation a couple have been traced back to contamination arising in the Radiopharmacy. Few product recalls have been needed for radiopharmaceuticals but examples include labelling errors, pyrogen contamination and particulate contamination.

<u>Monitoring for medical hazard</u> is mainly concerned with adverse reaction detection. In the United Kingdom a system exist for spontaneous reporting by doctors of suspected adverse reactions on postage-paid "yellow cards". Information from these cards and from other sources such as published papers or monitored release schemes are examined by the Committee on Safety of Medicines who advise the Licensing Authority if warnings need to be issued or modifications made to the product or its recommended use(s). In the case of radiopharmaceuticals input to the CSM on suspected adverse reactions is also provided by the special monitoring scheme operated by those working in the field of nuclear medicine.

Only a few serious problems have arisen with radiopharmaceuticals in the past. The agent which has probably caused the most problems is radiolabelled iron hydroxide precipitate used for lung scanning. This agent is no longer used as the risks were certainly found to outweigh the benefits particularly when other lung scanning agents became available. Problems have also occurred as a result of the use of preparations of unsatisfactory quality. Factors such as contamination with pyrogens and inadequate particle size control are examples of quality factors causing adverse effects. These are more correctly classified as product defects but such problems may first come to light as suspected adverse reactions. Improvements in quality control and analytical techniques have hopefully reduced such occurrences.

4. PHARMACOPOEIAL STANDARDS

Under the Medicines Act, British and European Pharmacopoeia monographs are given statutory force. These regulations make it an offence to sell or supply a medicine which is ordered or prescribed by reference to a name at the head of a monograph unless the medicine complies with the standards in that monograph.

5. ADMINISTRATION OF RADIOACTIVE MEDICINAL PRODUCTS

Under Article 5a of the European Communities Directive 76/579/Euratom and its latest revision 80/836/Euratom, a system of prior authorisation is required with respect to radioactive substances administered to persons for the purpose of diagnosis, treatment or research. In 1978 legislation was introduced in the UK which required doctors and dentists to hold appropriate authorizing certificates. Although this legislation was made under the provisions already existing in the Medicines Act, additional legislation was needed to extend these provisions to certain other radioactive substances and to cover administration to healthy humans for research purposes. Responsibility for granting the certificates lies with the Health Ministers advised by a Committee of experts – The Administration of Radioactive Substances Advisory Committee (ARSAC). Certificates are granted if the radiological hazards to patients from the products to be used are considered acceptable and the use of the products is within the competence and facilities of the proposed certificate holder. A list has been produced detailing the nature and maximum usual activity of particular radioactive medicinal products which ARSAC advise may be administered to humans under specified conditions. It is noted however that the fact that the radiological hazard of a product in the list is considered acceptable does not confirm pharmaceutical and toxicological safety which must be established for products which have not received clearance from the Committee on Safety of Medicines.

6. OTHER LEGISLATION

Radiopharmaceuticals are subject to controls operating with respect to all radioactive substances under the Radioactive Substances Act 1960 and the Health and Safety at Work Act 1974; advice given in the Code of Practice for the Protection of Persons against ionizing Radiations arising from Medical and Dental Use (1972) is also applicable. These cover measures necessary to safeguard against radiation hazard from the product during production, transport, storage and use and the requirements for disposal of waste. Inspections to ensure compliance with regulations are carried out by the appropriate Inspectorate. The need to comply with the basic safety standards for radiation protection set down in the Euratom Directive and with the recommendations of the International Commission on Radiological Protection (ICRP) have led to proposals for new legislation. The consultative document on "The Ionizing Radiations Regulations 198-" outlines this new legislation and the "Approved Code of Practice" which is intended to accompany it; guidance notes are also included.

7. CONCLUSION

Radiopharmaceuticals, generators or kits would normally be obtained from licensed manufacturers under the authority of Product Licences unless required for a clinical trial in which case a Clinical Trial Certificate or exemption would be needed. Any subsequent preparation undertaken in hospital is required to comply with Good Manufacturing Practice and is subject to inspection by the Medicines Inspectorate. Administration of the preparation must be undertaken by or under the responsibility of a practitioner holding an appropriate certificate authorizing the procedure or investigation to be undertaken and the dose levels appropriate. All operations involving radioactive substances are subject to inspection to ensure compliance with requirements to safeguard against radiation hazard.

REFERENCES
1. The radioactive Substances Act 1960, London, Her Majesty's Stationery Office

2. The Medicines Act 1968, London HMSO.
3. MAL 2 - Notes on Applications for Product Licences (Medicines for Human Use), 1981, London, DHSS.
4. MAL 99 - The Control of Medicines in the United Kingdom of Great Britain and Northern Ireland, 1981, London, DHSS.
5. DHSS Guide to Good Pharmaceutical Manufacturing Practice, 1977, London, HMSO.
6. DHSS Circular HSC(IS)128, Application of the Medicines Act to Health Authorities, 1975, London, DHSS.
7. DHSS Guidance Notes for Hospitals on Premises and Environment for the preparation of Radiopharmaceuticals, 1982, London, DHSS
8. DHSS Hazard Warning: Radioisotope Generator for Technetium - 99m, DS (supply) 23/74, 1974, London, DHSS.
9. DHSS Circular HSC(IS)41, Reporting of Accidents with and serious Defects in Medicinal products and other Medical Supplies and Equipment, 1974, DHSS, London.
10. British Pharmacopoeia 1980, London, HMSO.
11. European Pharmacopoeia 1980, France, Maisonneuve SA.
12. Statutory Instrument 1978 No 1004, The Medicines (Radioactive Substances) Order 1978, London, HMSO.
13. Statutory Instrument 1978 No 1005, The Medicines (Committee on Radiation from Radioactive Medicinal Products) Order 1978, London, HMSO.
14. Statutory Instrument 1978 No 1006, The Medicines (Administration of Radioactive Substances) Regulations 1978, London, HMSO.
15. DHSS Notes for Guidance on Administration of Radioactive Substances to persons for purposes of Diagnosis, Treatment or Research 1978, DHSS, London.
16. The Health and Safety at Work ACT 1974, London, HMSO.
17. Code of Practice for Protection of Persons Against Ionizing Radiations Arising from Medical and Dental Use 1972, London, HMSO.
18. Health and Safety Commission Consultative Document - The Ionizing Radiations Regulations 198-, 1982, London, HMSO.

20. REGULATORY ASPECTS IN THE FEDERAL REPUBLIC OF GERMANY
HANS DETLEV ROEDLER

1. INTRODUCTION

The demands on safety and efficacy of a radiopharmaceutical are related to its property of being a drug as well as a radioactive substance. For this reason, radiopharmaceuticals are subject to drug and radiation protection regulations. These are described in the following prior to a discussion of special problems of classification into drug and finished drug products, of clinical trial, approval for marketing and post-marketing surveillance. In addition, some experiences from the author's work will be described together with conclusions drawn.

2. DRUG LEGISLATION

The law on the reform of drug legislation of the Federal Republic of Germany (Arzneimittelgesetz 1976) (1), referred to as Drug Act, has brought a far-reaching conformity to international standards. This constitutes an essential contribution to the development of a uniform European Drug Legislation by converting the respective Council Directives of the European Community (2) into the national legislation and signifies a first step towards the goal of a common European market for drug products. At the same time a legal basis for converting the WHO Directives for the Manufacture and Quality Control of Pharmaceuticals (3) is hereby established.

For the protection of the consumer, only qualitatively unobjectionable, effective and safe drug products may be placed on the market in compliance with the Drug Act (1). In complying with numerous regulations, the safety of drug products is monitored at various levels. In the newly introduced approval procedure, the quality, efficacy and safety of drug products must be documented. By constant surveillance of all drug products on the market, errors should be detected which may have occured in spite of all precautionary measures during development, approval or manufacturing. By including all those having to do with drug products, the monitoring of drug-caused risks should be rendered as effectively as possible. Provision for immediate reactions to reports of such risks have been established.

Of the 16 sections of the Drug Act (1) particularly those described below under their respective headings - including some comments - are of special significance for radiopharmaceuticals:

I : "Purpose of the law and definitions": Definitions of drug products, finished drug products, radioactive drug products, marketing, pharmaceutical sponsor.

II: "Drug requirements": The marketing of radioactive drug products is prohibited unless authorized by ordinance of the Federal Minister. Labelling of finished drug products and flyleaves.

III: "Manufacture of drugs": Manufacturing authorization.

IV: "Approval of drugs for marketing": Obligation to have finished drug products approved for marketing, documentation required in applying for approval, expert assessments, decisions regarding approval, authorization to extend the regulations on approval to other drug products.

VI: "Protection of the individual during clinical trials".

VII: "Drug distribution"

VIII: "Quality assurance and control": Operating regulations (referring essentially to the GMP Directive (3) of the WHO) and the pharmacopoeia.

X: "Observation, recording and analysis of risks from drugs": Organization, phase plan.

XI: "Supervision"

XV: "Designation of the competent Higher Federal Authority and other provisions": For most drugs (including radiopharmaceuticals) the Federal Health Office is the competent Higher Federal Authority.

XVI: "Liability for hazards from drugs".

XVII: "Penal regulations and fines".

In addition to the Drug Act (1), the following regulations on drug products apply:

a)   The "Ordinance on marketing drug products exposed to ionizing radiation or containing radioactive substances" (4) which - due to considerations on radiation protection - essentially authorizes the distribution of any radioactive drug product to hospitals and research centers but restricts the release of these drug products to physicians for a certain number of specified radionuclides, not including e.g. iodine-123, thallium-201, gallium-67, indium-111 or radioactive gases.

b)   The European and German pharmacopoeias are issued in the "Pharmacopoeia Ordinance" (5) and are declared as binding for manufacturing and marketing drugs.

c)   The "Phase Plan"(6) representing general administrative regulations for observation, recording and analysis of risks from drugs.

d)   The "Operational regulations for pharmaceutical enterprises" (7), based essentially on the WHO GMP regulations (3), are still in preparation, but are already used as guidelines in daily practice.

Finally, the "Official explanatory comments of the Federal Health Office in reference to the application for approval of a drug product" (8) should be mentioned here. They include forms and data sheets for standardizing and expediting the procedures.

Competent for supervision and execution of the Drug Act (1) are the authorities of the Federal States of the Federal Republic of Germany; the competent Higher Federal Authority is the Federal Health Office which is reponsible for

- the approval of drug products for marketing, except questions of approval obligation;

- the recording and analysing of risks from drug products and the coordinating of measures to be adopted;

- the deposition of material documenting the pharmacological-toxicological tests prior to the clinical trial;
- the report of the pharmaceutical sponsor on experiences with certain drug products only to be supplied upon prescription;
- the chairmanship and management of the pharmacopoeia commission.

3. RADIATION PROTECTION REGULATIONS

The "law on the peaceful use of nuclear energy and protection against its hazards" (9) provides the authorization for an ordinance to protect life and health against the hazards of radioactive substances and ionizing radiation by surveillance and protection regulations.

This Radiation Protection Ordinance (10) refers to both the non-medical and medical use of radionuclides. In this context, four paragraphs are of special interest:

§ 3: Authorization for handling radioactive substances
§ 41: Use of radioactive substances for medical research purposes
§ 42: Use of radioactive substances in diagnosis and therapy
§ 43: Patient records

The guideline "Radiation Protection in Medicine" (11) -addressed to the competent Federal State Authorities and to those working with radionuclides and ionizing radiation in the medical field - specifies the relevant regulations of the Radiation Protection Ordinance (10) in more detail. For instance, it contains rules for protection of the patient, safety and organisational requirements for the use of radiopharmaceuticals as well as surveillance- and control measures. The competent authorities are those of the Federal States of the Federal Republic of Germany.

4. CLINICAL TRIAL OF RADIOPHARMACEUTICALS

Here, too, drug and radiation protection regulations must be observed. The former are contained in section VI of the

Drug Act (1) and specify the protection of the volunteer on the basis of principles having their origin in the jurisdiction for penal law and the ethical standards expressed by the Declaration of Helsinki. Some conditions to be fulfilled are:

- balancing the anticipated benefit and risk,
- informed consent,
- personal liberty status of the volunteer,
- minimum experience of the responsible physician concerning clinical trials (2 years),
- pharmacological-toxicological test,
- deposition at the Federal Health Office of documentary material on the pharmacological-toxicological test,
- information for the physician responsible for the clinical trial concerning pharmacological-toxicologial results and anticipated risks,
- insurance coverage of the volunteer.

The clinical trial of radiopharmaceuticals is not mentioned in the Radiation Protection Ordinance (10). This Ordinance addresses only the application of radioactive substances in medical research and clinical trials of pharmaceutical drugs labelled with radionuclides, whereby the following conditions must be fulfilled:

- evidence of urgent need for administration of radionuclides,
- benefit-risk assessment,
- lowest possible toxicity of radionuclide applied,
- administered activity as low as reasonably achievable,
- lowest possible number of volunteers,
- compliance with dose limits corresponding to 1/10 of those for occupationally exposed persons,
- qualification of the physician: 2 years of experience in the use of radionuclides administered to man, attendance of radiation protection courses,
- informed consent,
- sufficient technical measuring equipment,
- insurance coverage of volunteers,
- personal liberty status of volunteers,

- age of volunteers over 50, unless safety and the special need for younger volunteers has been documented.

The compliance with the above and additional radiation protection conditions must be evidenced - contrary to the above mentioned drug legislation requirements - by an application to the competent Federal State authority which, in turn, requires an expert assessment from the Federal Health Office in most cases, so that the procedure may be extended over several months.

The analogous application of radiation protection requirements for clinical trials of radiopharmaceuticals poses the following problems:

- the very restrictive dose limits may prevent the permission for clinical trial;
- the requirements of more than 2 years of experience in the use of radioactive substances (radiopharmaceuticals) in man and an equally long period of experience in the clinical trial of drugs (Drug Act) are, in a strict sense, only rarely fulfilled;
- the basic restriction to persons older than 50 years leads to difficulties in obtaining standard values and results for younger patients, in view of the more functionally oriented nature of radiopharmaceutical diagnosis;
- the classification into permit requiring medical research and into diagnosis not requiring special authorization may be difficult in case of radiopharmaceuticals administered to patients. Therefore, the intention of gaining scientific results from new procedures on the one hand and the expectation of a benefit for the individual patient on the other may be a criteria. However, which of these applies more readily, may be just as difficult to decide as where a new or a standard procedure is concerned, in particular since a well performed diagnosis and therapy always includes the aspect of assessing and evaluating the results.

5. DEFINITIONS OF DRUG PRODUCTS AND FINISHED DRUG PRODUCTS

The Drug Act (1) differentiates between drug products and

finished drug products. The definition of the finished drug product is an extension of that of the proprietary medicinal product given in the First Pharmaceutical Directive of the European Community (2) in as much as it does not require the characteristic of a special name, and thus includes the generics. The finished drug product is the collective term for proprietary medicinal products and generics. The respective definitions are:

Finished drug products are drug products which are manufactured in advance and then marketed in packages ready for distribution to the consumer (Drug Act) (1).

Proprietary medicinal products are ready-prepared medicinal products placed on the market under a special name and in a special pack (Council Directive 65/65/EEC) (2).

The essential consequence of a classification as drug product or finished drug product lies in the fact that the latter may be placed on the market not earlier than after approval by the competent Higher Federal Authority. The obligation for obtaining this approval is the most important revision of the Drug Act (1) in comparison to earlier laws.

6. APPROVAL OF RADIOPHARMACEUTICALS FOR MARKETING

6.1. Classification of radiopharmaceuticals

Neither the Radiation Protection Ordinance (10), nor the Drug Act (1) contain the term "radiopharmaceutical". The Drug Act (1) defines radioactive drug products as being drug products containing radioactive substances and spontaneously emitting ionizing radiation, which are intended to be used due to these properties. Therefore, the definition of radioactive drug products, additionally to radiopharmaceuticals, includes radioactive items such as gold seeds (Au-198) or derma plates (Sr-90) and radium applicators. The classification of radiopharmaceuticals, kits and generators as finished drug products (approval required) or as drug products (approval not required) has initially created uncertainties in recent years. This, essentially, may have been caused by the fact that for kits the term of finished drug products is particularly misleading. Since a kit requires labelling with a radionuclide prior to administration, a classification as finished drug product may, at first, hardly be understood. It does, however, agree with the definition given in the Drug Act (1). It should be noted that this definition does not imply that a finished drug product is ready for use. The Federal Health Office has authorized kits without the labelling radionuclide as finished drug products whereby, however, during the approval procedure, the clinical results, indications for use and radiation exposure for the final product (after labelling with the nuclide) are assessed.

Similar problems occur with the classification of generators. Considering these as items, they do not even constitute a drug product in compliance with the definition given by the Drug Act (1), since they are not intended to be brought into contact with the human body either on a temporary or a permanent basis. When referring to the mother radionuclide, this might be considered as being placed on the market, but it is not actually administered to the patient. When referring to the daughter radionuclide, it must be realized that it is mainly generated after the generator has left the manufacturer, whereby the manufacturer, in reality, has placed the mother nuclide on the market with only a small fraction of the totally generated daughter nuclide, so that the daughter nuclide in effect was not prepared in advance and thus does not constitute a finished drug product requiring approval.

Radiopharmaceuticals manufactured on individual request and not prepared in advance are, according to present regulations, not subject to the approval for marketing.

6.2. Approval procedure

For radiopharmaceuticals classified as finished drug products, the quality, safety and efficacy must be documented when applying for approval.The compliance with these criteria is reviewed by the Federal Health Office as the competent authority. The particulars and documents to be submitted for approval are specified in the Drug Act (1) and described in detail in the official Federal Health Office Explanatory

Comments (8) of approximately 50 pages, referring to the
application for approval including 13 forms and 10 data
sheets. The requirements are based on the Council Directives
of the Commission of the European Communities (2) and,
therefore, do no need to be discussed here. In the forms and
data sheets on safety and efficacy the usual aspects of
pharmacological-toxicological tests and clinical trials are
listed. In an individual case, however, it depends on the
requirements of the Drug Act (1) and on the state of the art
whether and how investigations are to be performed, results
presented and respective data listed in the data sheets.
Therefore, it may not be necessary for radiopharmaceuticals to
refer in detail to several aspects required in the
applications for other finished drug products: e.g.
pharmacodynamics, repeated dose toxicity, foetal toxicity,
harmful effects on progeny and reproductive function or
carcinogenicity for the non-radioactive components of the
radiopharmaceutical. Due to the specifics of radiopharmaceuticals (in general, single administration, small pharmacological doses), a well performed acute toxicity test is usually
considered as being sufficient. In addition to the
determination of LD_{50} values it should include observations
such as type, time of appearance and duration of toxic
symptoms, or include clinical, biochemical, and hematological
parameters, respectively (12). For unknown substances and
those under suspicion of risks, additional tests, such as
subacute toxicity for two weeks or teratogenicity, may be
appropriate. In any case, well founded data for the radiation
exposure of the patient must be submitted with the
application. Contents and amount of material submitted for
documenting safety and efficacy depend, within a certain
framework, on the state of the art and not on detailed and
rigid formal regulations.

At the Federal Health Office the material submitted is
checked and expert assessments referring to the following
aspects are prepared:
- formal pharmaceutical review,
- analytics,

- galenics,
- medicine (scientific results),
- clinical,
- pharmacological and
- toxicological.

Within a period of 4 - or 7 months in exceptional cases -the Federal Health Office decides on the application for approval. If necessary, the authority will supply the applicant with a written report on deficiencies which are to be corrected within a certain time period. Should these deficiencies not be corrected as required, the approval will not be granted.

7. POST-MARKETING SURVEILLANCE

In the interest of preventing hazard to human health, it is the responsibility of the Federal Health Office to record and analyse risks from drug application, in particular in respect to side effects, interaction with other products, contraindications and falsifications and to coordinate measures to be adopted in accordance with the Drug Act (1). For this purpose, the Federal Health Office acts in cooperation with the agencies of the World Health Organization, the Drug Authorities of other countries, the Health Authorities of the Federal States, the Drug Commissions of the Associations of Medical Professions as well as with others who, as part of their tasks, are keeping records on drug risks. By general administrative regulations, a Phase Plan (6) has come into force in 1980 specifying the execution of the tasks as indicated above. In this plan, the measures to be taken in the form of collaboration between the authorities and departments involved are detailed as to the various degrees of risks regarding side effects; the matter of intervention on the part of the pharmaceutical sponsor is clarified and the various measures to be taken in compliance with the regulations of the Drug Act (1) are determined.

8. COMMENTS ON RECENT EXPERIENCES

In general, the risk to the patient from the application of

radiopharmaceuticals is extremely small. This refers - as the relevant statistics show - to side effects of the administered substance as well as to the radiation risk which may only be assessed by computation and in reality cannot be proven for diagnostic radiopharmaceuticals (including, up till now, the radioiodine test). Radiopharmaceuticals are subject to manifold regulations in the drug and radiation protection legislation; their specifics, however, in some cases are not in harmony with the general basic structures of these regulations. This becomes particularly evident in drug legislation when classifying radiopharmaceuticals into drug products or finished drug products and in radiation protection legislation relating to clinical trials.

The quality of documentary material submitted with the application for approval of radiopharmaceuticals (up till now, essentially kits) varies considerably. The deficiencies seen were primarily of formal nature - e.g. incorrect names or insufficient documentation of available results - and not so much related to content. For instance, the biokinetic data used for estimation of radiation exposure were not given, and the instructions for use were either inadequately or erroneously translated into German (e.g.: "A sterile, pyrogenic solution to be injected" or: "The physician must possess a radiation protection ordinance" (instead of the required licence)).

One report only of 3 cases of unforseen side effects from radiopharmaceuticals was received by the Federal Health Office in 1979. It was related to iodine-131 aldosterone from one manufacturer: 5-10 min p.i. generalized erythema, shortness of breath, pain in the abdominal area, vomiting and slightly disturbed conscientiousness occured and persisted for 15-20 min. It should be noted that administrative regulations such as the Phase Plan (6) do not oblige the Drug Commissions of the Associations of Medical Professions and of the pharmaceutical industry to report risks from drugs to the Federal Health Office. However, it is to be expected that the respective commissions react to the regular inquiries of the Federal Health Office in a cooperative manner and give information about available reports or permit access to their files.

9. CONCLUSIONS

The present status of regulatory aspects on radiopharmaceuticals in the Federal Republic of Germany shows some need for further improvement, particularly with regard to the following:

a) It appears to be inappropriate to exclude the practizing physician from applying some of the newer radionuclides only because the respective ordinance (4) has not been revised during the past 12 years. A reform has been in preparation for some time, but unsuitably refers both to sealed radioactive substances and the radiation treatment of drugs.

b) For future drug regulations, the consideration of the specifics of radioactive drug products, particularly in regard to manufacture and marketing, should be more appropriate.

c) The future radiation protection regulations, especially for clinical trials of radiopharmaceuticals, should be formulated in a more appropriate and precise manner.

After a period of successfully propagating the consumer protection, the optimisation of this protection in view of a cost and benefit assessment under appropriate use of available resources should be an essential goal for future endeavours.

ACKNOWLEDGEMENTS

Thanks are due to my colleagues Dr. Blumenbach, Dr. Grase and Dr. Schmidt for helpful discussions, to Mrs. R. LeMar for assistance in translation and to Mrs. I. Zeitlberger for preparing the manuscript.

REFERENCES
1. Gesetz zur Neuordnung des Arzneimittelrechts vom 24. August 1976. BGBl.I, 2445.
2. Commission of the European Communities: The rules governing medicaments in the European Community. ISBN 92-825-0275/9. EEC: Brussels-Luxembourg, 1978.

3. GMP-Richtlinie: Official records of the World Health Organization. Nr. 226, Annex 12, 1975.
4. Verordnung über die Zulassung von Arzneimitteln, die mit ionisierenden Strahlen behandelt worden sind oder die radioaktive Stoffe enthalten. i.d.F. der Bekanntmachung vom 8. August 1967 (BGBl.I, 893) und der Verordnung vom 10. Mai 1971 (BGBl.I, 449).
5. Verordnung über das Arzneibuch i.d.F. der Bekanntmachung vom 25. Juli 1978 (BGBl.I, 1112) und der Verordnungen vom 6. Juni 1980 (BGBl.I, 668) und vom 22. Juli 1981 (BGBl.I, 670).
6. Allgemeine Verwaltungsvorschrift zur Beobachtung, Sammlung und Auswertung von Arzneimittelrisiken (Stufenplan) nach §63 des Arzneimittelgesetzes (AMG) vom 20. Juni 1980. Bundesanzeiger Nr. 114 vom 26. Juni 1980.
7. Betriebsordnung für pharmazeutische Unternehmer. In Vorbereitung. Referentenentwurf in DAZ, 1981: 882.
8. Amtliche Erläuterungen des Bundesgesundheitsamtes zum Antrag auf Zulassung eines Arzneimittels. Bundesanzeiger Verlagsgesellschaft mbH, Köln.
9. Gesetz über die friedliche Verwendung der Kernenergie und den Schutz gegen ihre Gefahren (Atomgesetz) i.d.F. der Bekanntmachung vom 31. Oktober 1976 (BGBl.I, 3053), geändert durch Art.9 Nr. 13 Ges.v.3.12.1976 (BGBl.I, 3281).
10. Verordnung über den Schutz vor Schäden durch ionisierende Strahlen (Strahlenschutzverordnung - StrlSchV) vom 13. Oktober 1976 (BGBl.I, 2905; berichtigt 1977, BGBl.I, 184 u. 269), zuletzt geändert durch die Erste Verordnung zur Änderung der Strahlenschutzverordnung vom 22. Mai 1981 (BGBl.I, 445).
11. Richtlinie für den Strahlenschutz bei Verwendung radioaktiver Stoffe und beim Betrieb von Anlagen zur Erzeugung ionisierender Strahlen und Bestrahlungseinrichtungen mit radioaktiven Quellen in der Medizin (Richtlinie Strahlenschutz in der Medizin). RdSchr.d.BMI v.18.10.1979 - RS II 5 - 515 032/2 GMBl. 1979, Nr. 31.
12. Bass R, Günzel P, Henschler D, König J, Lorke D, Neubert D, Schütz E, Schuppan D, Zbinden G: LD 50 versus acute toxicity. Arch Toxicol 1982;51:183.

21. REGULATORY ASPECTS - EXAMPLES FROM SWEDEN

BERTIL NOSSLIN

1. INTRODUCTION

I have been asked to describe the development in Sweden, to review my own experience during this work and to give my opinion on the effect to our new law on radiopharmaceuticals with regard to its effects on practical work within nuclear medicine. Up to 1982 there was no special legislation on radioactive drugs, since they were explicitly exempted from the Drug Act when it was introduced in 1962. Since no other rules were laid down at the same time, this field has in practice been without regulations from many years. Existing rules have mainly dealt with radiation protection, while very few prescriptions have existed regarding requirements as to pharmaceutical or biological properties. This has implied a great freedom in choosing products and methods in clinical work and also in developing and testing of new compounds. In spite of this lawlessness an extensive activity within nuclear medicine has taken place without serious incidents. To my knowledge, only one serious reaction has been reported, namely an aseptic meningitis after intrathecal injection of labelled albumin for cisternography. It must be admitted, however, that reporting of adverse reactions has certainly been incomplete just because of the exemption of radiopharmaceuticals from the Drug Act.

If, nuclear medicine has been practiced for many years in a way that seems to have brought about both safety and efficacy, one may ask whether special regulation is necessary. All physicians in Sweden are by law obliged to act according to "scientific knowledge and proved clinical experience", and this general guideline could be considered enough. The reason why this is not the case is formal. The patient has the right to be treated with the same safety and efficacy as with other drugs, and the responsible authorities can not accept that there is no special regulation that guarantees such a condition. The nuclear medicine doctor must of course accept this point of view, but he would at the same time like to stress that the rules must be as few and as simple as possible, well adapted to clinical activities, and executed by supervising authorities having a qualified staff at their disposal.

2. PREPARATION OF REGULATIONS

It is nearest at hand to believe, since the demand for safety and efficacy is the same as for ordinary drugs, that the rules and the supervising authority also should be the same. This question has been under lively discussion in Sweden for 15 years, and only recently has a final decision been taken by the parliament.

Politicians, administrators and pharmaceutical scientists have in general favoured a joint legislation and supervision, while most physicians and physicists have been of the opinion that the specific problems with radiopharmaceuticals necessitate separate rules and a separate controlling system. In 1971 a departmental committee proposed inclusion of radiopharmaceuticals into the Drug Act. This would mean that registration and supervision should be exercised by the Drug department of the National Board of Health and Welfare. Because of heavy criticism on several points the proposal was rejected, and a new committee was appointed. This committee stated in 1974 that the unique properties of radiopharmaceuticals necessitated a separate legislation under a separate authority. After several years of further discussions a Law on Radiopharmaceuticals came into action in 1982. The law implies a compromise between the two main lines of opinion in as much as radiopharmaceuticals are still exempted from the Drug Act, but the regulatory authority is the same as for ordinary drugs. The main reason for a separate legislation was that it was realized that radiopharmaceuticals have very special properties as compared to ordinary drugs. These properties have been mentioned several times earlier by different authors, but I would like to summarize them here once again as they were presented in the Swedish committee report.

3. SPECIAL PROPERTIES OF RADIOPHARMACEUTICALS

a) The main use is for diagnostic purpose, not therapeutic.

b) They are usually given only once to each patient, occasionally a few times but never continuously.

c) They often consist of a radioactive form of a normal constituent in the body, such as an ion, a protein etc.

d) The active substance is usually given in microgram quantities.

e) The dominating risk comes from radiation, not from pharmacological or toxic effects.

f) The use is controlled by a double set of regulations, one because they are drugs, another because they are radioactive compounds.

g) They are used only in hospitals and are administered by medical personnel; they are never left to the patient for self-medication.

h) Radiation safety regulations limit the number of hospitals and doctors involved; radiopharmaceuticals cannot be prescribed by every practitioner.

i) The short half-life of the radionuclide causes specific problems with regard to production, distribution and control. Semi-manufactured products like non-radioactive kits are common.

j) From a commercial point of view radiopharmaceuticals are "small" products compared to ordinary drugs.

4. DISCUSSION

The Law on Radiopharmaceuticals came into action in 1982. The transitionary regulations were gentle, and detailed application rules have not yet been laid down. All radiopharmaceuticals and methods in use before the law came into operation may still be used for the present, but they had to be reported to the central authority for consideration and approval. This work is still going on, and therefore no great changes in the working conditions for the nuclear medicine department have occurred so far.

Since we do not know what the final outcome will be, there is, however, still room for some fear about negative effects, and I will present some main points that have been raised in our discussions.

One point is about the rules for production and control. It can be argued that the risks are lesser with radiopharmaceuticals than with ordinary drugs because of negligible pharmacologic and toxic effects. Therefore, safety could be guaranteed with rules and procedures that are simpler than for ordinary drugs. Final control of ex tempore produced radiopharmaceuticals in the hospital is a special problem. Daily chromatography is expensive and takes time, thereby limiting the capacity of the department. Increased amount of free technetium or other defects in the preparation are easily seen on the scan, and the harm to the patient is negligible. In those few cases where it happens the patient can be reinvestigated within hours or the next day. Personally, I do not think it necessary to prescribe daily control of all kit preparations. As a rule, control measures in hospital should concern methods, not products.

With regard to "home-cooking" we have gone through several stages during the short history of nuclear medicine. First we used only a few ready-to-use compounds. Then, before industry entered the field, an increasing amount of home-made preparations came into use, especially since technetium became available. Later on radiopharmaceutical firms took over most of the kit production, at the same time as the total armoury of radiopharmaceuticals could be shrinked, also as a consequence of the technetium development. Hospital radiopharmacy to-day is mostly simple mixing and dilution, and I do not think there is a need for a pharmacist to perform these operations, but of course all methods used should be under supervision from the hospital pharmacy.

Another point for discussion concerns detailed rules about the medical use of radiopharmaceuticals. When an ordinary drug is registered in Sweden, it is also decided which diseases it may be used for, and no doctor may use them on other indications without special permission from the central drug department. A similar system would be unnecessarily stringent in the use of radiopharmaceuticals. After intravenous injection of pertechnetate, for example the harm to the patient is the same whether I plan to make a brain scan, a thyroid scan, a salivary gland scan, a search for Meckel's diverticulum or any other of the many possible investigations that can be performed. A definition like "Diagnostic investigation after intravenous injection" should be enough. "Scientific knowledge and proved clinical experience" is still a valid guide-line.

As already said, the supervising authority is the same as for ordinary drugs, i.e. the Drug Department of the National Board of Health and Welfare. It is organized in five divisions, concerned with pharmaceutical, pharmacological-toxic and pharmacological-therapeutic properties and with registration and inspection respectively. All divisions will be involved in some respect for each radiopharmaceutical under consideration. Only one of the divisions, that for pharmaceutical properties, has a radiopharmaceutical scientist on the staff. There is a certain danger that other officials, used to the rules for ordinary drugs, wish to apply the same routines for radiopharmaceuticals. This could lead to exaggerated demands, for example for tests for acute and chronic toxicity, or requirement of clinical trials to be performed in Sweden even if the substance has already been well tested and approved in other countries, and so on. This would in its turn lead to charges for the registration and for maintaining the product on the Swedish market of the same size as for ordinary drugs.

The question about increased costs of radiopharmaceuticals has been in the center of the discussion in Sweden. Radiopharmaceuticals are small products. To-day twelve foreign firms have announced about 300 products for registration. There are about 130 000 patient investigations performed during one year. If the charges for registration will be the same as for ordinary drugs, two things will happen. First, several of the products will be withdrawn from the market, which ·is especially serious since there is no Swedish production any more, and of course this will limit the possibility for the nuclear medicine department to offer a broad program of investigations. Secondly, the price for the remaining radiopharmaceuticals will increase considerably, which in a time of very limited hospital budgets will again mean a decreased capacity of the department.

Extended legislation will inevitably lead to increased bureaucracy. The extra paper work will take time, personnel and money from the productive work in the department. The increased number of supervising authorities, and the division between radiation protection and other control measures leads to duplication of some work. The rules for licence to use a non-registered compound are difficult to apply in routine work since they normally refer to use of a certain compound for an individual patient, not for a group of patients. Very hard rules have been laid down concerning the use of radiopharmaceuticals in medical research. Even if a registered radiopharmaceutical is used, and the study does not concern the radiopharmaceutical itself but is only used to get some desired information about the patient, special permission by the central authority for each patient is requested. Personally, I do not understand the meaning of this prescription, as long as we have no similar limitations in the use of other diagnostic methods in medical research, often carrying much greater risks than nuclear medicine methods. I think that such questions should be treated in exactly the same way as all other scientific work in the hospital, i.e. within a local ethical committee.

In conclusion I want to stress, that so far the introduction of the law has run smoothly and we have hopes that the application rules to come will be well adapted to the needs and the situation in the hospital. The final outcome of the new legislation will become evident in the nearest future.

22. LICENSING OF RADIOPHARMACEUTICALS IN EUROPEAN COUNTRIES 1982

KNUD KRISTENSEN

Licensing of individual pharmaceuticals has been used for many years as a mean of securing efficacy and safety of such products. During the last ten years a number of countries have introduced legislation in the field of radiopharmaceuticals (radioactive material intended for use in medical diagnosis or therapy). In order to obtain an up-to-date survey of the situation in European countries on the requirements for a licensing of radiopharmaceuticals letters were sent to authorities and individuals in all European countries. The following very short summary was written based on the replies received, and on information supplied by individuals. In the annex a list of adresses of relevant national authorities is given. In most countries regulations with the purpose of radiation protection with regard to workers and patients have been in force for many years. Such regulations are not reviewed here.

AUSTRIA: Legislation on radiopharmaceuticals is under preparation.

BELGIUM: According to a royal decree of February 28, 1963 a qualified pharmacist must approve radiopharmaceuticals. Royal decree's from June 6, 1960 and July 3, 1969 relates to the approval of manufacturers and to licensing of products. Radiopharmaceuticals for diagnostic use should be notified with the authorities, while products for therapy should be licensed. A recently created new control institution for radiopharmaceuticals is planning a reorganization of this field.

CZECHOSLOVAKIA:Radiopharmaceuticals (active and nonactive kits) are covered by the same legislation as nonradioactive drugs (regulation from 1969) and must be registered before marketing. Special explanatory material about preclinical testing of radiopharmaceuticals has been issued by the Commission for new drugs in 1980. All radiopharmaceuticals must be controlled by the state institute for drugs control.

DENMARK:Special regulations for the control of radiopharmaceuticals was issued in 1976. Radiopharmaceuticals may either be licensed by the National Board of Health and thereby distribution may take place direct to hospitals or they must be delivered through the Isotope-Pharmacy of the National Board of Health.

FEDERAL REPUBLIC OF GERMANY:The marketing of radiopharmaceuticals is regulated primarily by the Arzneimittelgesetz 1976 (Federal Drugs Act). The classification of medical products into essentially ready-prepared and products prepared on individual request, bears the following implications: for kits (radionuclide not included) and ready-prepared radiopharmaceuticals, an authorisation is required for marketing these products, as opposed to radiopharmaceuticals prepared on individual request - for instance due to the short physical half-life of the radionuclide used. For ready-prepared radiopharmaceuticals, the quality, safety and efficacy must be documented when applying for authorisation to place the radiopharmaceutical on the market.The compliance with these criteria is reviewed by the Bundesgesundheitsamt BGA (Federal Health Office) as the competent authority. An extension of the authorisation procedure to radiopharmaceuticals prepared on individual request is currently under consideration.

FINLAND:Radiopharmaceuticals may be sold by all companies

having a permission to sell pharmaceuticals (Apoteksvarulag
5.12.1935/374). There are no requirements for licensing of
individual radiopharmaceuticals. The organization of the
quality control of radiopharmaceuticals is at present under
discussion.

FRANCE:Radiopharmaceuticals are governed by the same
legislation as nonradioactive proprietary and are covered by
pharmaceutical monopoly. They are manufactured by
pharmaceutical firms whose establisment is subject to
ministerial authorisation. In addition, they are subject to a
further ministerial authorisation on the advice of the
Interministerial Committee on Artificial Radio-elements in
accordance with the Public Health Code article R 5230, R 5234
and 637. Special regulations (memorandum 24. June 1980 from
the Ministry of Health and Social Security) gives a
description of the minimum requirements for obtaining a
product license for preparation kits.

GERMAN DEMOCRATIC REPUBLIC:In addition to the Drug Law from
1964 a special regulation for radiopharmaceuticals was issued
in 1973. In another addition to the Drug Law the testing
system of new radiopharmaceuticals was regulated in 1976:
after toxicologic, pharmacologic, radiopharmacokinetic
checking in animals and quality control the examination of the
radiopharmaceutical in man has to be performed. Thereafter the
permission for application and sale is given by the "Institute
for Drugs". The application of radiopharmaceuticals for
treatment was regulated in a special law edited in 1974.

HUNGARY:Ministry of Health directives No 19/1970 gives
detailed requirements for production, quality control and
marketing of radiopharmaceuticals. Generators and preparation
kits are included. Only licensed products can be marketed.All
products must be quality controlled by the Institute of
Isotopes.

IRELAND:Radiopharmaceuticals placed on the market in Ireland are subject to the product licensing requirements which apply to medicinal products generally. However import and use of radiopharmaceuticals frequently occur without such licenses. In these cases the products are for use by medical specialists in radiology for the treatment of patients under their care.

ITALY:No radiopharmaceuticals are licensed and no pharmacopoeial monographs on such products are in force. National companies producing radiopharmaceuticals are licensed.

LUXENBOURG:No regulations providing detailed criteria for radiopharmaceuticals are in existence.

NETHERLANDS:At present no special regulations on radiopharmaceuticals are in force but such regulations are in preparation.

NORWAY:Radioactive pharmaceuticals are covered by the act of 20 June 1964 relating to Medicinal Goods and Poisons etc. They are however exempted from regulations on pharmaceutical specialities and the sole rights of the Norwegian Medical Department (Whole-saler) and the pharmacies to distribute drugs. They must be imported or produced by the Institute of Energy-Technology, Kjeller.

PORTUGAL:At present no special regulations on radiopharmaceuticals and no pharmacopoeia monographs in force.

SPAIN:Regulations on sterile material are applied. Spanish produced products are controlled by Nuclear Energy Commission. It is the intention of Ministry of Health to have special regulations for radiopharmacy and radiopharmaceuticals.

SWEDEN:A law on radioactive drugs was passed on April 23, 1981 followed by a decree on radioactive drugs of December 3, 1981. Both came into force on January 1, 1982. They require radiopharmaceuticals to be licensed. Generators and preparation kits may be included. A permission may be given to sell

unapproved radiopharmaceutical specialities. The regulations
follow those for nonradioactive pharmaceuticals closely.
Detailed regulations have not yet been issued.

SWITZERLAND:Radiopharmaceuticals   are   licensed   by   a
professional commission with members appointed by the Federal
office of Health (Radiation Protection) and the intercantonal
office for the Control of Medicine (IKS). The basis are
regulations by IKS from December 16, 1977. A number of
detailed notes for guidance have been issued. Besides ready
for use radiopharmaceuticals, generators and preparation kits
are included.

UNITED KINGDOM:A product licensing system for radiopharmaceuticals (including generators and kits) have been in operation
since 1971. No official quality control analysis are
performed. Guidance notes for hospitals on Premises and
Environment for the preparation of radiopharmaceuticals was
issued October 1982.

USSR:Marketing of radiopharmaceuticals requires a license from
the Pharmacological Committee of Medical Application.

LIST OF ADRESSES OF REGULATORY AGENCIES

AUSTRIA:
Federal Ministry of Health and Environmental Protection
Landstr. Hamptstr. 55-57
A-1030 Vienna, Austria
BELGIUM:
Ministere de la Sante Publique et de la Famille
Inspection Generale de la Pharmacie
Cite´ administrative de l´Etat
Quartier Ve´sale
1010 Bruxelles, Belgium
CZECHOSLOVAKIA:
Ministevstvo zdravotnictvi
Department of drugs regulation
Trida W. Piecka 98
120 37 Praha 10, Czechoslovakia
DENMARK:
The National Board of Health
The Isotope-Pharmacy
378 Frederikssundsvej
DK-2700 Brønshøj, Denmark

FEDERAL REPUBLIC OF GERMANY:
Bundesgesundheitsamt
Institut für Arzneimittel
Postfach 33013
D-1000 Berlin 33, FRG
FINLAND:
Läkemedelslaboratoriet
Lilla Robertsgatan 12 B
SF-00120 Helsingfors 12, Finland
FRANCE:
Ministere de la Santé
Direction de la Pharmacie et du Medicaments
1. Place de la Fontenoy
75700 Paris, France
GERMAN DEMOCRATIC REPUBLIC:
Ministerium für gesundheitswesen
Institut für Arzneimittel wesen
112-Berlin-Weisensee
GREECE:
Ministry of Health
State Drug Control Laboratory (K.E.E.F.)
Athens,Greece
HUNGARY:
National Inst. of Pharmacy
Zrinyi v.3
H 1051-Budapest, Hungary
ICELAND:
Lyfjanefnd
Laugaveguv 16
Reykjavik 105, Iceland
IRELAND:
National Drugs Advisory Board
Charles Lucas House
57 C Harcovt Street
Dublin 2, Ireland
ITALY:
Ministro della Sanita
L-1 Direttore Generale del Servicio Farmaceutico
Roma, Italy
LUXEMBOURG:
Direction de la Santé
Division de la Pharmacie et des Medicaments
28, Boulevard Joseph 11
1840 Luxembourg
NETHERLANDS:
Directory of Public Health (Drugs)
Postbus 439
2660 AK Leidschendam, The Netherlands
NORWAY:
Pharmaceutical Division
The Health Services of Norway
The Royal Norwegian Ministry of Social Affairs
Akersgatan 42
Oslo, Norway

RUMANIA:
Secretary to Romanian Dept. of Health
Commission for radiopharmaceuticals
Head Department of Nuclear Medicine and Clinical Physiology
Inst. of Physical Medicine
IK, Bd Cosbuc
Bucharest, Rumania
SPAIN:
Direccion General de Farmacia y
Medicamentos
Ministero de Sanidad y Consumo
Paseo del Prado 18-20
Madrid 14, Spain
SWEDEN:
National Board of Health and Welfare
Department of Drugs
Box 607
S-75125 Uppsala, Sweden
SWITZERLAND:
Intercantonal office for the Control of Medicines
Erlachstrasse 8
CH-3000 Bern 9, Switzerland
UNITED KINGDOM:
Department of Health and Social Security
Market Towers
1 Nine Elms Lane
London SW8,SNQ, United Kingdom
USSR:
Ministry of Health
Pharmacol. Committee of Medical Application
Rahmanovski Per D3
Moscow I. 51, USSR

Part 2

DESIGN OF LABORATORY FACILITIES FOR PREPARATION OF
RADIOPHARMACEUTICALS AT HOSPITALS

INTRODUCTION

The nature of the radioactive substances used in medicine particularly their short physical half-lives and the need for labelling of patient material requires that part of the production process of radiopharmaceuticals takes place at the hospitals. As for the industrial production this requires laboratory facilities designed to protect the working staff against radiation and to protect the product against contamination with microorganisms or other foreign substances. The traditional requirements of pharmacy and radiation protection may lead to conflicts. At the same time traditional pharmaceutical techniques designed for the production of large batches of sterile products to be used over a long period of time may be felt as "overkilling" in the case of a simple closed-procedure-preparation of a Tc-99m labelled product to be used within the next few hours. Discussion of these questions started more than 10 years ago and took place on many occassions during the seventies. The European Joint Committee on Radiopharmaceuticals of the European Society of Nuclear Medicine and the Society of Nuclear Medicine, Europe took up this question with the aim of giving advice on the subject. It was, however, soon realized that such advice if it should cover the situation in european countries would be very general and add very little to already existing publications in the field. It was therefore decided to take up the subject at the symposium and to have experts prepare reviews on this difficult aspects and also to review the existing recommandations. The following 3 chapters covers the present status.

It is obvious that although the scientific evidence has become more extensive in recent years, there still is a need for much more solid scientific knowledge about the relationship between environmental conditions and product quality as a basis for less stringent requirements than those based on pharmaceutical tradition. If a sterile product in the traditional sense is needed - and this may be questioned - the environmental conditions must be thoroughly controlled and bacterial contamination held at a low level. The standards for sterile products ($1:10^6$) was, however, also questioned and it was suggested that an index of harm parallel to what has been developed in radiation protection might be useful in order that different aspects of the whole process can be planned at the same level of safety (or risk).

Radiation protection were well developed before the introduction of pharmaceutical technique in the field of nuclear medicine. There might therefore have been a greater attention to this latter problem in recent years. The balancing of the two aspects where they are in conflict must be of continuous interest as new scientific evidence developes.This process will be of a political nature, also because different groups - staff/patients - are involved as risk groups.

The monitoring of radiation dosis in a number of departments illustrates that roughly two third of the radiation dose to the staff comes from handling of the radiopharmaceutical and one third from handling the patient. Radiation dose to fingers are often a most critical value to consider. Methods for monitoring of radiation doses are well developed and easy to perform while the microbiological safety is difficult to assess and to a much greater extent must rely on the testing of the whole system. The system must therefore also be build with several "barriers" in order to avoid steep gradients, which can cause heavy contamination if one of them fails.

In pharmaceutical technique as in radiation protection training is of paramount importance. Even the most sophisticated laboratories or laminar-air-flow techniques will be of no advantage if it is not used and maintained in the correct way. Training of staff in radiation protection and in pharmaceutical technique must therefore be a continuous operation and may be much more cost-effective than building new laboratories.

23. DESIGN CRITERIA IN RELATION TO PROTECTION OF THE PRODUCT

NEIL BELL

1. INTRODUCTION

The hospital preparation of radiopharmaceuticals over the last ten years has come to be dominated by formulations based on short-half-life injections assembled from commercially available kits. A survey of 80 United Kingdom hospitals showed that in 1977-78 short-lived injections accounted for 83 per cent of the doses they produced and that two-thirds of the respondents relied on commercially produced kits for over 90 per cent of their entire output (1). In this way much of the primary responsibility for quality assurance has been transferred to the manufacturers of radionuclide generators, non-radioactive targetting substances, saline injection used as diluent and even empty rubber-closed vials, all of which can be purchased as sterile products free from pyrogen. The manufacture of short-lived injections has thus been reduced to the ability to assemble eluate, diluent and targetting substance in appropriate proportions according to the instructions of the manufacturers of the components. The emphasis of quality control procedures lies now, therefore, on checking those factors likely to be at risk as a result, such as parent breakthrough in the eluate or inefficient labelling of the targetting substance (2). The prime responsibilities however are the measurement of radioactivity and the presentation free from foreign particulate matter of a sterile product. It is this latter requirement which has most effect on the design of production facilities and which has given rise to a great deal of discussion during the last five years.

2. LABORATORY DESIGN

In pharmaceutical terms, the method of choice for ensuring sterility of injections is terminal sterilization by autoclaving but the thermolability of some radiopharmaceuticals makes an aseptic facility necessary. Therefore to save time and also to avoid the complications of autoclaving radioactive materials, it is convenient to prepare all of the injections aseptically from the sterile components available. Thus the development of radiopharmacy design required primarily the merging of requirements for asepsis with those for radiological protection. In United Kingdom terms, this meant the reconciliation of the appropriate parts of the Guide to Good Pharmaceutical Manufacturing Practice (3) and the Code of Practice for the Protection of Persons against Ionising Radiations arising from Medical and Dental Use (4). This was attempted by The Hospital Preparation of Radiopharmaceuticals (5). A much more comprehensive work issued by the International Atomic Energy Agency set forth the principles of "Good Radiopharmacy Practice" (6).

Both publications showed that the simultaneous objectives of protection of the product from microbial contamination and protection of the personnel from radiation was achievable although at first sight the requirements might seem to be diametrically opposed. The basic plan of a laboratory with a changing room was common to both radionuclide and to aseptic laboratories. The materials and style of construction used to maintain a high standard of cleanliness within an aseptic suite were quite acceptable in radionuclide laboratory terms, although it was observed by Little (7) that the converse was rarely true.

The radiological protection requirement for a laboratory maintained at negative pressure against its surroundings was easily displaced by the aseptic requirement for positive pressure. This was because negative pressure would have been for an unlikely spillage event, made more unlikely still due to the special containment provided by the generator and the use of injection vials, whilst a positive pressure requirement provided by HEPA-filtered air was considered necessary for the routine maintenance of satisfactory clean room conditions. Those who prepared radiopharmaceuticals had little difficulty in adopting the scrub-up procedures and protective clothing routines when entering the facility and observing the radiation monitoring and careful clothing disposal procedures on leaving (8). Both disciplines were accustomed to the step-over bench in the changing room which provided the psychological barrier at which these events took place. Gloves and other protective clothing necessary for aseptic procedures, were, conversely, quite adequate to fulfil the requirement of protection from radioactive contamination.

The clean room standard which the Guide to Good Pharmaceutical Manufacturing Practice (3) prescribes as appropriate to aseptic procedures is Class 1, BS 5295 (9) which is approximately equivalent to Class 100 (U.S. Federal Standard 209B). In conventional pharmacy this has been achieved by maintaining room ventilation at a standard, in the occupied state, of Class 2 (Class 10 000) and providing unidirectional (laminar airflow) cabinets in which to perform the critical parts of the filling or transfer procedures. In a radiopharmaceutical context, this resulted in a rather more complex reconciliation of the two disciplines. The cabinets usually employed for aseptic work and the fume cupboards appropriate to radiological protection were each directly inimical to the requirements of the other. Aseptic cabinets gave no radiological protection to the operator and fume cupboards gave no aseptic protection to the product.

The problem was usually resolved by using a cabinet in which the filtered air was propelled vertically downwards to the working area and removed through ducts in the working surface. The speeds of the control fans were adjusted to ensure that an inflow of room air to the front of the worksurface provided protection to the operator against airborne radioactivity which might be generated in aerosol form. At the same time the major part of the worksurface was enveloped in sterile air which had passed through the HEPA filter in the ceiling of the unit. Lead glass at eye level guided the vertical airflow. Lead shielding fitted externally to the cabinet and up to chest level at the front satisfied the requirements of radiological protection without interfering with the even flow of air necessary for asepsis. In the United Kingdom, the radiopharmaceutical cabinet was, and still is, a conception not recognised by a British Standard Specification. It is the responsibility of the purchaser to verify from drawings such as Fig. 1 that, as well as the safety protection afforded by the Class II requirements of BS 5726 (10), the cabinet is capable of providing the clean room standard of air quality defined as Class 1, BS 5295. The most important requirement for the latter is that there should be a HEPA filter at the ceiling of the cabinet.

These cabinets have been much improved in recent years both as regards their ability to satisfy the protection factor requirements of BS 5726 and in those features of design relevant to their asepsis function. The cabinet illustrated provides a perforated worksurface which minimizes turbulence around the receptacles placed on it and therefore improves the air quality close to these objects. For reasons of radiological protection, it is considered desirable to provide a second cabinet to house the radionuclide generators. For this purpose or for centres with small workloads, an alternative method of providing the dual protection of product and personnel is by installing a small vertical laminar flow cabinet ("miniunit") inside an existing fume cupboard.

The radiopharmaceutical facility which results from the combination of the best asepsis and radionuclide facilities is an ideal which was not attained by many of the locations in United Kingdom hospitals used in 1978 for the purpose. Thus at least 35 centres carried out their production in an ordinary radionuclide laboratory without a unidirectional down-draught workstation (1). Workstations of this type were fitted in 45 of the centres and, in about a third of these, some kind of filtered air was supplied to the room. Some of the less well equipped centres produced as few as 300 short-lived injections per year and there was therefore a reluctance on grounds of cost to upgrade the facilities. This provided a stimulus to question the need for high grade aseptic facilities and has

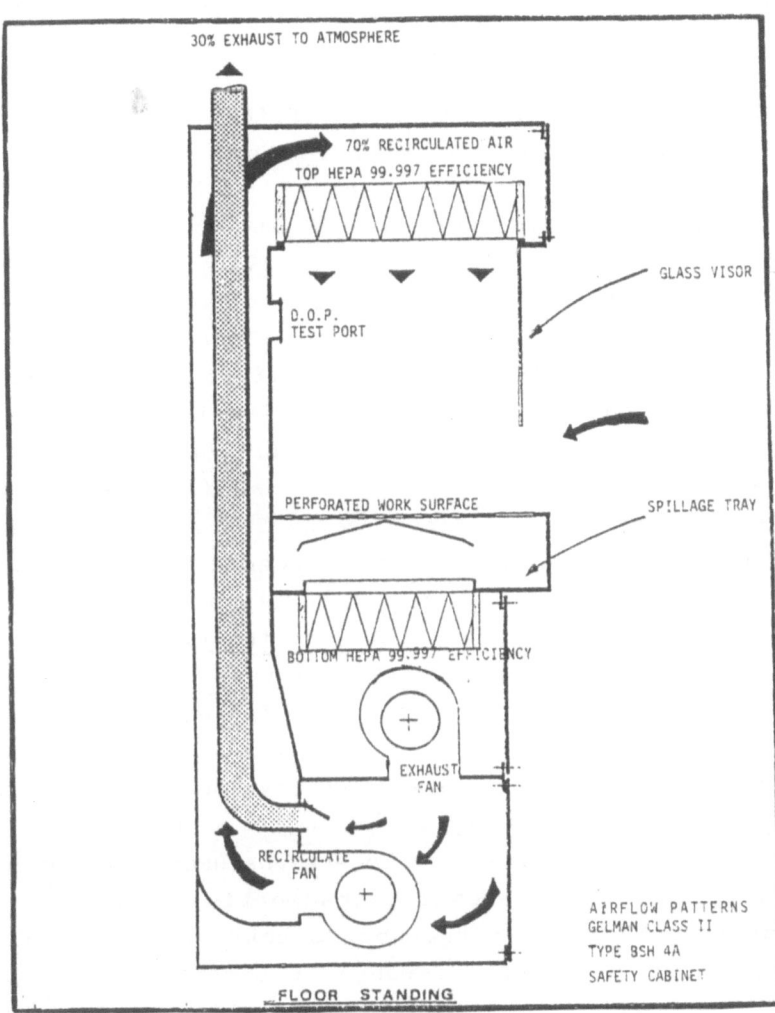

Fig. 1. Side elevation of a cabinet which provides a Class 1, BS 5295
environment and has a protection factor conforming to Class II,
BS 5726

resulted in a debate, not about the merging of conventional pharmaceutical asepsis facilities with those of radiochemistry but about the substitution of conventional asepsis facilities by some kind of lesser standard of clean room conditions which would be acceptable.

3. RADIOPHARMACEUTICAL QUALITY - STANDARDS

The reason most often advanced for supposing that the conventional standards for aseptic manipulations are not required is that there never seem to be any adverse patient reactions which could be traced directly to the presence of live organisms in the injections produced. Certainly the system set up to monitor such reactions in the United Kingdom has not received such a report since it was set up (11). The experience in the United States of America has been similar (12, 13) and no such adverse reaction in relation to radiopharmaceuticals has been reported. However, United Kingdom replies to a questionnaire by Abra et al (1) indicated seven possible instances in more than 230 000 doses of all types. There may be a genuine difficulty in identifying such reactions even if they do occur and the recent review of the clinical significance of microbial contamination in pharmaceutical products by Ringertz & Ringertz (14) suggests some of the ways in which symptoms might be masked. Indirect effects of microbial contamination have been reported in both countries as cases of aseptic meningitis. These were due to the presence of pyrogens in injections used for radionuclide cisternography (15). Such a contamination is due to faulty preparation of sterile components used for assembly of the injection. It is not of relevance to a consideration of any aseptic environment which might be used to assemble the injection. It is of interest to note that all of the implicated preparations tested by Cooper & Harbert (15) were strongly positive to the Limulus test but gave a negative result when tested by the rabbit method on a dose per weight basis. The authors took this as confirmation of animal experiments which showed that endotoxin is at least 1000 times more toxic intrathecally than intravenously and they understandably concluded that the pyrogen test of the United States Pharmacopeia was insufficient for intrathecal injections.

Any decision by regulatory authority to downgrade the asepsis facilities required specifically for the hospital preparation of short-lived radioinjections has to be made against a background of the long term effects which this may have on the nuclear medicine patient. In the last few years much more of this kind of information has become available but more requires to be done fully to elucidate the problems. Asepsis in this connection can be defined as the prevention of entry of organisms in numbers which are unacceptable in an injection which will not be terminally sterilized. Current versions of unacceptable numbers of contaminated containers for non-radioactive injections are 0.3 per cent (World Health Organization, 1973) and 0.1 per cent (Parenteral Drug Association, 1980). It has been suggested by Whyte (16) that these standards are based on what can be achieved rather than on what is necessary. The standards apply to what, in radiopharmaceutical terms, would be called "open" procedures. For reasons of radioactivity containment, most radioinjections are assembled in such a way that all transfers are made using syringe needles and rubber-closed vials. This "closed" procedure results in the presentation of an injection vial with a rubber closure which has already been pierced at least once. It is the method used particularly when short-lived radioinjections are made from kits and generatoreluates.

4. THE EFFECT OF AIR QUALITY ON PRODUCT QUALITY

Abra et al. (17) evaluated the comparative risks of contamination of closed and open procedures carried out in an artificially contaminated environment and showed that closed transfers were one sixth as liable to microbial contamination as open transfers between screw-capped bottles. A theoretical estimate of contamination rate based on the areas of needles, open bottle necks, needle hole areas and deposition rates gave an answer of 1:19 in favour of the closed type of transfer. Whyte et al (18) have shown that in order not to exceed the contamination standard of 0.1 per cent when open vials were filled with broth in factory conditions, it was essential to use a Class 1 environment and adopt the best possible hand protection methods. In this way a contamination frequency of 0.04 per cent was obtained. When the same exercise was carried out in Class 2 conditions (U.S. Fed.Std. 209B, Class 10 000), there was a contamination rate of 0.24 per cent. This does not suggest however that it would be possible to meet the Parenteral Drug Association standard in a Class 2 environment using closed procedures because each completed radioinjection represents a multiple transfer procedure involving generator elution, addition of eluate to kit vials, distribution of aliquots, etc. Abra et al. (17) saw no reason why aseptically assembled injections should be designed to be of a lower standard than the 0.0001 per cent proposed by the Pharmacopoeia Nordica (19) for terminally sterilized products and assumed that any advantage to be gained from the use of the closed procedure would be applied to an improvement of the product.

An investigation which compared broth transfers carried out in hospital radiopharmacies with their environment standards revealed a contamination rate of two in 2099 (20). No conclusions can be drawn from such small numbers of contaminants and in fact one of these came from a grade B radionuclide laboratory without a down-draught workstation, the other from a facility having such a workstation situated in a room provided with HEPA-filtered air. Settle plate data collected at the same time showed that the use of a unidirectional down-draught workstation produced a significant reduction in microbial fall-out. There was no significant difference (although there was an improving trend) when the workstation was sited in a room supplied with air through filters rated at 95% efficiency against 5 μm particles or in a room supplied by HEPA-filtered air.

Although there must obviously be a strong correlation between the quality of ventilation of an environment and the number of contaminations of transfers which result, there was also a statistically significant difference between the

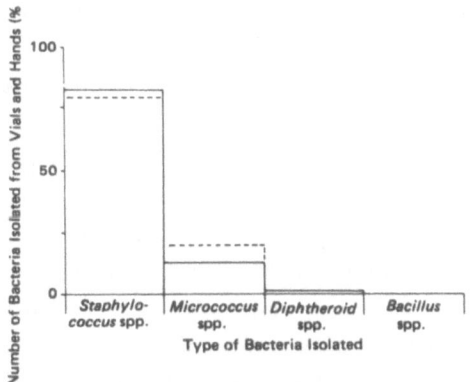

Identification of microbial contaminants by the contact route.
Solid line indicates the organisms isolated from the vials; broken line
indicates the organisms isolated from the hands.

Fig. 2. From Whyte et al. (18). Reproduced by kind permission
of the Journal of Parenteral Science and Technology.

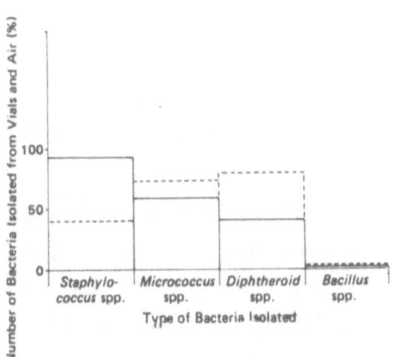

Figure 3   Identification of microbial contaminants by the airborne route.
Solid line indicates the organisms isolated from the vials; broken line
indicates the organisms isolated from the air.

Fig. 3. From Whyte et al. (18). Reproduced by kind permission
of the Journal of Parenteral Science and Technology.

contamination rates of open procedures in a Class 1 environment when three different hand treatments were used (18). These were a. a double scrub in chlorhexidine gluconate followed by application of an antiseptic barrier cream. Sterile surgical gloves were put on and sprayed regularly with isopropyl alcohol, b. same as a. but no gloves or isopropyl alcohol, c. no hand treatment. It is particularly interesting that there was a marked qualitative correlation between the organisms isolated from contaminated containers and the organisms isolated from the hands of the operator in experiments where the hand treatment was varied (Fig. 2) whereas the correlation is not so marked between container contaminations and aerial organisms when the air quality was varied (Fig. 3). It may be that the closed radiopharmaceutical preparation procedure with its emphasis on close individual handling of containers might be affected by the swabbing techniques employed and the state of preparation of the hands.

Whyte et al.(18) have suggested that the microbial concentration appropriate to Class 1 conditions is "less than $1/m^3$". Their results showed slit-sampler counts of $0.4/m^3$ for Class 1 in a unidirectional airflow cabinet, $85/m^3$ for Class 2, using the general room ventilation only, and $186/m^3$ when the aseptic suite was unventilated. By comparison, Favero et al. (21) found that an average production area not provided with specialized ventilation gave a value of approximately 600 organisms/m^3.

Since it is known (1) that many radioinjections must have been assembled in environments approximating to this last figure, apparently without mishap, it should be instructive not only to consider facility design criteria in this review but to try to establish some of the possible reasons for the absence of adverse reactions.

5. RISK OF BACTERIAL GROWTH

A further two features peculiar to short-lived radiopharmaceuticals should be considered, namely short shelf-life and the presence of radioactivity. Assuming that chance contamination at the time of preparation will never be large enough to constitute an infective dose to the patient, a dangerous situation will result from contamination only if substantial multiplication of a contaminant takes place. The addition of bactericides to short-lived radioinjections is not customary (European Pharmacopoeia (22)) so it is important to known what potential there is for subotantial microbial growth in these formulations. When Abra et al.(23) inoculated a selection of reconstituted but non-radioactive kit vials with five test organisms in numbers ranging from 70 down to less than ten, the numbers tended to remain very approximately constant over an eight-hour period (the expected maximum shelf-life). An exception was Escherichia coli which doubled in numbers in Diethylenetriamine pentaacetic acid (DTPA) and Macroaggregated albumin (MAA). The test organisms used were those recommended by the United States Pharmacopeia (1975) for its Antimicrobial Preservatives Effectiveness Test.

The radiation effect within a typical injection vial containing about 500 MBq will amount, in a period of eight hours to about 10 Gy (23). Decimal reduction doses of ionizing radiation vary greatly from one microbial genus to another, for instance from 40 Gy for Pseudomonas aeruginosa to more than 15 kGy for Sarcina rubens (24). In the case of Pseudomonas this would result in a reduction of about 40 per cent of any contamination.

Holmes & Allwood (25) have reported that while they found little consistency in the growth of E. coli, Gram-negative organisms of the Klebsiella-Enterobacter group could multiply by up to three or four log cycles within 48 hr in such a simple chemical fluid as physiological saline. This period of time would be well outside the shelf-life of short-lived injections. Organisms of the Klebsiella-Enterobacter-Serratia group (the tribe Klebsielleae) have been found to multiply rapidly in simple glucose solutions (26) and a member of the genus Pseudomonas is known to multiply in distilled water (27). In the former case, a doubling of numbers would be possible in eight hours although it is unlikely that radiopharmaceutical formulations would provide such a readily available carbon source while in the latter case the time-scale is outside the shelf-life of a short-lived radiopharmaceutical. In addition to that, it is true as a broad generalization that while Gram-negative organisms are less fastidious in their growth requirements than Gram-positives and are therefore more likely to proliferate in simple solutions, they are not often found on the skin of personnel and rarely in the room environment (18). The Gram-positive organisms which predominate in the atmosphere are also the ones less likely to multiply in simple formulations. Ringertz & Ringertz (14) reported that thrombophlebitis and endocarditis of the right side of the heart are quite common in narcotic addicts, usually due to access of the Gram-positive Staphylococcus aureus.

Clinical reactions resulting from the introduction of comparatively small numbers of organisms at injection site are associated frequently with the greatly extended contact times associated with the placing of intravenous cannulae but again this is fortunately not relevant to radiopharmaceuticals. Whyte et al., using volunteers, have simulated the skin piercing appropriate to the administration of radiopharmaceuticals. Results (to be published) show that saline subsequently ejected through the needles used was contaminated in 2.4 per cent of the cases and a further 2.8 per cent of needles were found on withdrawal to be contaminated externally. The volunteers did not suffer any adverse effects.

6. FUTURE STANDARDS

It is proposed that the third edition of the (United Kingdom) Guide to Good Pharmaceutical Manufacturing Practice will state, in relation to the assembly of short-lived radioinjections prepared from kits and generator eluate, that "it may be acceptable to carry out this work under environmental conditions less demanding" than those described for conventional aseptic transfers elsewhere in the guidance. This less demanding standard is not defined and its use is on condition that all transfers will be of the "closed" type and that the product will be administered within a few hours of preparation. Recently issued guidance notes for hospitals (28) define the facility to be used for this type of preparation as a cabinet, conforming to Class 1, BS 5295 and to the protection standards of BS 5726, set in a room with a good standard of hygiene preferably supplied with filtered air to the Controlled Area or Class 3 standard of BS 5295. The definition of a closed procedure is extended by this guidance document to include the withdrawal, in one amount, of a solution from an ampoule opened within the workstation. The guidance is consistent with the findings of Abra et al. (20) that settle plate counts in unidirectional down-draught workstations are not significantly altered by the outside environment. The guidance makes it clear that the immediate environment in which the transfers take place should be of Class 1, BS 5295 standard. The contamination rates demonstrated by Whyte et al. (18) between Class 1 and Class 2 conditions are of the same order as the advantage which closed procedures have over open procedures but this would not allow the Parenteral Drug Association standard to be achieved in Class 2 conditions. This is because of the multiple transfers needed in the assembly of radioinjections. The standard of one contamination in a thousand injections implies that substantial numbers of injections have a live organism present. It implies that even those who employ the highest standards at the point of transfer must be depending on the complex microbiological factors described to avoid adverse reactions.

REFERENCES
1. Abra R M, Bell N D S, Horton P W, McCarthy T M. A survey of radiopharmaceutical manufacture in United Kingdom hospitals. J Clin Hosp Pharm 1980;5:11-20.
2. Bell N D S, Horton P W. Radiopharmaceuticals - present and past. J Clin Pharm 1978;2:137-154.
3. Guide to Good Pharmaceutical Manufacturing Practice. London: HMSO. 1977.
4. Code of Practice for the Protection of Persons against Ionising Radiations arising from Medical and Dental Use. London: HMSO. 1972.
5. Hospital Preparation of Radiopharmaceuticals. Scientific Report Series No. 16. London: Hospital Physicists' Association. 1977.
6. Kristensen K. Preparation and control of

324

radiopharmaceuticals in hospitals. Technical Reports Series No. 194. Vienna: International Atomic Energy Agency. 1979.

7. Little, W.A. Radiopharmaceuticals. In Allwood M C, Fell J T. Eds: Textbook of Hospital Pharmacy. Oxford: Blackwell Scientific Publications. 1980:170-198.

8. Bell N D S. Radiopharmaceuticals and the pharmacist. Pharm J 1977;219:503-504.

9. British Standards Institution. Environmental cleanliness in enclosed spaces. BS 5295:1976. London: BSI. 1976.

10. British Standards Institution. Specification for microbiological safety cabinets. BS 5726:1979. London: BSI. 1979.

11. Keeling D. Chapter 16 of this book.

12. Rhodes B A, Cordova MA. Adverse reactions to radiopharmaceuticals: Incidence in 1978, and associated symptoms. Report of the Adverse Reactions Subcommittee of the Society of Nuclear Medicine. J Nucl Med 1980;21:1107-1110.

13. Cordova M A, Rhodes B A, Atkins H L, Glenn H J, Hoogland D R, Solomon A C. Adverse reactions to radiopharmaceuticals. J Nucl Med 1982;23:550-551.

14. Ringertz O, Ringertz S. The clinical significance of microbial contamination in pharmaceutical and allied products. In Bean H S, Beckett A H, Carless J E. Eds: Advances in Pharmaceutical Sciences. London: Academic Press. 1982;Vol.5:201-26.

15. Cooper J F, Harbert J C. Endotoxin as a cause of aseptic meningitis after radionuclide cisternography. J Nucl Med 1975;16:809-813.

16. Whyte W. Settling and impaction of particles into containers in manufacturing pharmacies. J Parenteral Science Technol 1981;35:255-261.

17. Abra R M, Bell N D S, Horton P W. An evaluation of some radiopharmaceutical transfer techniques. J Clin Hosp Pharm 1980;5:3-9.

18. Whyte W, Bailey P V, Tinkler J, McCubbin I, Young L, Jess J. An evaluation of the routes of bacterial contamination occurring during aseptic pharmaceutical manufacturing. J Parenteral Science Technol 1982;36:102-107.

19. Pharmacopoeia Nordica. Edito Danica Addendum 1964-1975. København: Nyt Nordisk Forlag Arnold Busck. 1975.

20. Abra R M, Bell N D S, Horton P W. Product quality and environmental standards in the hospital assembly of radiopharmaceuticals. J Clin Hosp Pharm 1980;5:299-306.

21. Favero M S, Puleo J R, Marshall J H, Oxbarrow G S. Comparative levels and types of microbial contamination detected in industrial clean rooms. Appl Microbiol 1966;14:539-551.

22. European Pharmacopoeia. Sainte-Ruffine, France: Maisonneuve S A. 1975;III:385.

23. Abra R M, Bell N D S, Horton P W. The growth of micro-organisms in some parenteral radiopharmaceuticals. Int J Pharm 1980;5:187-193.

24. Stapleton G E, Engel M S. Cultural conditions as determinants of sensitivity of Escherichia coli to

damaging agents. J Bacteriol 1960;80:544-551.

25. Holmes C J, Allwood M C. The microbial contamination of intravenous infusions during clinical use. J Appl Bacteriol 1979;46:247-267.

26. Maki D G, Martin W T. Nationwide epidemic of septicemia caused by contaminated infusion products. IV. Growth of microbial pathogens in fluids for intravenous infusion. J Infect Diseases 1975;131:267-272.

27. Carson L H, Favero M S, Band W W, Peterson N J. Morphological, biochemical and growth characteristics of Pseudomonas cepacia from distilled water. Appl Microbiol 1973;25:476-483.

28. Department of Health and Social Security. Guidance notes for hospitals: Premises and environment for the preparation of radiopharmaceuticals. 1982.

24. DESIGN CRITERIA IN RELATION TO PROTECTION OF THE
PERSONNEL AND THE ENVIRONMENT

KLAUS R. ENNOW

1. INTRODUCTION

Handling of dispersible radioactive substances ("unsealed sources") is generally required to be carried out in an "isotope laboratory" for the purpose of radiation protection.

The classification and construction of isotopelaboratories has for many years followed the principles given by IAEA (1) which are very general in order to allow handling of all possible radionuclides.

If the radioactive substances are used for in-vivo studies on humans by intravenous injection, the radioactive compounds have to be considered as pharmaceuticals: radiopharmaceuticals, which have also to be handled in accordance with the rules of "good manufacturing practice" -GMP, GRP (2) for the preparation of pharmaceuticals.

About 50% of all investigations with radiopharmaceuticals are carried out with Tc-99m and almost all preparations carried out in hospital departments are labelling of various compounds with Tc-99m.

Therefore, instead of constructing general purpose isotopelaboratories in hospitals, it would be better to separate the radiochemical work from the preparations of radiopharmaceuticals, and then change the principles for the design and construction.

2. RADIATION PROTECTION

Protection of personnel and population against unnecessary exposure and optimization of the radiation protection are general requirements in all legislation, based on the recommendations given by the International Commission on

Radiological Protection.

A general problem to be dealt with is the allocation of limited resources for design and construction of premises, for personnel protection and monitoring and for prevention of accidents.

For the handling of radionuclides in hospitals and for preparation of pharmaceuticals, the construction of the premises is of importance in order to achieve a constant level of safety - for the personnel and for the patients.

It is therefore wise to "reconcile" radiation protection and GMP as soon as possible in the stage of design of facilities and premises. In radiation protection the purpose of the design of working places is given as (3):
- minimizing the exposure of the personnel
- protecting visitors and workers in the vicinity
- controlling the dispersal of radioactive material into the working environment
- controlling and minimizing the spread of radioactive material and waste into the environment of man.

2.1 Protection of the personnel

The routes of exposure of personnel by handling of dispersible radioactive substances are: (1) external exposure, (2) airborne radioactivity and (3) spills and incidents.

2.1.1. External exposure. Modern Tc-generators are effectively shielded at delivery, although some generators need additional shielding. The dose rate at 0.5 meter is less than 1 μGy/h (e.g. Tecegen S, IRE + 5 cm lead bricks) and do not contribute significant to the irradiation of the personnel. The use of short-lived radionuclides, like Tc-99m, prepared as ready-for-use pharmaceuticals in the morning to fulfil the needs for the whole day means handling of excess activity of the order of four times the activity to be injected.

Tc-99m is easily shielded by few mm of lead but to be able to measure the activity, the Mo-99 content, to label vials and to administer the dose to the patient, the Tc-99m solutions have to be handled unshielded. This leads to irradiation of

the staff and the dose records in Denmark 1982 as well as
other measurements (4,5) shows that the average whole-body
doses is 2 mSv annually for those involved in the work with
Tc-99m but only few persons exceeding 15 mSv/year. The
collective dose is of the order of 1 mSv per Ci Tc-99m
injected (0,001 manSv/Ci).

More detailed measurements of the whole body dose have
shown that, on average, the annual doses are due to 1/3 from
elution and preparation, 1/3 from injection and 1/3 from
scintigraphy (exposure from the activity in the patients),
this means that a considerable part of the exposure (from the
patients) is unavoidable, but this assumes that all vials are
shielded during the compounding of the radiopharmaceuticals.
An advantage of the kit preparation - from a radiation
protection point of view - is the easy shielding of all vials
in small lead pots and the short handling time.

Handling of unshielded vials and syringes could give doses
to fingers and hands exceeding the dose limits and use of
shielding and tongs is required.

The external exposure during hospital preparation of radiopharmaceuticals can be limited to an acceptable level by
proper shielding and the laboratories should therefore be
equipped with adequate space for shielding of generators, for
storage of lead pots and with lead glass shieldings e.g. for
reading of labels. Lead shielding should be well painted and
easily washable and the lead pots should be so constructed
that safe injections through rubber stoppers are possible.

2.1.2. Airborne radioactivity. The internal exposure by
inhalation of airborne radioactivity is a problem of special
concern in construction of isotope laboratories in which a
fume hood is required (1). In order to protect the personnel,
work with volatile materials has to be carried out in the fume
hood and the ventilation is provided mainly by the exhaust
system of the fume hood.

It is well known that work with iodine (I-125, I-131)
labelled pharmaceutical can give contamination of the air but
measurements of Tc-99m in the air and in personnel during
normal operation have shown that no internal contamination

took place through airborne route (6-9). Even if a down-floow
work-station is used outside the fume hood, airborne
contamination of Tc-99m do not present a radiation hazard,
although activity in the air could be measured.

2.1.3. Spills and incidents. Measurements of partial and
whole body contents have shown that internal Tc-99m
contamination in personnel do occur but mainly in persons
working with "open" preparations and far below the dose limit
(6-9).

For Tc-99m as well as for I-125 and I-131 the internal
contaminations can not be explained by airborne activity and
spills followed by ingestion are believed to be the reason for
most contaminations. It is not unusual that handling of great
numbers of small vials leads to accidental release of Tc-99m
solutions (droped vials, disconnections etc.) in which cases
high levels of contamination of premises and personnel is
found. In these situations it is very important that all
surfaces in the laboratory is easily decontaminated and that
washing and changing facilities for personnel is located close
to the working place.

2.2. Protection of workers in the vicinity

Exposure in neighbouring rooms is a problem today where
hospitals are built of light materials (Gypsum boards). It is
important to construct all storage areas with either shielded
walls or shelves strong enough to withstand the weight
(200-300 kg/m^2) of leadshielding e.g. pots around all
solutions; also for waste temporarily stored for decay. In
radiochemical work and preparation of iodine labelled
compounds it is required to protect the vicinity from airborne
radioactivity by maintaining a lower pressure in the
laboratories than in the neighbour rooms. As airborne activity
of Tc-99m is very rare this could be disregarded in locations
solely used for kit preparations.

2.3. Dispersion of radioactive materials into the environment

During normal work no activity of Tc-99m will be dispersed
into the outdoor air through the ventilation system. Mo-99 and

Tc-99m can easily be stored for physical decay for few months and only the activity in the patients excreta should be allowed to be disposed off to the sewage system. Generators can contain some long-lived impurities (e.g. Co-60) and precautions should be taken to measure the content before incineration of old generator columns.

3. CLASSIFICATION AND DESCRIPTION OF ISOTOPELABORATORIES

It is well known that isotopelaboratories are classified into three types (A, B and C) and that the type of laboratory suitable for a certain application depends on the activity to be handled. Activity limits are given for 4 toxicity groups in which all radionuclides are classified according to their radiotoxicity (Annual Limit of Intake (ALI) or Derived Air Concentration (DAC) by inhalation). Laboratories for handling of low levels of radioactivity are described as type C and for type C the upper limit for group 4 radionuclides, like Tc-99m, is 100 mCi for "Simple wet operation".

This limit will often be exceeded for preparation of Tc-99m radiopharmaceuticals which then would require a type B lab. This is described as the real Isotopelaboratory (sometimes called "a hot laboratory") and it has been recommended that new laboratories for "medical care" should be planned as type B. It has been stated above that airborne radioactivity and internal contamination do not take place during normal work with Tc-99m. Therefore instead of following a general activity limit based on internal contamination by inhalation it would be better to give separate recommendations for the locations where Tc-99m labelled radiopharmaceuticals are prepared.

Instead of constructing a type B isotopelaboratory with space for Tc-99m preparations it would be better to separate the location for this work from the laboratory for general radiochemical work (if this is needed) and then take into consideration also the requirements for aseptic preparation. The resources needed for facilities for GMP could then be limited to the smaller area for Tc-99m preparations and not necessarily used for the whole isotopelaboratory.

3.1. Ventilation

Theoretically the only possible conflict between radiation protection and GMP would be on the ventilation of the type B laboratory. Type B laboratories shall be kept at reduced pressure relative to the surroundings and the air change should be at least ten times per hour in order to protect personnel from any contamination from the "product". On the other hand the product (and then the patients) has to be protected against contamination from the great amount of replacement air needed. This would require that all replacement air should be filtered but this would only be possible if the pressure in the laboratory was higher than in the surroundings. Therefore the ventilation should be designed in agreement with GMP rules and down-draught work stations should be allowed for storage of generators and for kit preparations. In isotopelaboratories the down-draught unit could be placed in the fume hood.

3.2. General recommendations

It has been emphasized that external radiation and decontamination in case of incidents is the most important problems by preparations with Tc-99m (and other short-lived radionuclides). The working place should then be designed, constructed and prepared for shielding e.g. by lead-glass plates. The entrance should be through an anteroom with washing and changing facilities. All surfaces, floor walls, benches, tables etc. should be easy to keep clean and decontaminated. The outline of the premises should be in agreement with the GMP rules but it is believed that all measures taken to assure a good aseptic standard will also assure a good protection of the personnel. A common requirement is good personal hygiene by all personnel.

4. SCHEDULE FOR PLANNING OF PREMISES
- the location in the building taking into consideration fire protection, connection to sewage system and sitting of exhaust vents,
- the location of individual rooms to give the best

manufacturing facilities,

- the construction of isotope laboratories and clean rooms,
- details like surfaces, furnitures, sinks etc.,
- inspection and testing.

REFERENCES
1. Safe Handling of Radionuclides, 1973, IAEA Safety Series No 1.
2. Kristensen K. Preparation and Control of Radiopharmaceuticals in Hospitals, IAEA Technical Reports Series No 194, Vienna 1979.
3. Radiation Protection. Recommendations in the Nordic Countries, Liber Tryck Stockholm 1976.
4. Ahlgren L et al. Radiation doses in connection with handling of Tc-99m in hospitals. 6th meeting Nordic Society of Radiation Protection, Iceland 18-20 June 1981. (in Swedish-Radfys report 81:04).
5. Emrich D et al. Strahlenexposition des Personals bei Nuklearmedizinischer in-vivo-diagnostik mit Tc-99m. Strahlenschutz in Forschung und Praxis - Stuttgart. Georg Thieme Verlag 1982;25:92-99.
6. Nishiyama H et al. Survey of Tc-99m contamination of laboratory personnel:Its degree and routes. Radiology 1980;135:467-71.
7. Eadie A S, Horton P W, Hilditch T E. Monitoring of air-borne contamination during the handling of technetium-99m and radioiodine. Phys Med Biol 1980;25:1079-87.
8. Falk R, Eklund G, Magi A, Schnell P-O. Internal radiation of hospital staff during work with radionuclides. SSI-1977-034 Stockholm National Institute of Radiation Protection 1977 (in Swedish).
9. Sorantin H, Angelberger P. Qualitetskontrolle von Radiopharmaka. Strahlenschutz in Forschung und Praxis, Stuttgart, Georg Thieme Verlag 1982;25:11-24.

25. PRESENT STATUS OF RECOMMENDATIONS FOR THE DESIGN OF LABORATORY FACILITIES

COLIN R. LAZARUS

1. INTRODUCTION

The design of laboratory facilities for the hospital preparation of radiopharmaceuticals must achieve two major aims:- (i) to protect the product from microbial contamination from the environment, the operator and other products, and (ii) to protect the operator from radioactivity and pathogenic organism hazards where these may be involved, e.g. the handling of blood and blood products. Various guidelines, recommendations, Codes of Practice, and regulations must be borne in mind during the design stage of laboratory facilities so that the above aims can be achieved. The requirements for facilities for sterile production and radiation protection are similar in many ways, but conflicting requirements do occur. Recommendations on the design of radiochemical laboratories are readily obtainable from Codes of Practice and other guidance, which are interpretations of the regulations laid down under national Radioactive Substances Acts. Similarly Guidelines for Good Manufacturing Practice (GMP) published by national and international bodies, assist in the design of laboratories for the production of sterile products. Radiopharmaceutical preparation presents some difficulties, peculiar to this type of product, and over the years many discussions have tried to resolve, to the satisfaction of all the professional disciplines involved, the design of the facilities to cope with these difficulties. Many publications have given guidance on the design of facilities, but the lack of any official status, particularly in the U.K., has not helped to resolve the arguments. However some guidance notes recently produced by the Department of Health and Social

Security (D.H.S.S.) in the U.K. will be invaluable to persons
designing laboratories.

This paper will review the recommendations available and
examine their status and their acceptance in various
countries. Emphasis will be placed on the situations in the
U.K. and Europe, but other countries will also be considered.

2. RECOMMENDATIONS AND THEIR STATUS

Many of the publications giving recommendations are based
on the views of the authors or the current practice at the
time they were written. These recommendations do not carry any
official status but are still consulted by the designers of
facilities and should therefore be considered. More recent
recommendations have been based on standards, regulations and
guidelines, not all of which may carry official status, but
may be the interpretation of official national regulations by
recognised authorities.

2.1. British Standards Institution (B.S.I.)

2.1.1. Environmental Cleanlines in Enclosed Spaces. Three
British Standards, BS5295, Parts 1, 2 and 3; 1976 (1, 2, 3)
are available concerning environmental cleanlines. Part 1
classifies environments into four classes in terms of size and
maximum number of airborne particles, and gives the
specifications for each of these classes in clean rooms and
work stations. In addition a controlled area is defined (see
Table 1).

In addition to specifications for particle size and numbers,
Part 1 also recommends the type of airflow for each class, and
the periodicity for air sampling and counting. No such
recommendations or specifications are given for the Controlled
Area which is defined in the Standard as "any work space or
room which cannot be classified as a clean room, but in which
the air is required to be cleaner than that of the outside
environment". Such an area allows selected environmental
conditions to be laid down locally to meet specific
requirements. Controlled areas are specified in two of the
current published recommendations for specific types of
preparation procedure. Part 2 of the Standard gives guidance

on the construction and installation of clean rooms and
workstations, and Part 3 the operational procedures in these
environments.

Table 1. Specifications for controlled environment clean
rooms, work stations and clean air devices. BS.5295, 1976.

Controlled environment	Maximum permitted number of particles/m^3 (equal to or greater than stated size)					Final filter efficiency %
	0.5µm	1µm	5µm	10µm	25µm	
Class 1	3000*	N/A	Nil	Nil	Nil	99.995
Class 2	300,000	N/A	2000	30	Nil	99.95
Class 3		1,000,000	20,000	4000	300	95.00
Class 4			200,000	40,000	4,000	70.00
Controlled Area	-	-	-	-	-	-

N/A Not applicable
*   Subject to a maximum particle size of 5µm

2.1.2. <u>Microbiological Safety Cabinets</u>. British Standard,
BS5726, 1979 (4) describes three Classes of Microbiological
Safety Cabinet. A Class I cabinet has a front opening for
operator manipulations, and air is continuously exhausted from
the cabinet at such a rate that escape of airborne
contamination from within the cabinet is prevented. A Class II
cabinet is a partially enclosed cabinet with a unidirectional
(laminar) downward airflow, and designed such that particles
generated within the cabinet are prevented from escaping by an
inward airflow through the working aperture. A Class III
cabinet separates the operator from the work by a barrier,
such as gloves, and from which the escape of airborne
particles is prevented by an exhaust system. These three types
of cabinet are recommended for the handling of different
Categories of organisms, but Classes II and III are also
recommended for some types of radiopharmaceutical preparation
procedures. Guidance on the siting, installation, maintenance,

testing and use of these cabinets is also given in this Standard.

2.2. Guide to Good Pharmaceutical Manufacturing Practice (GMP)

These guidelines, which are produced by many countries, outline steps which should be taken by manufacturers of medicinal products to ensure their products are of the nature and quality intended. The current GMP, 1977 (5) as used in the U.K., has no statutory force and should not be regarded as an interpretation of the requirements of any Act, Regulation or Directive. The Guide was compiled by the Department of Health and Social Security (D.H.S.S.) in the U.K. and reference is made by the Medicines Inspectors to the guidelines given during their official visits to premises manufacturing radiopharmaceuticals. The latest GMP, 1983 (25), published by the D.H.S.S. has an appendix specifically referring to the manufacturing of radiopharmaceuticals, and environmental conditions considered necessary.

2.3. Codes of Practice

The design of laboratories and necessary requirements for the safe handling of radioactive materials are given in these Codes. In the U.K. the current Code of Practice for the Protection of Persons against Ionising Radiations arising from Medical and Dental Use, 1972 (6), was prepared under the Radioactive Substances Act 1948 (7), and is the third edition. The Code itself has no statutory force, but sets out the basic principles of radiation control and gives general guidance on good practice, and puts into practical terms the regulations imposed by the Act. Many of the recommmendations are based upon the requirements given in international publications such as the International Atomic Energy Agency (I.A.E.A.) and the International Commission on Radiological Protection (I.C.R.P.).

Standards of laboratory facility and equipment can be classified into three grades, A, B and C (or types, 1, 2 and 3, in some publications), each grade being appropriate for

particular ranges of activity for different toxicities of
radionuclides. These grades are defined by the I.A.E.A. in
Safety Series No. 1., 1962 (8) and the types of laboratory in
the I.A.E.A. report on Radiation Protection Procedures, 1973
(9) and can be summarised in Table 2. The levels of activity
may have to be modified with appropriate factors depending on
the type of procedure to be carried out in the laboratory.

The four classes of radionuclide are based on their
radio-toxicity per unit of activity according to the
recommendations of the I.C.R.P., 1964 (10) and I.C.R.P., 1977
(11). Some examples of the radionuclides commonly used in
nuclear medicine and their toxicity classification are shown
in Table 3.

Table 2. Grade of laboratory required for various activities
of radionuclides of various toxicities

Classification of Radionuclide (Toxicity)	Grade of laboratory required for unsealed radionuclides at levels of activity specified		
	C (Type 1)	B (Type 2)	A (Type 3)
Class 1 (High)	<10 µCi	10 µCi – 1 mCi	>1 mCi
Class 2 (Medium)	< 1 mCi	1 mCi – 100 mCi	>100 mCi
Class 3 (Medium)	<100 mCi	100 mCi – 10 Ci	>10 Ci
Class 4 (Low)	<10 Ci	10 Ci – 1000 Ci	>1000 Ci

Table 3. Classification of some radionuclides commonly used in
nuclear medicine.

Toxicity	Class	Examples
High	1	None
Medium	2	Na-22, Ca-45, I-125, I-131, Cs-137
Medium	3	C-14, F-18, P-32, Cr-51, Fe-59, Ga-67, Se-75, I-123
Low	4	H-3, Tc-99m, In-113m, Xe-133

2.4. Design of Laboratory Facilities

One of the earliest guides to the design of a radiopharmacy was described by Kawada et al., 1974 (12), where the
design was based on a planning guide which consisted of
operational planning and architectural planning. Architectural

planning was influenced by operational planning which in turn depended on the type of radiopharmaceutical to be provided and the level of service offered. Although descriptions of radiopharmacy layout and equipment, including sterile air laminar flow hoods, were described, air filtration into the rooms themselves was not proposed. These recommendations did not carry official status. A paper by Hill and Smith 1977 (13) described the structure and operation of the radiopharmacy at Bristol General Hospital, which included a full aseptic suite but again with no official status.

2.4.1. <u>British Institute of Radiology Report</u>. A report published by the British Institute of Radiology, 1975, and revised in 1979 (14), defined basic facilities required for the preparation of various types of radiopharmaceuticals under conditions which comply with the obligations imposed by the Medicines Act, 1968(15), and the Radioactive Substances Act, 1960 (16). The guidelines were produced by a multidisciplinary working party, and the recommendations express the views of the authors and not of the British Institute of Radiology. The facilities described in the B.I.R. report fall into two main categories of laboratory; a high grade (Class HG) and a minimum grade (Class MG), with the addition of an Aseptic Area for some operations. The High grade laboratory conditions are those described as clean conditions in Appendix 1 to GMP, 1977 (5) and are suitable for those products which can be terminally sterilised after processing under clean, but not necessarily aseptic conditions. Such products include those sterilised in their final containers by autoclaving or assembled from sterile ingredients and used within 8 hours of preparation and stored at 4°C. Other products should be manufactured under clean conditions up to the sterilisation stage and then processed and filled into their final containers under aseptic conditions. Preparations which cannot be sterilised at all must be handled under aseptic conditions throughout their preparation. The clean conditions are those described in the GMP, 1977 (5). The Minimum grade facility are those found in a radionuclide Class C laboratory described in the Code of Practice, 1972 (6), with modifications to make them pharmaceutically acceptable for the storage and elution of radionuclide generators and preparation of radiopharmaceuticals from kits. This facility does not provide any filtered air, but if the modifications are not available then a unidirectional airflow station must be used. An additional requirement for this facility to be suitable for kit radiopharmaceuticals is that the product be used within 8 hours and stored at 4°C. Oral preparations can also be prepared in Minimum grade laboratories but may require a fume cupboard to protect the operator from radioactive contamination. The report also describes the achievement of aseptic conditions but using a unidirectional airflow cabinet situated in a clean room, or if placed in a Class MG laboratory, its use must be restricted to certain agreed procedures.

2.4.2. The Hospital Physicists Association Report. This report, published by the Hospital Physicists Association in 1976 (17), recommends laboratory facilities of a high pharmaceutical standard. These high standards are recommended in order that the higher risks associated with increasing production of radiopharmaceuticals can be coped with. In order to comply with GMP statement that "products which are terminally sterilised should be processed under clean, but not necessarily aseptic, conditions", the report suggests a clean grade B radionuclide laboratory. All other preparations, long-lived, short-lived, closed kit and open procedures should be prepared aseptically in a down-draught workstation after the sterilisation stage of preparation. An aseptic area for kits is recommended because the act of adding a reagent to a closed container puts the sterility of the product at risk, and data on the evaluation of the risk was not available. The HPA report described the necessity to maintain laboratories at an air pressure slightly in excess of surroundings in order to maintain clean conditions. This is contrary to the practice in high activity radionuclide laboratories where a negative pressure is maintained in order to confine airborne radioactivity. However, it was considered that with short-lived radiopharmaceuticals, the protection of the product against airborne microbial contamination is more difficult than protection of the operator against airborne radioactive contamination, and the pharmaceutical requirement of positive pressure should be followed. The report also recommends that the clean rooms should be ventilated and the air filtered through high-efficiency sub-micron particulate air (HESPA) filters into the room such that the particle count in the room is within the limit for Class 2 (BS 5295). The room should also be entered through a double-door changing room to avoid drops in overpressure due to the passage of personnel entering and leaving. Other recommendations as to surfaces, use of sinks, storage areas are also made. A balanced-air down-draught workstation sited in a clean laboratory provides an aseptic area of Class 1 (BS 5295) standard suitable for certain radiopharmaceuticals. The report, prepared by authors of different specialities, has no official status, but represents their interpretation of the regulations and official guidelines current at the time of preparation.

2.4.3. The International Atomic Energy Agency Technical Report. The general principles for the design of premises are described in this I.A.E.A. report, 1979 (18). The influence of the similarities and differences between the pharmaceutical and radiological requirements on design are explained. In general the room design should be based on radiation protection requirements and levels of radioactivity, and then pharmaceutically modified. Using I.A.E.A., 1973 (9), definitions a type 1 or type 2 radioactive laboratory is required, and the type of radiopharmaceutical to be prepared will further determine the design of the facility. The report defines three types of hygienic zone or class of room necessary to manufacture radiopharmaceuticals. These zones are colour coded according to the form of the radiopharmaceutical. Particle control of the environments are those specifications laid down in BS 5295, 1976. Aseptic rooms, where required, may be Class 1 (BS 5295, 1976) with changing rooms, and transfer hatches, with a high standard of finish. The individual requirements of premises, facilities and equipment for the

preparation of different types of radiopharmaceutical are
described in detail.

2.4.4. Radiopharmacists Sub-Committee Report. A group of
practising radiopharmacists forming a sub-committee of the
U.K. Regional Pharmaceutical Officers Committee produced a
report in 1980 (19), basing their recommendations for design
on the GMP, 1977 (5), modifying the requirements for the
handling of radioactive materials. The recommendations carry
no official status, but represent the views of the authors
based on their collective experience in radiopharmacy. The
standards of facility recommended should depend on the type of
product prepared, and not on the scale of production or status
of the nuclear medicine department. Further, where a range of
products is to be prepared, the facilities must be designed
to suit the products most at risk from contamination. The
report then describes specific recommendations for the various
types of radiopharmaceuticals to be prepared. Radiopharmaceuticals for oral use should be prepared under conditions
similar to those required for non-sterile pharmaceuticals
(GMP, 1977, section 6 (5)), and modified in accordance with
the Code of Practice, 1972 (6). For Radioactive gases and
volatile products, the radiation protection requirements
should be observed. Radiopharmaceuticals prepared using
non-sterile ingredients or containers which are terminally
heat sterilised, and intended for parenteral administration,
should be prepared in a room supplied with air filtered to BS
5295 Class 2 with conventional airflow. Those parenteral
products prepared by an open procedure, that is where the
contents are exposed to the atmosphere, and are not terminally
heat sterilised must be handled and filtered whenever possible
into their final containers in a unidirectional downdraught
workstation. This workstation must be in a room supplied with
air filtered to BS 5295 Class 1 with conventional airflow. The
requirements of grade B radionuclide laboratory must also be
met. Those injections prepared by closed procedures, such as
from kits, and involving the addition of sterile ingredients
to presterilised closed containers may be prepared in a
unidirectional downdraught workstation within a Controlled

Area (BS 5295). A BS 5295 Class 1 environment in the workstation is necessary, and the Controlled Area must be finished to grade B radionuclide laboratory standards. The use of BS 5295 Controlled Area allows for flexibility at a local level, and as the majority of radiopharmaceuticals prepared in hospitals fall into this group, the recommended standard should not be too onerous or expensive to achieve. Radionuclide generators are recommended to be stored and eluted in a BS 5295 Class 1 environment. This can be achieved by a unidirectional workstation of appropriate design in a Controlled Area, or on an open bench in a room ventilated with air filtered to BS 5295 Class 1 standards.

2.4.5. The Department of Health and Social Security Guidelines. These guidance notes, in the form of a letter from the Chief Pharmacist at the DHSS to the Regional Pharmaceutical Officers, October 1982 (20), make a clear distinction between `open` and `closed` procedures. The guidelines are mainly concerned with premises for preparation of radiopharmaceuticals by `open` procedures. Advice on short-lived preparations produced by `closed` procedures, including kits, and on blood component labelling is given in appendices for those seeking guidance. The hope expressed in these guidelines is that only a few hospital will use `open` procedures, and that all `open` procedures will be confined to these premises. The Medicines Inspectorate will refer to the Notes when inspecting premises and making their recommendations to the Licensing Authority. Initially their inspectors will concentrate on premises using open procedures. These guidelines are the official guidelines which hospitals in the U.K. will now have to work to when designing premises. The recommendations in these guidelines are similar to those recommended in the radiopharmacists report (see 2.4.4.). Radiopharmaceuticals for parenteral use, which are prepared aseptically by `open` procedures, and are not terminally sterilised, should be handled in an aseptic room with air filtered to BS 5295 Class 1 in a contained workstation. Preparatory work prior to the aseptic procedure should be performed in an adjacent clean room with air filtered to BS

5295 Class 2, with connection to the aseptic room via an airlocked hatchway. Similar conditions should also be used for those parenteral radiopharmaceuticals, prepared by `closed` procedure, but not intended for use on the same day of preparation. The handling of blood and blood components involves an additional risk to the operator and other products of viral contamination. A suitable separate area is advisable, but where this is not available, a `closed` procedure should be used in a workstation providing air filtered to BS 5295 Class 1, and also complying with the requirements of a Class II or Class III microbiological safety cabinet, BS 5726, 1979 (4).

3. RADIOLOGICAL PROTECTION

The implementation of Article 5 (a) of the European Communities Directive (Euratom, 1976) (21) on basic safety standards for health protection against the dangers of ionising radiation,has necessitated countries in the European Community introducing new legislation. Countries are at different stages in the process,and the U.K. Health and Safety Commission has recently produced a consultative document entitled The Ionising Radiations Regulations 198-(22), in compliance with its duty under the Health and Safety at Work Act, 1974 (23). A draft Approved Code of Practice has been produced in the same document. The National Radiological Protection Board has produced draft guidance notes (24) which are intended to replace the Code of Practice (6), and to supplement the forthcoming Ionising Radiations Regulations, 198-, and associated approved code of practice. Certain sections of these regulations are particularly relevant to work with unsealed sources, viz. Regulation 21 on requirements for premises, equipment and fittings. The guidance notes make recommendations on the design of laboratories which, unlike the present Code of Practice, include aseptic facilities, clean areas, changing rooms, vertical laminar flow cabinets, and an over-pressure in the radiopharmacy. These recommendations will add weight to the recently produced Guidance Notes from the DHSS, and should lead to an increased standard in premises in the U.K.

4. STATUS AND ACCEPTANCE OF THE RECOMMENDATIONS

Most national and international organisations publish guidelines for good pharmaceutical manufacturing practice (GMP). These guidelines are similar and form the basis for good radiopharmacy practice. In most countries including the U.K., the GMP has no statutory force and should not be regarded as a interpretation of the requirements of any Act, Regulation or Directive. The purpose of the Guides is to outline steps which should be taken to ensure the products are of the nature and quality intended. Methods other than those described in the Guides may be equally acceptable if they achieve the same ends. The 3rd edition of the GMP, 1983 (25), to be published in the U.K. will contain a section on the Manufacture of Radiopharmaceuticals. The guidance given is a summary of those Guidance Notes for Hospitals on the Premises and Environment for the Preparation of Radiopharmaceuticals, produced by the DHSS, 1982 (20).

In the U.K. the National Health Hospitals enjoy Crown exemption whereas privately owned institutions do not, and this exemption is safeguarded in Section 133 (3) of the Medicines Act (1968) (15). This means that bodies and persons acting for the Crown are not bound by statute, but these legal constraints are replaced by recommendations given in official reports and advice in Notes and Circulars issued by the DHSS or Scottish Home and Health Department (SHHD). Compliance is a matter of employee discipline and not law enforcement. In these circumstances it is the responsibility of local Health Authorities to interpret the requirements of the Medicines Act and to ensure that suitable standards are introduced. A circular, HSC (1S) 128, 1975 (26) (Application of the Medicines Act to Health Authorities and Administration of Radioactive Substances to Persons) recommended that Health Authorities introduce arrangements in hospitals corresponding to the Act, and that Medicines Inspectors visit hospitals with a view to ensuring that standards in hospitals are maintained.

In Denmark specific guidelines are issued by the Isotope

Pharmacy (Copenhagen) which is the official body dealing with pharmaceutical aspects of radiopharmaceuticals (Guidelines for the Preparation of Radiopharmaceuticals in Hospitals 1975) which now appear in the IAEA's Technical Report Series No. 194 (18), on behalf of the Danish Health Service. Again the GMP forms the basis of the recommendations and the conditions described are those which are considered to be desirable and therefore strongly recommended, or requirements that are considered indispensable. As with the U.K. the premises must be approved and regular inspections for pharmacy and radiation hygiene are undertaken by the Isotope Pharmacy, National Board of Health.

The recommendations for premises in Holland are again based on the GMP and modified to cope with the requirements for handling radioactive materials. The hospital premises require prior approval by an Inspectorate for Health and Environmental Protection, a requirement under the Nuclear Energy Law. Regular inspection under the same Law is also required.

Switzerland does not have a GMP, but again hospital premises must be approved by the radioprotection unit of the Federal Bureau of Public Health, and regular inspections by the bureau are undertaken.

In the U.S.A. there are no official guidelines dealing specifically with radiopharmacies, although guidelines for the handling of radioactive materials are in existence. The relevant sections of Good Manufacturing Practices are used as Guidelines.

In Canada the regulation of hospital radiopharmacies is dependent on the hospital administrative organisation and provincial college of Pharmacy requirements. If a radiopharmaceutical is prepared with no intention of distribution, then the requirements of the Food and Drugs Act are not relevant. Radiopharmacies which compound and distribute radiopharmaceuticals to non-affilicated institutions are considered to be manufacturing for the purpose of distribution, and must comply with all of the regulatory requirements. Manufacturing includes aliquoting from one container to another, preparation of radiopharmaceuticals using commercial kits and synthesis of radiopharmaceuticals from basic raw materials. Thus a hospital radiopharmacy must be in possession of a Canadian Food and Drug licence, and a pre-licencing inspection is undertaken to verify claims made in the licence application. One of these claims is a description of the facility including the area for the protection of sterile, pyrogen free products.

Prior to 1978 radiopharmaceutical products in Australia were supplied by the Australian Atomic Energy Commission direct to Nuclear Medicine department, and sterile dispensing and pharmacy involvement was not required. Radiopharmacy departments are now being established on a regional basis, and must satisfy the requirements of radiation protection and sterility. The control of the dispensing of radiopharmaceuticals is by the Director of Pharmacy Services, and adherence to policies set out for sterile manufacturing and quality control of pharmaceuticals is required. Advice is given by the Australian Atomic Energy Commission, the Division of Occupational Health and Radiation Control, and Hospitals with radiopharmacies. It is considered that most nuclear medicine departments would seek guidance from the IAEA Technical Report No. 194, and HPA and BIR reports, as well as the Code of Good Manufacturing Practice for Therapeutic Goods, Appendix B, Supplementary Notes for Hospital Pharmacists.

ACKNOWLEDGEMENTS

I should like to acknowledge the invaluable discussions with John Turner, Principal Medicine Inspector, Department of Health and Social Security, and the many pharmacists in different countries who provided information.

REFERENCES
1.   British Standards Institution, Environmental Cleanlines in Enclosed Spaces, 1976, Part 1. Specification for controlled environment clean rooms, work stations and clean air devices. BS 5295, Part 1.
2.   British Standards Institution, Environmental Cleanlines in Enclosed Spaces, 1976, Part 2. Guide to the construction and installation of clean rooms, work stations, and clean air devices. BS 5295 Part 2.
3.   British Standards Institution, Environmental Cleanlines in

Enclosed Spaces, 1976, Part 3. Guide to operational procedures and disciplines applicable to clean rooms, work stations and clean air devices. BS 5295, Part 3.

4. British Standards Institution, 1979. Specifications for Microbiological safety Cabinets. BS 5726.

5. Guide to Good Pharmaceutical Manufacturing Practice. Department of Health and Social Security, HMSO, London. 1977.

6. Code of Practice for the Protection of Persons against Ionising Radiations arising from Medical and Dental Use, HMSO, London. 1972.

7. Radioactive Substances Act, 1948, HMSO, London.

8. International Atomic Energy Agency Publications Safety Series No. 1. Safe Handling of Radioisotopes, First Edition. IAEA, Vienna. 1962.

9. International Atomic Energy Agency, Radiation Protection Procedures, Safety Series No. 38, IAEA, Vienna. 1973.

10. International Commission on Radiological Protection. Report of Committee 5 on the Handling and Disposal of Radioactive Materials in Hospitals and Medical Research Establishments, ICRP Publication 5, Pergamon Press, London. 1964.

11. International Commission on Radiological Protection. The Handling, Storage, Use and Disposal of Unsealed Radionuclides in Hospitals and Medical Research Establishments, ICRP Publication 25, Ann ICRP 1977;1:(2).

12. Kawada T, Wolf W and Seibert S. Planning a Radiopharmacy. Amer J Hosp Pharm 1974;13:153-157.

13. Hill PMM, Smith RNB. Establishing a Radiopharmacy, Report, Bristol General Hospital. 1977.

14. British Institute of Radiology. Guidelines for the Preparation of Radiopharmaceuticals in Hospitals, 1975 (Revised 1979), Special Report No. 11, B.I.R., London.

15. Medicines Act, 1968, HMSO, London.

16. Radioactive Substances Act, 1960, HMSO, London.

17. Hospital Physicists Association. The Hospital Preparation of Radiopharmaceuticals, 1976, Scientific Report Series -16.

18. International Atomic Energy Agency. Technical Report Series No. 194. Preparation and Control of Radiopharmaceuticals in Hospitals. IAEA, Vienna. 1979.

19. Facilities for the Hospital Preparation of Radiopharmaceuticals, Nucl Med Commun 1980;1:54-57.

20. Guidance Notes for Hospitals. Premises and Environment for the Preparation of Radiopharmaceuticals. Department of Health and Social Security, London. 1982.

21. Council Directive 76/579/Euratom Off J Eur Communities 1976;19:No.L187.

22. The Ionising Radiations Regulations, 198-. Consultative Document, 1982, Health and Safety Commission, HMSO, London.

23. Health and Safety at Work etc., Act, 1974, HMSO, London.

24. Draft Guidance Notes for the Protection of Persons against Ionising Radiations arising from Medical and Dental Use. Consultative Document, National Radiological Protection Board, HMSO, London. 1983.

348

25. Guide to Good Pharmaceutical Manufacturing Practice, 1983. Department of Health and Social Security, HMSO, London (in preparation).
26. Application of Medicines Act to Health Authorities. Health Service Circular (Interim Series) 1975, HSC (IS) 128, HMSO, London.

Part 3

QUALITY CONTROL OF RADIOPHARMACEUTICALS PREPARED FROM
GENERATORS AND KITS

INTRODUCTION

A very large part of nuclear medicine procedures to-day is based on radiopharmaceuticals prepared from Tc-99m generators and preparation kits. Modern generators and kits are in general considered to be effective and simple to operate. They are supposed to give products of adequate quality. Generators and kits may come from different origins and thereby we are faced with the problem of compatibility. The final radio-pharmaceutical may involve two different manufacturers and further the radiopharmacist or technician at the hospital doing the necessary steps of preparation. From this follows the problem of divided responsibility and the question: to what extent must quality control programmes be part of good radiopharmacy practice at the hospital. In view of the increasing awareness of quality requirements and of responsibilities for quality assurance it is certain that more resources will be used both by manufacturers and by hospitals in the future. It is therefore relevant to discuss where in the system this will be most cost-effective. These questions are reviewed in the following 5 chapters (23-27) by experts from manufacturers, hospitals and regulatory authorities.

These papers were discussed at the symposium. No consensus were obtained or aimed at. It was however obvious as can be seen from the following chapters, that there were much general agreement about principles among the participants irrespectively of their professional working place.It was stressed that there are very important methodological problems regarding methods for determination of radiochemical purity. Fast and simple in-vitro methods may not correlate very well with biological distribution in humans. At present animal distribution studies may be necessary for the manufacturer as a batch release method. More proper chromatographic methods may also be relevant. In-vivo stability should be established by the manufacturer and here are relevant animal models indispensable. It is a wish from hospital users that manufacturers along with their specifications give relevant quality control methods. Some manufacturers found it difficult to give limits for radiochemical purity as the analytical results will depend on the operators skill and equipment. Reference was made to monographs in the European Pharmacopoea where minimum specifications and analytical quality control methods are given for some few Tc-99m radiopharmaceuticals.

Compatibility problems between generators and kits are not often found. Changes in the production of a generator must be accepted by the licensing authorities but is not always made known to kit-manufacturers or to the users. This problem may have to be dealt with, for each individual country, by the relevant national authority. Quality control at the hospital should primarily take care of problems that may occur due to transport, storage and the final preparation. It was generally accepted that parameters that could not be influenced, could be left out. It was also generally accepted that some (simple) quality control methods should be available at the hospitals. To be able to use these methods it is necessary to practice them now and then. Some felt that the main use of these methods was in trouble-shooting when unexpected biological distribution were seen in patients. They felt that daily use would not be cost-effective. These methods should also be used when first introducing the product in the department. Safety and efficacy should be built into the products during manufacture and during the hospital preparation whereby daily analytical quality control could be limited to a minimum. Others felt that daily quality control should be performed. Either as a release criteria or as a basis for answering possible questions about unexpected biological distribution in the patient. Methods and technique used should give correct results. A comparative evaluation of methods used at different hospitals might therefore be relevant.

26. GENERATOR QUALITY - INDUSTRY POINT OF VIEW

YVES JEAN-BAPTISTE

1. INTRODUCTION

The generator of radionuclide or milking system allows the obtention at the hospital of a solution of radionuclide for medical use.This system has greatly participated to the development of Nuclear Medicine over the past fifteen years. Although many couple of radioisotopes can be used, the most widespread generator of radioisotope is the 99Mo/99mTc generator system

2. QUALITY OF A GENERATOR - DEFINITION

The quality can be defined as the fitness for use. In the special case of a generator which deliver a pharmaceutical product the quality concerns the physician who will eluate the generator and the patient who will receive the eluate direct as an injection or after labelling as a labelled compound.The common concept of quality covers in the physician´s point of view:the delivery in time, the accuracy of the elution yield, the chemical strenght and biological potency of the eluate. The patient is only waiting for an effective and safe drug.

3. THE PARAMETERS OF THE QUALITY

The parameters defining the quality of a generator can be attained by the manufacturer in two steps :

      The Research and Development step (R+D)

      The production step

The quality is reached in the R and D stage through an important analysis to define the parameters of the generator;

by this one must understand the definition of the intended
usage. From this study the following parameters can be fixed :

        Nominal activities available

        Day of calibration

        Minimal elution volume

        Mode of elution

        Protection against radiation

        Security of the generator

        Convenience of handling

    Some parameters are imposed by the pharmacopoeia :

        Radionuclidic purity

        Radiochemical purity

        Content in alumina

        pH

        Sterility

    Some parameters such as pyrogenicity and toxicity which are
not included in the pharmacopoeia can be taken into account by
the manufacturer.An issued document will describe all these
parameters and it will be considered as a reference quality
standard document.

    4. QUALITY ALONG THE MANUFACTURING PROCESS

    From this document the manufacturing process and quality
control analysis will be elaborated including the purchase,
receipt and control of all the raw materials.To keep the
quality of the product during its life cycle the manufacturer
has to establish a Quality Assurance program to prevent any
deviation from the quality standard. Furthermore the analysis
of customer's complaint - if so -will greatly help in taking
the necessary actions to correct or improve the failing
points.The implementation in the manufacturer's facilities of
good manufacturing practices and quality control will be the
most effective and less expensive ways to secure the quality
of the produced generators.Among the quality controls which
are performed during the manufacturing processes one must
emphasize the importance of the control of the manufacturing
environment as regard to the cleanliness and the control of
the sterilization cycle to be sure to provide the users with a

sterile generator.Furthermore the elution of each generator before shipment allows the producer to check for generator integrity, eluted volume, clarity, elution yield and breakthrough of Aluminium ions.

5. LEGAL RESPONSIBILITIES AND HOSPITAL POINT OF VIEW

The legal responsibilities of the manufacturer seems to lie in the respect of the good manufacturing processes and the quality standard.At least the generators have to deliver eluates which respect the required parameters of the pharmacopoeia.This statement should not make a control at the hospital unnessessary.Hospitals have to check the received product -generators, kits and radiopharmaceuticals- and for the generator to measure the eluted activities, to check the volume and clarity of the eluates, to search for breakthrough of Aluminium ions.

What about the particular problem of labelling kit? Two questions lies here.
The compatibility of the generator's eluate and kit composition.
The responsibility of the hospital which labels the kit.

It seems that there is no universal answer to the question of compatibility. However we can notice that there's no publication relating incompatibility between kit and generator eluate.Furthermore most of the labelled molecules used at the hospital are now described in the pharmacopoeia. This provide the manufacturer and the user with a reference quality standard and analytical methods to check up this question.Furthermore the generator and kit manufacturer will generally test their generator's eluate or kit formulation with products coming from other companies.
From this statements the legal responsibility of the hospital is to have a good record keeping, to respect the prescribed instruction for the utilisation of both the generator and the kit and to prepare injection following the good hospital practices.

27. GENERATOR-HOSPITAL POINTS OF VIEW

STEN-OVE NILSSON

My comments on generators from hospital points of view are restricted to the most widely used generator model being based on the column chromatographic process, having in mind that there also are other so-called generator systems. Most generators used in nuclear medicine today are available as licensed radiopharmaceuticals, delivered ready for use by a commercial manufacturer. The national authorities should see to, that the producer set up a proper quality program to ensure that only safe and efficient generators are delivered thus reducing the extent of further testing at the hospital or by the radiopharmacy to a relevant level.

The Tc-99m generator is the most widely used generator in nuclear medicine and its predominant role will probably not be significantly changed in the immediate future. The problems with the Tc-99m generator are nowadays wellknown for the manufacturers, users and I hope the authorities. The last few years have brought some new technical and quality aspects which are important for the hospital in the choice of the right, i.e. safe and efficient generator. Many other useful generator systems for different clinical applications have been and will be developed in the future. A most interesting area is the development of generators for production of ultra-short-lived radionuclides for many dynamic studies. The ultra-short-lived radionuclide generator complies with the desirability of obtaining the highest photon yield with a minimum of radiation exposure. Such radionuclides can and must by directly injected intravenously as a bolus for kinetic studies which can be repeated numerous times on a patient or may be given direct as a continuous infusion or inhaled.

Special problems concerning sterility and apyrogenicity arise in the case of direct injection and infusion.

The quality control program at the hospitals is focused on the resulting eluate and may include tests for radionuclidic purity and identity, radiochemical purity, chemical purity, breakthrough, sterility, apyrogenicity, toxicity and of course assessment of radioactive concentration. The extent of the quality control program is dependent on several factors, often combined:

The half life of the daughternuclide.

The way the eluate is used (for labelling of kits or other compounds, for injection without labelling, direct infusion or injection, inhalation, intrathecal injection etc.).

Sterile or non-sterile generators (Radiopharmaceuticals or radiochemicals).

Commercially manufactured or in-house produced generators.

National laws and directions.

Cost-benefit.

Quality control of the resulting eluate including all relevant parameters are time consuming and often not cost-effective. The time constraint aspect is stressed when the eluate is used for kit labelling and in the field of ultra-short-lived radionuclides. Another reason for not performing all tests is the radiation protection aspect.

When a generator is commercially produced many of the tests can be left to the manufacturers. Generator safety must be based on the research work done during development of the product as well as on the complete production scheme. The generators should have been correctly controlled before shipment and tested on a random basis for some of the parameters e.g. radionuclide and radiochemical purity, pH etc. I could stop at this point with the comment that in-hospitals, quality control can be limited to assuring that the correct radiopharmaceutical in the required amount is administered to the patient and that additional tests at the hospital are not necessary and not cost-effective unless they are pointed out by the package insert. In my opinion the extent of such a quality control in the hospital, as can be seen in some literature, is not satisfactory. The quality control for the Tc-99m generator should consider following parameters:

Inspection of the package/generator on arrival

Clarity, which can reveal Al-breakthrough and subsequent Mo-99 breakthrough

Mo-99 breakthrough (maximum 1 µCi per 1 mCi Tc-99m according to the European pharmacopoiea)

Elution volume

Activity/Elution yield (a low elution yield can indicate defects of the generator)

Sterility (random samples)

Apyrogenicity (e.g. intrathecal route of administration)

Record keeping for all data concerning the generator including results of different tests

Documentation including written instructions and the records

Some of these statements can be applied to other generator systems after some modification. However, when a new generator is introduced or when staff changes, additional quality control tests may be necessary to assure that unforseen problems have not been introduced due to changes. It must be pointed out that the ultimate responsibility for the quality of the eluate is in charge of the hospital or the radiopharmacy because of the possible risk of jeopardizing the safety of the eluting system, for example with respect to the possibility of external contamination if the instructions for use is not complied with(Use of incorrect aseptic technique.) Furthermore, compatibility between generators and kits cannot allways be assumed. The radiopharmacist should be aware of radiopharmaceutical defects and where they can arise, as all troubleshooting begins with this knowledge.

Some generators used as radiopharmaceuticals are not proved for sterility and apyrogenicity, e.g. the Ga-68 generator. The resulting eluate has to be sterilized by autoclaving or membrane filtered and then tested for sterility and sometimes

Table 1. Characteristics of some commercially available
generators

System	Halflife Daughter	Sterile	Pyrogen free	Eluant	Route of administration
Mo–99/Tc–99m	6 h	Yes	No	0,9% NaCl	i.v. injection intrathecal inj. labelling
HG–195m/Au–195m	30,5 s	Yes	Yes	$Na_2S_2O_3$ $NaNO_3$	Direct injection
Rb–81/Kr–81m	13 s	Yes	Yes	5% Dextrose	Direct injection Inhalation
Ge–68/Ga–68	68 min	No	No	0,005 M EDTA	Intrathecal injection i.v. injection labelling

for apyrogenicity. All testing for sterility and apyrogenicity
of the resulting eluate must of necessity be determined before
the product come into use or for the individual preparation
after use. If however, the procedure of establishing a sterile
and pyrogenfree system for producing short lived radionuclides
is employed such prospective or retrospective testing is
adequate and serves merely to verify the performance of the
system. In some cases, the eluate or the final product
prepared from generators and kits are administered as an
intrathecal injection as for example Tc-99m DTPA (using single
photon thomography) and Ga-68 EDTA (using positroncamera) for
cisternographic procedures used at the Karolinska Hospital in
Stockholm. These radiopharmaceuticals requires the highest
possible purity as for example apyrogenicity. A delicate
problem is the direct injection or infusion of the eluate into
the patient, as for example the Au-195m and the Kr-81m
generator. Special care has to be taken in the production and
use of such generators as usual testing methods cannot be
applied. Whatever different tests that are carried out it must
be emphasized that the outmost goal is safe and effective
radiopharmaceuticals to the patient (and the nuclear
physician).

28. KIT - INDUSTRY POINTS OF VIEW

DEREK E. LOVETT

The symposium secretariat guidelines for this Panel Discussion emphasise two factors having a significant bearing on batch quality control of kits:

Increasing resources needed for quality control and its cost effectiveness.

Division of responsibility between manufacturer and hospital user.

I would like to add a third factor to these:

Variations in the make and size of generator used by the hospital.

To tackle the second, and in my view, more important factor first, my opinion is that the manufacturer must simulate what the hospital will do in reconstituting his kit and control the finished active injection as part of final batch release. This obligation applies irrespective of whether hospitals have a quality control programme or not. At the same time the manufacturer should encourage hospitals to do independant quality control on the principle of "belt and braces" and should assist the hospitals with information on suitable testing methods. In a Panel Discussion such as this we can easily have too much quality control philosophy and not enough practical detail, so my next comments relate to the actual testing needed. Animal biodistribution has emerged as the main safeguard of product efficacy and the right attitude in 1983 should be that there has to be animal dissection and counting of organs and tissues of interest, using the 2 out of 3 animals specification, unless it can be clearly demonstrated that there is no suitable animal model or that results are misleading. In other words a manufacturer needs a flawless excuse for NOT doing physiological distribution testing.

Rosemary Smith has the last paper in this Panel Discussion (Chapter 30), giving the regulatory point of view. She is likely to advise that in law these kits are not medicines but they are controlled as ingredients of medicine. This has to be so since the most important ingredient is not in the bottle supplied by the kit manufacturer. It doesn't alter the reality of the fact that what _is_ in the bottle vitally affects the efficacy of the radioactive ingredient added by the hospital. This is particularly true in relation to radiochemical purity which is the next important test parameter after animal biodistribution. It is a test that hospitals can and often will recheck but the manufacturer cannot anticipate this and must make radiochemical purity determination part of his batch release.

The third type of testing that we have to discuss is tin -in some cases just stannous tin, in others total tin, or both. I view the tin measurement as an efficacy parameter rather than safety and the manufacturer's batch specification requires a limit of both maximum and minimum for efficacy of the kit. The tin and the technetium are common to bone, lung, liver and other kits, but what might be called the "specific-organ-seeking" ingredient is specific to a particular kit. It does not follow that this ingredient must be quantitatively determined for each batch of kits in all instances. It may be practical and relevant to have a maximum and minimum vial content of this specific ingredient but organ uptake may be influenced far more by the stannous content, the pH, the rubber of the bottle cap or various other things rather than the content of the "Identifying" ingredient. We therefore return to the suggestion that animal biodistribution is the No. 1 test. I must admit to having made provocative comment about the need to assay ingredients such as MDP and HIDA in order to stimulate questions in the discussion session. Another testing procedure that is applicable only to 2 kits, lung and liver kits, is physical methods of sizing. Microscope measurements of particles in lung kit testing is well established and quite straight forward. It is far from established or straightforward in colloid measurements and staff at the Isotope-Pharmacy and at Amersham have laboured for years trying to "get a handle" on this. If I may add a few more provocative comments for our discussion session, I would add that these physical measurements are only "belt and braces" with the animal test anyway, they can be very misleading, and they are much more valuable when a kit is some months old and approaching expiry rather than at the time the manufacturer surveys his test results in order to release a batch. The remaining test parameters are pH, sterility, pyrogens and clarity of reconstituted injections. These are common to other parenterals, i.e. are not peculiar to radiopharmaceutical kits and not particularly exciting. Manufacturers are well aware however that the normal expectations of batch testing criteria must apply.

At the outset of this talk I added variations in make and size of generator to the quality control guidelines. We come now to the distinction between testing that is necessary to prove satisfactory development of a kit and testing that is necessary for each batch of kits. Since competitor manufacturers of generators may modify their generator slightly without publicity, it is clearly impractical to do compatibility testing with all generators continously with each batch of kits. Some checking of variations is required at intervals and the general philosophy is to look for the worst possible case in testing.

Last year Amersham had to produce a large amount of supporting data in order to obtain registration of a new kit. This was not in our own country and I hope that our hosts will not mind me revealing that it was the competent licencing officials of Denmark. Their questions were very fair and I am presenting this because it is an excellent example of the manufacturer's need for increasing resources. We had to "validate" statements and claims in respect of:

Maximum and minimum mCi Tc-99m that could be added

Maximum and minimum millilitres that could be added (hence radioactive concentration variations).

Maximum and minimum time between reconstitution and

administration of injection.

Not to be outdone, Amersham went one further and volunteered additional variations between the kit as supplied and:

Simulated hospital sub-division of reconstituted kit into unit-dose syringe presentations with and without saline dilution.

I should add that further variations were incorporated through using different manufacturer brand names of generator in item 1.If the statisticians here work out the permutations combining maxima and minima of all these variables it will total a staggering number of kits and would obviously use up the whole of a batch so that the manufacturer would have none to sell. This clearly is testing appropriate for product development but the principles need to be incorporated as far as possible in the regular quality control of kits.

29. KIT - HOSPITAL POINTS OF VIEW
JØRGEN MARQVERSEN

1. INTRODUCTION

Radioactive materials given to patients for the purpose of diagnosis are pharmaceuticals and are expected to give the same degree of safety as other pharmaceuticals. This means that when producing such pharmaceuticals only ingredients with certificate of origin and of pharmaceutical grade are used and all procedures are outlined in order to secure a final product meeting the demand of the user. This also include that possible risks can be estimated and compared with the benefit of the investigation.

The use of radiopharmaceuticals involves several risk factors such as Radiation, Toxicity, Adverse reactions, Bacteria, Pyrogens, Abnormal biodistribution (leading to doubtful or wrong diagnosis).

2. RADIATION DOSIMETRY

The risk from unexpected radiation due to radionuclidic impurities in generator eluate are the responsibility of the producer of the generator, as discussed in chapter 26 and 27. Effective dosis-equivalent calculations on Tc-99m-chelates and pertechnetate (1-2) indicate only insignificant changes in radiation doses from products containing radiochemical impurities.

3. TOXICITY

Test for toxicity means animal studies for several weeks and use of doses of the components exceeding the total content of the kit (3). The label with its product-code and batch-number is a certificate of origin, and implies test for toxicity.

4. ADVERSE REACTIONS

The number of adverse reactions from radiopharmaceuticals is low, but all ingredients including the reduction and chelating agent, stabilizers and bactericide should be indicated in the prospect in order to minimize the risk (4-5).

5. BACTERIA

Preparation of radiopharmaceuticals from kits by adding generator eluate require the use of an aseptic technique, but the closed procedure minimize the required facilities. Laminar air flow cabinets can assist but not replace well-trained personnel and the sterility of the preparation must be regulary tested. In our laboratory sterility test has been done using membrane filter technique (Millipore XX10, 0,22μ filters, 1 ml sample and incubation 7 days 33°C on 10% bloodager). Out of a production of 750 generator eluates and a similar quantity of kit-preparations/year 671 preparations has been tested. Results are shown in table 1.

Table 1. Bacteriological control of Tc-99m preparations

year	number of samples	non-sterile
1978	199	0
1979	173	3
1980	122	7
1981	47	0
1982	130	2
	671	12 < 2%

Table 2. Details of sterility testing in 1982

	number of samples	non-sterile
Generator eluate	77	2
Diphosphonate	25	0
Alb.microspheres	9	0
Tincolloid	11	0
Glucoheptonate	8	0

Preparations are done without LAF and the test has been performed after 2-6 patient-doses were given. Colonies in connection with the filter has been counted as unsterile. Less than 2% unsterile preparations has been detected.

6. PYROGENS

Pyrogens are a minor problem as radiopharmaceuticals are used in small quantities and kit preparations with short-lived isotopes are used within one day, usually for intravenous injection. Limulus lysate test poses a useful test method for special applications, and can be applied on most radiopharmaceuticals (6) but some additives i.e. Benzylalkohol in excess of 1% inhibit gelation (7).

7. ABNORMAL BIODISTRIBUTION

Unexpected biodistribution could be due to radiochemical impurities or physical factors such as particle size. Methods for testing radiochemical purity or labelling efficiency is usually chromatographic methods: Thin-layer paper- or column chromatography and electophoresis. A lot of methods are reported. (8, 9, 10, 11). Nucleopore filtration are recommended for particle size measurement (22).

How serious is this problem? A frequency of one inappropriate biodistribution per 500 administrated doses which means only 0,1 % were reported. Danish Hospitals reported 18 unexpected biological behaviour out of 50.000 technetium-99m radiopharmaceutical doses given in 1979, most of which was related to the kit rather than to the generator used. (12). Imaging artifacts are not only related to the radiopharmaceutical. In their catalogue of "radionuclide Imaging Artifacts" Wells and Bernier (13) state that artifacts do indeed occur. Out of 93 possible reasons, only seven were due to the radiopharmaceutical, four of these were caused by improper injection technique, one due to the patient and only two due to the preparation itself.

Does the fact that an examination fails in a few occasions invalidate our work? Few clinical test procedures including test methods in Nuclear Medicine are specific. Using Bayes Theorem on Nuclear Medicine (14) post test probability can be estimated. In the example following assumptions have been

made: sensitivity 90%, specificity 90%, prevalence for disease
50%, this gives a predictive value for a positive test

$$PV+ = \frac{0,9 \times 0,5}{(0,9 \times 0,5) + (1- 0,9)(1- o,5)} = 0,90$$

Assuming 2% failures due to the radiopharmaceutical

$$PV + \text{including prep} = \frac{0,9 \times 0,5 \times 0,98}{(0,9 \times 0,5 \times 0,98) + (1- 0,9 - 0,98)(1 - 0,5)} = 0,87$$

These calculations describe "worst case" and in practical work
an abnormal biodistribution due to the radiopharmaceutical
will not always lead to a wrong diagnosis because the
biodistribution of common impurities (pertechnetate or reduced
but not bound Tc) is known and can be outlined on the
scintiphotoes. Fault from low labelling efficiency is
therefore not the major problem, human factors and electronic
factor taken into account (15). In case of doubt it is
essential that tests on the preparation could be done
immediately due to the short halflife of the nuclide and the
chemical instability of the complex. Test procedures and
equipment should be ready "in house", but for such purpose a
simple chromatographic test may be useful.
Why not test all preparations before in vivo application?
Because only few in-vitro analyses directly can be compared to
in-vivo behavior. Pauwel has compared several methods and
state that the radiochemical purity is unique for the method,
and needs to be defined when stated (16). Interaction between
the radiopharmaceutical and the solvent or the chromatographic
material gives higher amount of pertechnetate when saline is
used as liquid phase than methylethylketon. At least a part of
retained activity is a result of such interaction in some
cases. Sophisticated chromatographic analyses of
Tc-99m-diethyl-IDA (17) giving multiple peak pattern were
found not significantly to alter the rate of biliary
excretion, suggesting rapid equilibration in vivo to common

chemical forms. In vitro analyses of radiopharmaceuticals therefore do not completely exclude abnormal biodistribution, and differences in results from in vitro analyses do not automatically lead to differences in biodistribution.

When interpretating results from quality control analysis, the time schedule must be taken into account. Labelling efficiency has been reported to increase with time in Tc complexes of Diphosphonates (18) Fibrinogen (19) and possibly HIDA (17, 20, 21).

Particle size increases by time due to aggregation of small particles (22, 23). Limits for safe use should be stated by the manufacturer. Amount of free pertechnetate increases rapidly as a function of time interval between application and elution of chromatograms (14). Reduced Tc can be oxydized by peroxide and similar radicals present in generator eluate as a function of radioactive concentration (24). This (4) forms a better explanation for poor labelling from generator eluate with low specific radioactivity due to intervals between elution of the generator, than the molar amount of Tc present. The same increase of free pertechnetate can be observed in products exposed to oxygen in air. A number of kit manufacturers recommend that the Tc-99m solution for preparation should contain no oxidizing substances. No test for this has been recommended and the most commonly used method is to test the radiochemical purity of the Tc-labelled product. Even though compatibility problems between generator and kit are not often seen (11) such testing should be dealt with when introducing a new kit, changing size or manufacturer of generator, but are not recommended in daily routine. Chemical testprocedures can only add safety to radiopharmaceuticals but not total exclude unexpected biological distribution. Animal models for testing biodistribution of labelled compounds are used by manufacturers as a final test before releasing kits for clinical trials and as a final check of each batch. Even this cannot totally secure quality of the

8. CONCLUSION

The cost of kits is high, and the difference in price between the rawmaterial and the final product should indicate reliability because a lot of know-how should be built into the kit during the manufacturing process.

Quality cannot be established by testing alone, it must be built into the product during the whole manufacturing process and maintained during transportation, and storage (8).

The radiopharmacist at the hospital must secure that kits are handled in such a way, that quality are maintained.

Prospects following the kit should include:

Indication for use.

Content of the kit.

Instructions for storage and labelling.

Data and methods for testing radiochemical purity.

Recommended dose and estimated radiation dose by normal distribution.

Contraindications and possible sideeffects.

Preinvestigative precautions for the patient.

Known artifacts.

REFERENCES
1. ICRP Publication 26, Pergamon Press 1977.
2. Johansson L, Mattsson S, Nosslin B. Stråledoser från radioaktive ämnen i medicinskt bruk. Statens strålskydds institut. Box 60204, 104 01 Stockholm. 1981.
3. Barker S L. Safety testing. In Rhodes BA eds. Quality Control in Nucl. Med. The C.V. Mosby Company, Saint Louis. 1977.
4. Kristensen K. Quality Control Analysis at the Hospital. Radiopharmaceuticals II, Proceedings 2nd International Symposium on Radiopharmaceuticals, Seattle, Washington. Soc Nucl Med, New York. 1979.
5. Blaha V, Colombetti L G. Adverse Reactions to Radiotracers. Principles of Radiopharmacology. CRC Press Inc 1979;II:165-177.
6. Sullivan J D, Watson S N. Factors affecting the sensitivity of limulus lysate. Appl Microbiol 1974;28:1023.
7. Murata H et al. Sensitivity of the limulus test and rehability factors in the Radiopharmaceuticals. J Nucl Med 1976;17:1088-1092.
8. Kristensen, K. Preparation and Control of Radiopharmaceuticals in Hospitals. Technical Report series no. 194, IAEA Vienna. 1979.

9. Saba G B. Fundamental of Nuclear Pharmacy, New York. Springer Verlag. 1979.
10. Frier M, Hesslewood S R. Quality Assurance of Radiopharmaceuticals. Chapman and Hall in ass. with The British Nuclear Medicine Society. London. 1980.
11. Purity testing of Technetium 99m-preparations in the Clinical Laboratory. Hoechst. 1982.
12. Kristensen K. Quality Control of Radiopharmaceuticals in Medical Radionuclide Imaging. Vienna IAEA 1981;2:59-78.
13. Wells E D, Bernier R D. Radionuclides Imaging Artifacts. Chicago. Year Book Medical Publishers. 1980.
14. Hamilton G W. Medical Decision marking and cost analysis in Cardiology. Proceedings of the third World Congress of Nuclear Medicine and Biology, Paris, Pergamon Press. 1982:1187-1190.
15. Rhodes A. Quality Control in Nuclear Medicine. The CV Mosby Company, Saint Louis. 1977.
16. Pauwels E K J, Feitsma R I J. Radiochemical Quality Control of Tc-99m-labelled Radiopharmaceuticals. Eur J Nucl Med 1977;2:97-103.
17. Fritsberg A R, Huckaby D. Development and Results of Routine Quality Control Procedures for Tc-99m-Iminodiace-tate Hepatobiliary Agents. Radiopharmaceuticals II. Proceedings 2nd International Symposium on Radiopharmaceu-ticals, Seattle, Washington. Soc Nucl Med, New York. 1979.
18. Unterspann S, Finck W. Chemical Structure and Pharmacokinetics of Tc-99m-labelled Aminomethane Diphosphonic Acid Derivatives. Eur J Nucl Med 1981;6:527-530.
19. Deacon J M, Eu PJ, Anderson P, Khan O. Tc-99m-plasmin, a new test for the detection of deep vein thrombosis. Brit J Radiol 1980;53:673-677.
20. Nicholson R W, Herman K J, Shilds R A, Testa H J. The Preparation and Composition of HIDA. Eur J Nucl Med 1980;5:313-317.
21. Pauwels E. K. J, Feitsma J I R, Vermey P. Composition of Tc-99m-HIDA as a Function of Time after Kit Preparation. Eur J Nucl Med 1981;6:433-434.
22. Pedersen B, Kristensen K. Evaluation of Methods for Sizing of Colloidal Radiopharmaceuticals. Eur J Nucl Med 1981;6:521-526.
23. Frier M, Griffiths P, Ramsey A. The Physical and Chemical Characteristics of Sulfur Colloids. Eur J Nucl Med 1981;6:255-260.
24. Der M, Ballinger J R, Bowen B M. Decomposition of Tc-99m Pyrophosphate by Peroxides in Pertechnetate used in Preparation. J Nucl Med 1981;22:645-646.
25. McLean J R, Rockwell L J, Welsh W J. Comparison of the Rat and Mouse Model for Monitoring the Radiochemical purity of Tc-99m Human Serum Albumin. Radiopharmaceuticals II. Proceedings 2nd International symposium on Radiopharmaceu-ticals. Seattle, Washington. Soc Nucl Med New York. 1979.

30. QUALITY CONTROL OF RADIOPHARMACEUTICALS PREPARED FROM KITS
AND GENERATORS IN HOSPITALS - UNITED KINDGOM DRUG CONTROL
POINT OF VIEW

ROSEMARY J. SMITH

1. INTRODUCTION

Many of the generators and kits used in hospitals hold full
Product Licenses and will have been fully assessed for safety,
quality and efficacy. It is proposed therefore to consider
briefly the information relating to quality that would need to
be supplied to support an application for a Product Licence in
order to illustrate how the quality of a licensed product is
established. Consideration will then be given to the question
of the quality control of radiopharmaceuticals prepared in
hospitals from such licensed generators and kits taking into
account the standards and guidelines which operate in the
United Kingdom. However, since the licensing status of one or
both components may be different, the quality control
necessary for such products will also be discussed.

2. QUALITY ASPECTS OF A PRODUCT LICENCE APPLICATION

Unless the product to be licensed contains a "new"
substance or radionuclide the quality evidence required would
normally be restricted to pharmaceutical data on the dosage
form as indicated in notes for guidance published by the
Department of Health and Social Security. A typical
application would require full details on the following:

Composition of active and inactive ingredients.
Method of manufacture.
Quality control for constituents, in-process controls
and finished product specification with tests and
limits applied.
Development pharmaceutics and biological
availability.

Stability testing.

Containers.

The published advice to applicants is of a general nature designed to cover most types of medicinal products; for radio-pharmaceuticals additional data relating to the radioactive component would need to be included. The specification of the radionuclide would need to reflect the impurities arising as a result of the method of production which may therefore have to be given. For other ingredients synthetic routes may also be necessary for components which, although not new, have not been used in medicine before. For generators and kits, data supplied would need to support the quality of the product as marketed and the quality of the radiopharmaceuticals prepared according to the instructions for use of the marketed product. The requirements of the European and British Pharmacopoeias apply where appropriate. Activity, radionuclidic purity and radiochemical purity are additional factors which need to be included in the specifications for radiopharmaceuticals. Evidence from development work would need to be included in order to demonstrate that the formulation was adequate for its intended use. Biological distribution work from other parts of the application relating to animal and clinical studies may be linked to this data. Attention would need to be given to physico-chemical factors which could influence biological distribution and controls applied where appropriate. The manufacturer of a kit is not in a position to ensure that the eluate actually used is compatible with the kit but development work related to possible problems arising from different eluate formulations can be undertaken to provide additional assurance. Stability testing would need to demonstrate that the formulation was stable for the purposes stated and would meet the finished product "check" specification throughout its shelf-life at all concentrations of radio-activity likely to be used. The suitability of added stabilizers would need to be demonstrated. Testing would also need to cover extreme conditions of use, for instance using a kit at the end of its shelf-life with a high activity eluate or one from an "old" generator. Containers would need to be adequate to maintain stability and quality. Finally it must be noted that full details including evidence of identity, method of manufacture, impurities, quality control and stability would need to be supplied for a new ingredient.

3. QUALITY CONTROL IN HOSPITALS

Turning our attention now to the subject of quality control for hospital production of radiopharmaceuticals prepared from generators and kits, it was already stated in Chapter 19 that the preparation of radiopharmaceuticals in hospitals is specifically included in the activities to which Good Pharmaceutical Manufacturing Practice is applied and the units where production takes place are subject to inspection by the Medicines Inspectorate. The Guide to Good Pharmaceutical Manufacturing Practice (hereafter referred to as the Guide) outlines those steps which should be taken to ensure that the products are of the nature and quality intended. The requirements have no statutory force and methods which achieve the same ends may be equally acceptable. The Guide defines Good Manufacturing Practice (GMP) as "that part of quality assurance aimed at ensuring that products are consistently manufactured to a quality appropriate to their intended use. It is thus concerned both with manufacturing and quality control procedures." This definition is based on the principle that quality cannot be established by testing alone but must be built into the product during its production. In order to achieve this proper facilities must be provided, including:

> appropriately trained personnel
> adequate premises and space
> suitable equipment
> correct materials
> approved procedures
> suitable storage and transport

General guidance on all these aspects is given in the Guide and in the additional guidelines prepared specifically for hospitals on premises and environment for preparation of radiopharmaceuticals; the latter publication details the modifications needed to take account of the special problems caused by radiation hazard.For aseptic procedures, use of a properly designed workstation in a suitable environment overcomes the conflict between the need to exclude micro-organisms and the need for operator protection. Good Manufacturing Practice also requires that documentation is kept for the procedures undertaken, the specifications applied and the results of tests undertaken.

Effective control of quality requires testing of starting materials, intermediates and finished product and where appropriate testing of the environment. These tests are required to be approved by the appointed Quality Controller who is not the person responsible for production. Approval for release and the retention of samples for subsequent testing is also the designated responsibility of Quality Control. This is satisfactory for other pharmaceuticals but the short half-life and the stability problems of radiopharmaceuticals would make such a practice difficult for hospital production; for this reason the producer will usually undertake those tests required immediately himself but this does not relieve the Quality Controller of all responsibility for the quality control applied. Furthermore, since some radiopharmaceuticals need to be administered shortly after preparation, the results of a number of tests may not be available before the preparation is given. Nevertheless, it is essential that testing is carried out to ensure that the production process is kept under proper control; strict compliance with GMP is of paramount importance and environmental monitoring essential.

In considering the testing to be applied to starting materials and finished products, Good Manufacturing Practice requires that tests with limits are included for identity, purity and assay. However where the starting material consists of a kit which is the subject of full product licence, these testing requirements would not apply since the manufacturer is responsible for the product meeting its specification. The user would need to ensure that the eluate to be used was compatible with the kit and if necessary testing would need to be undertaken in order that this might be established. In the case of a generator, even when the subject of a full product licence, testing must be undertaken on the first eluate to establish that the generator has not been damaged in transit, has been set up properly and is functioning correctly. Subsequent use requires testing to ensure elution is satisfactory and at the end of use it is generally considered wise to recheck sterility as a control on aseptic technique.

In the earlier consideration of quality standards of licensed generators and kits it was noted that the supporting data with an application extended to radiopharmaceuticals produced according to the instructions supplied with the components. Therefore responsibility for quality of the final product is shared between the manufacturers and the user. The actual testing to be carried out in the hospital to ensure compliance with the finished product specification can be modified to reflect this situation; provided that the compatability of the components has been established and the manufacturers' instructions have been followed the testing programme required should reflect the production process in the hospital and any special factors that require control. Activity must, of course, be rechecked.

It is important that the documentation clearly states the tests which are required on a routine basis and the circumstances or intervals which apply to other tests. In addition, the tests for which results will only be available after the product is used must be specified. Sterility and, where appropriate, pyrogen requirements as laid down in the European Pharmacopoeia are applicable to injections although problems related to sample size and non-availability of results before use are recognised. It is also noted that a test employing limulus amoebocyte lysate may be useful in circumstances where the official test for pyrogens may not be sufficiently sensitive for preparations intended for administration by any route giving access to the cerebrospinal fluid, or when testing after release for use may be unacceptable. This test does not replace the official test and its limitations must be recognised.

Consideration of quality control applicable to preparation

of radiopharmaceuticals in hospitals has been related solely to the circumstances operating when fully licensed generators and kits are used. If one or both of these components is not supplied under the authority of a full product licence or clinical trial certificate the responsibility of the hospital with respect to quality control increases. The most common situation to be encountered is the one where the product(s) concerned hold Licence(s) of Right; although these products have never been formally assessed for safety, quality and efficacy they have been used safely for a number of years and will have been manufactured in accordance with GMP standards. The user should verify that the specification applied by the manufacturer is satisfactory after which the licensing provisions applied to the manufacturer should ensure that quality of components is maintained. If however the kit is made in the hospital the quality control applicable would need to be up to the standard applied to the commercial manufacturer which will usually necessitate evidence from animal studies of biological distribution. The final category of product that may be encountered in a hospital in the United Kingdom is the unlicensed one manufactured or imported to the order of a physician for administration to a particular "named patient". Although the physician is responsible for using the product, control procedure should be carried out to confirm that the product is of satisfactory quality unless the physician has agreed to use the product in the absence of such assurance.

4. CONCLUSION

The use of fully licensed generators and kits for production of radiopharmaceuticals prepared in accordance with standards of Good Manufacturing Practice in hospital reduces the burden of quality testing to be applied by the hospital. The use of other components does not give the same advantage and this must be reflected in the quality control procedures applied.

REFERENCES
1. The Medicines Act 1968, HMSO, London.
2. MAL 2, Notes forGuidance on Applications for Product Licences (Medicines for Human Use) 1981, London, DHSS.
3. MAL 99, Notes for Guidance on the Control of Medicines in the United Kingdom of Great Britain and Northern Ireland, 1981, London, DHSS.
4. DHSS Guide to Good Pharmaceutical Manufacturing Practice, 1977, London, HMSO.
5. DHSS Guidance Notes for Hospital on Premises and Environment for the Preparation of Radiopharmaceuticals, 1982, London, DHSS.
6. British Pharmacopoeia 1980, London, HMSO.
7. European Pharmacopoeia 1980, France, Maisonneuve SA.
8. DHSS Circular HSC(1S)128, Application of the Medicines Act to Health Authorities, 1975, London, DHSS.
9. DHSS Health Notice HN(77)64, Application of the Medicines Act to Health Authorities: Quality Control, 1977, London, DHSS.

SUBJECT INDEX